Fighting for Our Lives

Critical Issues in Health and Medicine

Edited by Rima D. Apple, University of Wisconsin–Madison,
and Janet Golden, Rutgers University, Camden

Growing criticism of the U.S. health care system is coming from consumers, politicians, the media, activists, and health care professionals. Critical Issues in Health and Medicine is a collection of books that explores these contemporary dilemmas from a variety of perspectives, among them political, legal, historical, sociological, and comparative, and with attention to crucial dimensions such as race, gender, ethnicity, sexuality, and culture.

Fighting for Our Lives

New York's AIDS Community and the Politics of Disease

Susan M. Chambré

Rutgers University Press

New Brunswick, New Jersey, and London

Library of Congress Cataloging-in-Publication Data

Chambré, Susan Maizel.
    Fighting for our lives : New York's AIDS community and the politics of disease /
Susan M. Chambré.
        p. ; cm. — (Critical issues in health and medicine)
    Includes bibliographical references and index.
    ISBN-13: 978-0-8135-3866-2 (hardcover : alk. paper)
    ISBN-13: 978-0-8135-3867-9 (pbk : alk. paper)
    1. AIDS (Disease)—New York (State)—New York—History. 2. AIDS (Disease)—
Social aspects—New York (State)—New York. 3. AIDS (Disease)—Political aspects—
New York (State)—New York. 4. AIDS (Disease)—Patients—Services for—New York
(State)—New York—History. 5. Community health services—New York (State)—
New York—History.   I. Title.   II. Series. [DNLM: 1. Acquired Immunodeficiency
Syndrome—history—New York City. 2. Politics—New York City. 3. Consumer
Advocacy—New York City.   WC 503 C447f2006]
    RA643.84.N7C43 2006
    362.196'97920097471—dc22   2005035909

A British Cataloging-in-Publication record for this book is available from the British Library.

Manufactured in the United States of America

The battle with AIDS is not one of liberals against conservatives or even of right against wrong—it is the fight of life against death.

—Randy Shilts, writing in the *San Francisco Chronicle*, June 1989

Contents

Abbreviations

ADAP	AIDS Drug Assistance Program
ADAPT	Association for Drug Abuse Prevention and Treatment
AHP	Advancing HIV Prevention
AI	New York State AIDS Institute
AIDS	Acquired Immunodeficiency Syndrome
AZT	Azidothymidine
BLCA	Black Leadership Commission on AIDS
CARE Act	Ryan White Comprehensive AIDS Resource Emergency Act
CDC	Centers for Disease Control and Prevention
DSAS	New York State Division of Substance Abuse Services
ESRD	End Stage Renal Disease
ETHA	Early Treatment for HIV Act
FDA	Food and Drug Administration
GAO	General Accounting Office
GLWD	God's Love We Deliver
GMHC	Gay Men's Health Crisis
GMWA	Gay Men with AIDS
HAF	Hispanic AIDS Forum
HHS	U.S. Department of Health and Human Services
HIV	Human Immunodeficiency Virus
IDUs	Injection Drug Users
IOM	Institute of Medicine of the National Academies
KS	Kaposi's sarcoma
MMWR	Morbidity and Mortality Weekly Report
MTFA	Minority Task Force on AIDS
NAACP	National Association for the Advancement of Colored People
NORA	National Organizations Responding to AIDS
NYT	*New York Times*
PCP	Pneumocystis carinii pneumonia
PWAs	Persons with AIDS
RFP	Request for Proposals
SAFE	Serostatus Approach to Fighting the Epidemic
SEPs	Syringe Exchange Programs
T & D	ACT UP's Treatment and Data Committee
TAG	Treatment Action Group
WARN	Women and AIDS Resource Center

In the late spring of 1987, my father spent two days waiting to be assigned a bed in a major New York City hospital after a heart attack. When he was finally placed in an intensive care unit, the bed opposite him was occupied by a person with AIDS. This was a vivid introduction to the growth in the number of AIDS cases in New York City; when I began to write this book, I realized why he waited so long for a bed. As the book neared completion, my then-widowed mother was fighting cancer. As her only child, I served as her major advocate. This experience, and the process of grieving as I reviewed the copyedited manuscript, gave me an even deeper understanding of how and why the AIDS community formed to respond to a complex medical condition and to the limitations of the contemporary health care system.

This book has evolved slowly. Hundreds of people have helped me along the way as I did the research. My greatest debt goes to the more than two hundred persons who spent time explaining their experiences as volunteers, as staff members, and as activists in AIDS organizations and in several major hospitals in New York City. They shared their fears, their concerns, and their successes, and helped me to understand how and why they were doing what they could to respond to a new disease that might take their lives and the lives of friends and family members. Most were enthusiastic about a project that has taken me a very long time, because they believed, as I do, that this is a story worth telling in all its complexity. People faced a new disease with courage and conviction, and, while one might in retrospect question some decisions, one cannot question people's sincerity and commitment.

It is customary for authors to thank by name the many who assisted them. I will in the interests of space simply express my gratitude to colleagues, friends, and an army of research assistants. A few people, however, deserve particular mention. Kathleen McCarthy, Director of the Center for Philanthropy and Civil Society at the City University of New York, provided seed money for the first phase of this project and encouragement at various stages of my career. The PSC-CUNY grant program and the Indiana University Center on Philanthropy gave me a number of small grants, and the Nonprofit Sector Research Fund and its then director, Elizabeth Boris, provided a major grant that underwrote the cost of a sabbatical to help launch this project. My home college, Baruch, provided two sabbaticals that gave me the time to expand the focus of the project and to begin to write the book. In addition, the Baruch College Fund underwrote the cost of several research assistants and the Weissman School of Arts and Sciences provided reassigned time to reduce my teaching responsibilities. Libarians and archivists—especially Louisa Moy and Rich Wandel—helped me to obtain thousands of documents. Fred Lane sent me at least one or two articles a week for over fifteen years. Michael Seltzer, David Nimmons, and Bert Hansen gave me access to their private papers, and Naomi Fatt allowed me free rein in searching the ADAPT files. Ana Oliviera and Krishna Stone assisted me to locate a photo for the cover. My editor Audra Wolfe, copyeditor Paula Friedman, and two anonymous reviewers helped me clarify my argument and write a far better book. Finally, my husband, Bob, and my children and grandchildren—Ephraim and Shlomit, Yoni and Shonnie, Daniel, Esther (my last research assistant), Chana B., Moshe and Michal—are constant reminders of why it is important to fight for one's life.

Fighting for Our Lives

Introduction

The epidemic became apparent slowly, and its potential impact was unclear. Toward the end of the 1970s and the early part of the 1980s, gay men in New York, Los Angeles, and San Francisco began to realize that their friends and lovers were becoming very, very sick, "dying before our eyes and no one had the vaguest idea of what was going on."[1] One man overheard a conversation in his doctor's office and called Dr. Lawrence Mass, a physician and regular contributor to his city's gay newspaper, the *New York Native* (hereafter: *the Native*), to tell him that there were "three—maybe [it's] five—gay men in New York City intensive care units. They've all got some weird pneumonia or something."[2] Mass called the city department of health to investigate, and published an article called "Disease Rumors Largely Unfounded" on 18 May 1981. The article reported that city health officials did not think that there was an "exotic new disease" in the gay community.[3]

The article was wrong and the rumors were true.

These were the first cases of the AIDS epidemic, one of the defining events of the late twentieth century.[4]

Two weeks later, on 5 June 1981, the federal government's *Morbidity and Mortality Weekly Report* (MMWR) described the cases of "5 young men, all active homosexuals" in Los Angeles, who each had three infections at once: Pneumocystis carinii pneumonia (PCP), cytomegalovirus (CMV), and mucosal candidiasis infection. A second *MMWR* article, in early July, reported that twenty-six gay men in New York and Los Angeles had another disease, Kaposi's Sarcoma (KS), a curious occurrence since the men were in their thirties and KS was a disease that occurred in older men. The article also mentioned that four more cases of PCP had been diagnosed in Los Angeles, and that there were six PCP cases in San Francisco. The article urged that "Physicians should be alert for Kaposi's sarcoma, PC pneumonia, and other opportunistic infections associated with immunosuppression in homosexual men." By the end of August, seventy additional cases of KS or PCP in gay men had been reported to the Center for Disease Control (CDC).[5]

Some doctors in New York City were not surprised. Gay men with night sweats and enlarged lymph nodes had been diagnosed with fevers of unknown origin for several years; there were also scattered cases of KS and PCP.[6] Dr. Donna Mildvan remembered that the pieces of the puzzle began to fit together in the early part of 1981 when "All of a sudden we knew. All those lymphadenopathy patients were part of this. The shingles epidemic we were seeing must be part of this. And the this must be part of it and the that must be part of it."[7] The disease was conceptualized as a "gay plague" even though it was occurring in other groups. Doctors, staff, and clients in drug treatment programs were noticing that drug addicts had been dying of "junkie pneumonia," and Dr. Arye Rubinstein, a Bronx pediatrician, realized in 1979 that there was a rise in "inexplicable infections among the children of drug users."[8]

The *New York Times* broke the story on the Friday just before the July 4 weekend. Titled "Rare Cancer Seen in 41 Homosexuals," the article took up a single column on page twenty.[9] One gay man recalled reading the article on the deck of his house on Fire Island and thinking that the idea of a homosexual illness was "insane. There's no heterosexual illness. And I turned the page . . . No one gave this a moment's thought."[10]

What at first seemed like a "gay plague" was to become epidemic in the United States and pandemic throughout the world. Its impact has been significant not only in terms of the past and future death toll, but also in the broad range of social policies and scientific advances that it has brought. Epidemics are natural experiments that require societies to respond on several levels. They are biological and medical events that evoke cultural, political, behavioral, and emotional responses. As relatively rapid sources of social change, epidemics provide a context for understanding how societies respond to events that expose the inadequacies of existing social arrangements and stimulate cultural and institutional changes. Existing policies and programs prove inadequate in the face of new demands, and what may begin as a temporary measure to ameliorate an emergency may become a permanent feature of a society.

AIDS caught Americans unaware. The slowness of defining the disease, identifying treatments, and searching for a cure, was thought due to enormous indifference, homophobia, inefficiency, and perhaps intent. But it was also due to disbelief, since Americans generally thought that contagious and infectious diseases were curable. At a conference early in 1983, the eminent physician Lewis Thomas pointed out: "At a time not long ago, I was totally confident that the great infectious diseases of humankind were coming under control and would soon—maybe within my own lifetime—vanish as threats to human health. . . . I take it back."[11] In fact, new lethal infectious diseases continue to be created, and, despite the existence of antibiotics, they began to account for more deaths beginning in 1980.[12] AIDS marked a turning point in this greater trend.

Numerous books have chronicled aspects of the AIDS epidemic. It is both appropriate and meaningful to look back at the social response to this epidemic in its epicenter in the United States, as the epidemic reaches the quarter-century mark. This book is a social history of the AIDS community in New York as a window into understanding the politics of health policymaking. The study starts at the very beginning of the epidemic and describes how the AIDS community, a diverse group of people—both those who were infected and those others who were affected—individually and collectively responded to "fight" AIDS. The AIDS community includes gay men, current and former drug users, substance abuse professionals, elite women, researchers, and people concerned about the epidemic because of strong religious or humanitarian convictions. Its members created organizations, designed programs, and influenced policies to care for the dying, to prevent the spread of the disease, and to prolong the lives of the living.

Previous histories of the AIDS epidemic consider the social and political forces that were responsible for our failure to effectively mount policies to serve people with the disease and to prevent the spread of the infection. But, the story is more complex than a tale of blame for those who became ill or who failed to recognize what was needed and did not respond. The factors are hard to untangle. The nature of the disease and its impact became apparent slowly. The fragmented and decentralized public policy system in the United States failed to respond for several years as a result of: organizational inertia;[13] limitations of the existing public health, medical care, and social service systems;[14] a lack of understanding of the potential impact of the disease, perhaps exacerbated by limited coverage by the mass media;[15] indifference to the kinds of people initially affected by the disease; and an inability to take action on the basis of fairly clear epidemiological data, with those who might initiate action awaiting, instead, more definitive scientific information. Once scientists agreed on the cause, in early 1984, nearly three years after the first cases were reported, values and beliefs deeply held by policy makers and people in the affected communities continued to slow down the response to preventing the spread of the new disease until, in many cases, too late to save lives.

The book describes a broad range of social, cultural, and political factors that influenced AIDS policy, but focuses on three distinct social forces: the growth of an AIDS community that designed programs and policies, engaged in advocacy, and drew upon the support of institutional advocates and elite allies; the effectiveness of the AIDS community's framing of public policies and public funding as having the capability to "save lives"; and a political context where the epidemic spurred a sense of urgency through its close association with a host of inner city problems, including drug use and crime.

The AIDS community combined institutional and noninstitutional politics, operating as both insiders and outsiders who engaged in advocacy, lobbying, and direct political action utilizing strategies that included policy research, lobbying and persuasion, candlelight marches, demonstrations, and civil disobedience. The rhetoric of the AIDS community was also powerful and persuasive. It stressed the uniqueness of the disease and the need for distinct policies and funding to fight the epidemic. A master frame in its ideology was that spending money would save lives, which resonated with a central feature of American political culture, the fact that politicians and the public are indeed highly committed to spending money to save lives. While the members of the AIDS community were claiming government indifference and parsimony, AIDS funding was rising rapidly, and by 1990, there were claims that AIDS was receiving more than its fair share of money for research and services. Funding expanded once it became evident that money spent for AIDS services and treatment would, in fact, sustain people's lives.

But, as social movement scholars note, the political context or political opportunity structure is also significant in explaining the impact of, to use William Gamson's term, challenger groups. The association of AIDS with the growth of an urban underclass is also significant. The efforts of the AIDS community were reinforced by the recognition of local and national elites that there was a need to fight AIDS as part of a broader response to a host of inner city problems that threatened the business climate of American cities. The objective nature of the disease and its social construction both shifted. No longer a short-term acute illness mainly confined to gay men, AIDS became a disease of the underclass in large American cities; it was embedded in a host of urban problems that signified a growing urban disorder. By the end of the 1980s, the fight against AIDS gained a greater sense of urgency. The expansion of public resources to fight AIDS was one manifestation of a broader set of public policies designed to reimpose moral order on cities that were becoming increasingly out of control.

This book focuses on the AIDS community in New York. Far from a typical American city, New York has been the center of the epidemic in the United States, and the place where many organizational models and policies were created. The city was hit early and hit hard by the epidemic. Half of the reported cases in the nation before 1983 were in New York. By the early 1990s, the disease was the third major cause of death for men in the city, and the fifth for women. Its effect was so enormous that it actually played an important role in reducing, between 1983 and 1992, life expectancy at birth for white men in the city by 1.1 years.[16] In 1993, New York City had more cases than the next forty cities combined, and individual neighborhoods had more cases than many states. In 2001, New York City's AIDS case rate of 65.9 per 100,000 people was nearly double San Francisco's (34.6), six times the rate in Boston (10.8), and four times the U.S. average (14.9).[17] A total of 128,141 people in New York City were diagnosed with AIDS during the first two decades of the epidemic, more than one in eight of the nearly 800,000 people diagnosed with AIDS in the United States during this period.[18]

New York's AIDS community emerged early and, given the size and diversity of the affected population, the community included the largest number, and most specialized, of formal and informal AIDS organizations in the nation. New York–based organizations were often the first of their type, like the Gay Men's Health Crisis (GMHC), the first AIDS organization in the world. New York was also the birthplace of the AIDS Coalition to Unleash Power, ACT UP, probably the best known health advocacy organization, whose dramatic and often brash form of activism contributed to some of the significant successes of the AIDS community. Many of the organizations in the city, including those described in this volume, served as models for groups in the United States and throughout the world. A great number of AIDS organizations were founded in the city, an estimated 188 between 1981 and 1997. These new organizations, as well as AIDS advocacy and service programs in existing organizations, benefited from the private funding available from foundations, corporations, and new AIDS charities located in the city. Many also relied heavily on funds from New York State's AIDS Institute.[19]

The implications of this book, however, go well beyond AIDS and beyond New York City since the events it describes form a case study of how American society responded to a major social problem at the end of the twentieth century. At the same time, the narrative outlines a profound tragedy, a story of the deaths of numerous people, most of them young. Noting some enormous fault lines in American society, both governmental and civil, it is written in the hope that, in the future, we will respond more effectively and sensitively. Although it is tempting to offer clear guidelines and to cast blame on government, the gay community, the African American and Hispanic communities, or American society in general, perhaps the most profound lesson of this book is the enormous complexity of the issues it covers and an inability even now to grasp and to recommend what might have been done.

The work of the AIDS community has another important implication. It illustrates the growing influence of a broad array of health organizations that represent health care consumers and patients for whom, according to Ulrich Beck, a sense of shared risk is an important mobilizing force.[20] In most instances, these organizations are based on specific diseases and health conditions. They are especially evident in the United States but exist in Europe and include a small number of international health policy organizations.[21] In a complex health care system where government, health professionals, and corporations—especially drug companies—are involved in the legislation, regulation, and delivery of a large segment of the American economy and a central set of institutions ensuring the well-being of citizens, the role of health care "consumers," patients and advocates, merits serious consideration. This study of nearly the first quarter century of the AIDS community provides a unique opportunity to understand the role of consumers in the dynamics of health policy.

A diverse range of organizations and individual actors influenced HIV policies, using a broad array of strategies. Many accounts of the AIDS community focus on the major role of ACT UP; they describe AIDS politics before ACT UP as preliminary to the emergence of the AIDS movement. ACT UP itself stresses its own key role. A closer look at the history of AIDS advocacy leads to a different interpretation: the fact that a broad range of organizations and actors together orchestrated the response often attributed to ACT UP. In fact, by the time ACT UP was founded in 1987, members of the AIDS community were already taking their place at a series of metaphorical tables of political influence. The culture of the AIDS community and what Tarrow calls the "repertoires of contention" that ACT UP used—the symbols and practices of the AIDS movement—were developed by the "early risers" (to use Tarrow's term) of the AIDS community.[22] ACT UP raised the ante and increased the volume of AIDS discourse; it was a highly visible and important part of the AIDS community; but, without the "insiders" taking their place at the table, ACT UP's effectiveness would have been greatly diluted. Reflecting back on the impact of the AIDS community in 1997, Tim Sweeney pointed out that it "utilized an arsenal of tactics to foster change—we pushed the media, we lobbied the legislators, and we rallied in the streets."[23]

By the mid-1980s, the growing number of new groups and organizations in New York City and throughout the nation led to the idea that there was an identifiable AIDS community with a distinctive culture that framed collective action.[24] Patients, especially those with long-term illnesses, develop a sense of community and a culture when they begin to share their experiences in coping with their illness and to view themselves as having a common fate. Often, these efforts become formalized into patient-initiated organizations that provide information and services. In other instances, particularly when people believe that it may be possible to find a cure for a disease, patient organizations raise money and begin to influence public policy.[25] In the very early days of the epidemic, when AIDS was baffling and seemingly impervious to medical intervention, GMHC volunteers and others who became part of an evolving AIDS community focused their attention on caring for the sick and for the dying. Members of the AIDS community created an impressive array of artworks to express their range of emotions and to mobilize opinions and concerns, and symbols and a shared rhetoric reinforced its permeable boundaries. This emerging community included people who became involved through their own AIDS diagnosis or the diagnosis of a friend, lover, or relative. Many people, however, particularly gay men and lesbians, voluntarily joined the AIDS community, from a sense of shared fate. Although the AIDS community was open to all who chose to join it, it was mainly created by gay men and lesbians.

Three qualities of the epidemic shaped the development of the AIDS community: uncertainty, stigma, and the disaster-like impact. For several years, certainly until 1984, the uncertainty was enormous. At first, the nature of the disease and the way it was transmitted were unknown, and those at risk were frightened.[26] HIV testing, which became available after 1985, enabled individuals to learn if they were infected but created a different uncertainty, the idea that an individual could be infected with HIV but that survival could be long-term. AIDS stigma was also huge. It was fueled by the claim that gay men and injecting drug users were responsible for being infected, in contrast to women infected by sexual contact, children born to infected women, hemophiliacs, and persons infected through a blood transfusion, who were viewed as innocent victims. Finally, the uneven distribution of AIDS cases created a sense of disaster in some communities, a sense that promoted a feeling of frustration at the indifference of the society and the state. The emotions that fueled the collective action of the AIDS community, as Deborah Gould discusses in detail, are a vivid illustration that collective action combines rational concerns and powerful emotions.[27]

But, even as various levels of government became more responsive and funding increased, anger escalated, since the programs, the research, and the funding seemed not to have an impact: people were continuing to die. Attaining the ultimate goal of the AIDS movement—to end the epidemic—was impossible. The growth of organizations was a painful reminder of the paradoxical success of the AIDS movement, which expanded systems of caring for people in an effort to either save their lives or keep them alive long enough for a cure.

This book traces the AIDS community's evolution. It is based on ethnographic research in the AIDS community, including 255 formal and informal interviews and 210 formal presentations. In addition, I did an extensive review of archival, published, and visual material, including 25 videos and oral history interviews.

Part I describes the development of the New York's AIDS community and its role in creating models for AIDS services and prevention. Chapter 1 describes the early years of the Gay Men's Health Crisis, which created a template to respond to the uncertainty and the "madness" of the epidemic. Chapter 2 outlines a second strand of the community's development, the creation of the PWA Coalition, which provided the ideology for the AIDS community and framed its actions by stressing the importance of individual and communal empowerment; one manifestation of that empowerment was the desire to stop the transmission of HIV, a complex endeavor that struck at the very heart of gay identity. The actions of the AIDS community put a "face" on the epidemic, which contributed to the idea that public support might save identified lives rather than a group of nameless and faceless "statistical lives." Chapter 3 follows the history of the development of "safe sex" and some of the contested aspects of this strategy. As the epidemic began to expand and affect a broader range of people, the AIDS community came to encompass additional people affected by the disease or concerned about its impact. Chapter 4 identifies another dimension of the AIDS community's evolution, the support of allies and patrons, particularly elite women and people in the city's faith community.

Part II describes certain features and implications of the expanding epidemic. Chapter 5 outlines the impact of the "changing face of AIDS," the increase in the numbers of African Americans, Hispanics, women, and injecting drug users infected by the disease. The mobilization of people in these communities was more belated and less forceful than in the gay community. This was due to enormous internal obstacles, notably an unwillingness to "own" AIDS, but also to the limited economic and social capital in these communities. Organizations founded to respond to this changing demographic of AIDS began to receive a significant infusion of public funds once the epidemic began to be linked to a "synergism of plagues" indicative of disorder in American cities. Initially most apparent in New York, these problems were recognized in many American cities and led to a more concerted federal response, with the 1990 passage of the Ryan White CARE Act (chapter 7).

Part III focuses on the evolution of AIDS advocacy. It traces the beginnings and the evolution of organized advocacy, with chapter 8 describing the important complementary role of both advocates and activists. Chapters 9, 10, and 11 focus on the AIDS community's role in three policy areas: finding a cure; reducing HIV transmission among drug injectors by providing access to sterile syringes; and refocusing prevention policies at the turn of the century. Chapter 12 looks at the nature of the AIDS community at the time of this writing, noting how much more of its work was directed toward maintaining AIDS exceptionalism at a time when AIDS was beginning to be mainstreamed in public policy with a focus on health disparities.

Part I

Uncertainty, Stigma, and the Creation of an AIDS Community

Chapter 1

Managing the Madness

The feeling was that everything was on fire and that we had to do something about it. We couldn't turn our backs to it and say "I am going to do something else." It was so compelling, so compelling! . . But it was also burning us out. And the impact went well beyond our awareness.

—Alex Carballo-Diéguez, GMHC volunteer,
   interview with the author, 4 January 2000.

When Larry Kramer read the 3 July 1981 *New York Times* story about the "rare cancer" among gay men, he "instantly understood that the new mystery disease might be contagious." Kramer, a well-known gay writer, went to see Dr. Alvin Friedman-Kien, one of the authors of the second *MMWR* report, to find out what he could do. At Friedman-Kien's suggestion, Kramer, Lawrence Mass, and two other men organized a fundraising meeting at Kramer's apartment on August 11 to raise money for research on the new disease. Kramer recalls that hundreds of men were invited to the event, including all of the known gay doctors in New York. About eighty men came. Friedman-Kien told the men that these early cases were just the beginning, the "tip of the iceberg." Writer Nathan Fain recalled "each man had swallowed his panic and—if you were there, you remember the exact moment—found himself shocked into action."[1] The meeting was historic: it was the first fundraiser for the Gay Men's Health Crisis (GMHC), the first organization in the world founded to "fight" a disease that had not yet been named.[2]

GMHC's early years capture the history of the epidemic in New York City. Its volunteers established ways to care for the sick and attend to the dying, transmitted a growing body of information on the epidemic, and taught people how to protect themselves. Its early volunteers—human service professionals, laypeople who took on professional roles, and people with communications, fundraising, and organizational skills—responded to the enormous uncertainty of the disease by gathering and disseminating information and developing services. They established the baseline of the social response in the city that would respond to the enormous fear and uncertainty about the disease and, within a year or two, to the beginning of an unending series of deaths.

Two decades later, the efforts of this handful of volunteers had grown into a major organization, the largest AIDS organization in the world, with a yearly income of $21 million. Its name reflected the organization's roots but did not capture the diversity of its volunteers, donors, and clients. Nearly one third of its clients defined themselves as heterosexual, and one in five were women.[3] By the end of 1991, the group had served a total of 13,441 persons.[4] Even after many other AIDS organizations were established and the AIDS community had expanded, GMHC continued to be its nexus and the model for other organizations. The history of New York's AIDS community, then, begins in GMHC.

With the recognition that there was a new disease among gay men, doctors became more alert, and the number of diagnosed cases increased rapidly. By the end of the year, 321 people had been diagnosed with the new disease, and half had died. The small critical mass of men working with Kramer set to work. Encouraged by their success at the group's first fundraiser in Kramer's apartment, they quickly organized themselves to raise money and to alert the thousands of gay men from New York City who would be vacationing on Fire Island over Labor Day weekend. The group distributed a six-page brochure under the doors of houses in The Pines and Cherry Grove, the island's two main gay resorts. The brochure included the reprint of a recent *New York Native* (hereafter: *Native*) article by Larry Mass and information about where they could donate money. The volunteers also set up tables at the ferry dock and at the Ice Palace, a popular disco. The response was baffling and distressing: they raised $769 from the fifteen thousand or so gay men who were on Fire Island that weekend. Although Kramer recalled that "All that people seemed to talk about were the latest intestinal parasites going around," another man remembered that there was little talk about the illness and that "we never discussed it as a group. We partied and had a fabulous summer."[5]

For the next several months, the small group of volunteers faced an uphill battle. Staff in the mayor's office were unresponsive, as were the mainstream press and most gay men. By the end of the year, however, the epidemic was impossible to ignore. Nathan Fain recalled that, by the winter of 1981, "many of us knew that our lives had been changed forever. We buried the dead, and we set to work. To do otherwise was out of the question. There was no choice about it."[6] Within the year, many of the men who were initially indifferent refocused their lives from partying to caregiving.[7] Never again would they celebrate Labor Day weekend in the same innocent state as in 1981.

On 4 January 1982, six men met at Larry Kramer's apartment and established a new organization they named the Gay Men's Health Crisis. The name was an acknowledgment of the health crisis that gay men were facing.[8] In the first six months of 1982, they raised about $106,000. A large portion came from GMHC's first major public fundraising event, the "Showers," that April 8. The date had been postponed several times because they had difficulty locating a venue. They decided on the Paradise Garage, a "legendary dance place" that mainly catered to African Americans. The organizers were concerned that few people would come, because it was the second night of Passover and was also Holy Thursday, but they need not have worried. The event was enormously successful. It raised over thirty thousand dollars and attracted two thousand people. GMHC's president, Paul Popham, told the crowd that things were going to get worse. The Gay Men's Chorus sang one of its signature songs, "He Ain't Heavy, He's My Brother," which took on a new meaning that night since increasing numbers of men were caring for friends and lovers. An article on the "gay plague" in *New York Magazine* described an incident that reflected a major area of contention:

> At the Paradise benefit, a saucy three-woman disco ensemble called the Ritchie Family closed its set with some motherly advice, counseling the men to stay out of the bathhouses, out of the back rooms, "and, this is the cardinal rule, fellas: one lover per person."
>
> The audience formed its own impromptu chorus chanting back, "NO WAY!"
>
> Everyone enjoyed a healthy laugh. It was, however, a laugh informed with fear.[9]

It rapidly became apparent that there was much more to do than to raise money for medical research. GMHC volunteers began to develop services in the spring of 1982. It was clear that the crisis was not one only of gay men's health. Essentially making it up as they went along, the founders were responding to a crisis with three interconnected aspects—a crisis in the gay community, a crisis in social institutions, and a crisis in individuals' lives.

The first step was to provide information. Gay men needed to be educated about the new disease: how to recognize what it was, and what to do about it if they thought they had it. A variety of techniques were used, including brochures, announcements in gay publications, and several informational forums. GMHC hosted the first forum on 12 May 1982 at New York University, with presentations by the three physicians who had been treating many of the early cases in the city, Alvin Friedman-Kien, Linda J. Laubenstein, and Daniel C. William.[10] At a second forum the following November, the auditorium was only able to accommodate two thousand people and five hundred were turned away.[11] The lessons were not abstract. A voice from the balcony cried out "Oh no!" when a slide of a KS lesion was shown on a movie screen at one of the early forums. [12]

GMHC's printed material, including weekly notices in the *Native*, reached an even larger audience. There was an initial run of twenty-five thousand copies of the first newsletter, a 36-page booklet called "A.I.D.," the name of the disease at that time. This newsletter commented, "As though the situation weren't confusing enough, our health emergency still seems to be shopping for a name."[13] Called "gay cancer," "Gay Related Infectious Disease," "Kaposi's Sarcoma and Opportunistic Infections," "Community Acquired Immune Deficiency," and "A.I.D." before the term AIDS was adopted in September 1982, the disease—its very nature and the way it was transmitted—was just beginning to be understood.

The first GMHC newsletter, appearing in 1982 and distributed widely throughout the country, captures the anguish and uncertainty of the time. Little was known about the disease—its cause, mode of transmission, or treatments. One new AIDS case was being reported every day and, Lawrence Mass told the readers of the *Native,* "It hasn't gone away."[14]

The first article, "Who We Are and What This Is," noted "We are Gay Men's Health Crisis. We are volunteers concerned about a growing threat of diseases in our community. Some of these diseases have killed nearly 200 Americans. Medical investigators do not know why. More than a year has passed since they began trying to tell us why."[15] It summarized available information and offered practical advice about symptoms and about possible diagnostic tests and treatments, information about contagion and lowering risks, a list of forty-five physicians "familiar with AID management," tips on selecting a doctor, and lists of other organizations, services, and publications.

Gay communities throughout the country were beginning to mobilize as more and more men were experiencing AIDS panic. Some was due to the growing number of cases, but perhaps even more important was the evidence that AIDS was sexually transmitted. GMHC's first newsletter pointed out that there were four hundred cases throughout the country and that "many men face a terrifying dilemma. Panic is now spreading among all of us. Nobody knows for certain what has brought on this outbreak of disease. . . . Suspicion has been cast on virtually every aspect of our lives, yet no firm proof has been established so far to help us choose what to do or what not to do."[16] One article, written by Marty Levine, who described himself as "a sociologist who writes about New York's gay ghetto and is very much a part of it," was called "Fearing Fear Itself." The article began with descriptions of three men who were so fearful of contracting AIDS that they had become social isolates. Levine underscored the epidemic's powerful impact on gay men and the gay community, noting that "Hospital visits and funerals are becoming as commonplace as Levi's 501 jeans. Friends who never before showed the slightest interest in gay causes are now besieging us for donations to Gay Men's Health Crisis." At the same time, he pointed to major shifts in behavior as a result of this caution: dating, fewer men going to gay bathhouses, and a rise in stable monogamous relationships.[17]

The newsletter also announced that GMHC would begin to provide services. Noting that because "The victims of AID disorders often find themselves swamped by a tide of problems over and above the desperate problems of health, . . . GMHC has organized a Patient Services Committee to help these men through what must be, in the best of circumstances, a terrifying moment in their lives." The first service was the hotline, which began when Rodger McFarlane, who worked as a health care consultant, listed his telephone number in GMHC's first newsletter.

The most distinctive feature of GMHC's early history is that the services were designed and delivered by volunteers. Some were professionals; most were not. Together they fashioned a set of programs emulated by organizations all over the world. Mel Rosen became GMHC's first Executive Director in the fall of 1982. He was, in fact, a volunteer; GMHC served as his field placement while he finished a graduate degree in social work. His arrival marked the beginning of what he called the group's second phase, when it evolved from being an all-volunteer fundraising group to a volunteer-dominated human service organization with a small paid staff. His vision of the organization's future was quite different from that of Larry Kramer, who had devoted himself almost full-time to getting GMHC off the ground. Kramer thought that GMHC ought to primarily be involved in advocacy, pressuring government agencies and existing social service organizations to serve people with AIDS. Rosen and GMHC's first president, Paul Popham, thought the group ought to become "a top notch social service organization in the gay community that had all the respect from other social service agencies in the city . . . in the country."[18]

Notices in the *Native* called for more volunteers, including doctors, social workers and psychiatrists, typesetters, "concerned individuals," and "people who don't mind hard work." The response was overwhelming, and more volunteers stepped forward than could be handled.[19] Prospective volunteers viewed AIDS as a personal and as a communal issue. Their involvement helped many to cope with what they realized was a communal tragedy and disaster.[20] Philip Kayal, a sociologist and GMHC volunteer, pointed out that the early volunteers were a self-selected group who overcame the internalized homophobia that many gay men experienced; their participation represented an important change in the gay community. Like Popham, who was initially unwilling to have himself publicly identified as the group's president, Rosen was reluctant to be interviewed on television because "I was afraid that my parents would see me. But after a while there were so many sick people that the principle became more important than my being seen on T.V."[21] Judge Richard C. Failla, a board member and early volunteer, pointed out on his retirement from the board in 1990 that his involvement "has made me more proud to be an openly gay man than anything I've experienced in fifteen years of community activism."[22]

GMHC was truly a grassroots organization, where volunteers were able to channel their concern about their own lives and the lives of their friends and family. Participation was highly personal and was the result of a complex set of emotions and concerns. One of GMHC's distinctive features was that the donors, the volunteers, the clients, and the staff had strong links to one another and, in many cases, people were involved in more than one role. People started out as volunteers, changed careers and became staff, and sometimes became clients. Nearly all of the group's early board members, including the first three presidents, died of AIDS.

Many of the gay volunteers became involved because they feared that they would become sick. Others saw it as an important health issue in the gay community or as an opportunity to help. Just doing something was a way to deal with anxiety and powerlessness. Lewis Katoff, a volunteer who became the director of client services, first became involved "because the epidemic was so difficult to comprehend or accept. I wanted to be where there were caring and informed people doing something about what was happening."[23]

Numerous volunteers moved into paid jobs as the agency grew. Volunteering was often described as transformative. GMHC volunteer Arthur Myers told a group of potential volunteers in 1989 that they would no longer recognize themselves after they became involved with the organization. Mitchell Cutler, the first coordinator of the buddy program, concluded that it had been "the most important work I'd ever do. . . . Years later, I'm acknowledged by people for doing this."[24] Early volunteers and staff engaged in magical thinking, hoping that their involvement protected them. When three key GMHC staff members were diagnosed with AIDS, one volunteer noted that "Somehow I felt that those working in AIDS should be exempt from the epidemic."[25]

Working out of donated space in a welfare hotel at 318 West 22 Street, Rosen and his volunteers began to construct an organization. Their immediate objectives were to recruit more volunteers, continue the hotline, start a buddy program, publish a second newsletter, establish fundraising committees, and obtain support from foundations.[26] About a month after Rosen started, 150 people attended a volunteer orientation. For him, the volunteers were the "manpower [that would] put many of our long-term plans into effect." Some volunteers became crisis intervention workers. Trained therapists provided counseling and led support groups, and buddies were assigned to do household chores and visit patients in their homes.[27] By the beginning of 1983, GMHC had a hotline, crisis intervention counseling, a buddy program, and a financial assistance department to provide help with welfare, food stamps, and Social Security. That year, they added recreation services, support groups, and patient advocacy.[28]

Starting with one tiny room in a basement, the office expanded as rooms in the hotel became vacant. The situation was a bit strange: rooms occupied by GMHC were alongside those occupied by the hotel's residents, including homeless and mentally ill people.[29] Volunteers worked at home, and support groups were held in the homes and offices of group leaders. Rosen recalled: "It was just complete pandemonium, but it was organized pandemonium."[30] There weren't enough phones, and, on a typical weekday in the spring of 1983, "as many as a dozen people [are] in the office answering telephones, running the xerox, typing letters, coordinating mailings, stuffing envelopes, or simply keeping the coffee pot perking."[31] A visitor from the AIDS Committee of Toronto observed that the office was small and smoke-filled, and "overrun with people, cockroaches, and files. Nonetheless, a steady stream of activity, extremely organized, somewhat messianical, continues to flow from there. . . . For the most part . . . there is an informal formality—a friendliness and dedication that is admirable and a definite hierarchy."[32] The office was a gathering place for people who volunteered and for people who needed help. Hotline callers would be invited to come into the office to get additional information. Some people simply walked in off the street. Sandi Feinblum went there to get information for a close friend and wound up volunteering because she was "very moved by how they talked to people over the phone and how kind they were to me giving me information."[33]

Services evolved quickly and the array of programs, referred to as the GMHC Service Model, was in place by June 1983.[34] They could barely meet the demand. Rodger McFarlane estimated that the hotline logged over one hundred calls its first night: "All these secret AIDS cases, all of these people who had been living in this fear and shame not knowing what was wrong with them . . . calling us because there's something with GRID or AIDS or whatever."[35] By 1985, there were twenty thousand calls per year, and the number more than doubled, to fifty thousand, two years later.[36]

Many calls were requests for information. Others involved deeper issues: gay men who wanted to know how to come out to their parents; bisexual men who led double lives; and brothers, sisters, and parents who were concerned about a gay relative. Barry Davidson, the coordinator during much of the 1980s, recalled that "The anonymity of the telephone was wonderful to get people to open up and talk."[37] The hotline was the gateway to the agency and calls provided clues about the work that needed to be done. Ken Wein, the first director of clinical services, remembered that "As the calls came in, we started to realize the extent of this nightmare epidemic."[38]

Some people called the hotline when they were neglected in hospitals or faced eviction from their apartments. Crisis intervention and buddy services were developed toward the end of 1982 to provide help. The early AIDS cases were confronted with a host of difficulties inside and outside hospitals. Robert Cecci, a long-term survivor and GMHC'S ombudsman, pointed out:

> For many, every contact with the system is a confrontation. . . . Voluntary ambulance and ambulette drivers . . . have refused to transport AIDS patients, leaving some to die at home, and humiliating others in front of neighbors. . . . Emergency room staff have overreacted to the diagnosis, isolating and neglecting patients and mistreating their families, giving misinformation such as "Go home and burn everything the patient has touched." . . . Once admitted, AIDS patients have been treated carelessly: They often are not properly medicated, fed, bathed, shaved nor are they spoken to with compassion by nursing staff. . . . Welfare staff refuse to see people with AIDS, so public assistance, Medicaid and food stamps are delayed. As the number of AIDS cases grows, it gets harder to handle the numerous complaints—repeated daily—case by case.[39]

Sandi Feinblum, a social worker who served as a crisis intervention team leader, recounted an incident that illustrates the complexity of some clients' problems. One of the buddies she supervised got a call from a client who told him that he was planning to commit suicide and then hung up the phone. The buddy called Feinblum, who called the police and also went to see him. The police were unable to intervene because this was a suicide threat, not an actual attempt. Feinblum counseled the patient, with the help of the director of clinical services, whom she called every hour. After several hours, she helped the client to express his fears and concerns, and he decided to move out of the YMCA where he was living and back into his mother's home.[40]

GMHC volunteers also responded to instances of discrimination against people with AIDS and against gay men perceived to have AIDS. People had difficulty obtaining dental care.[41] The New York State Funeral Directors Association urged its members not to embalm people with AIDS, a surprising move in light of the fact that they knew how to handle cases of Hepatitis B, a disease transmitted in similar ways. The Salvation Army allegedly refused to accept clothing that had belonged to a person who had died of AIDS.[42]

One early success was a court case where the Lambda Legal Defense Fund, with financial support from GMHC, fought the eviction of Dr. Joseph Sonnabend, a physician who cared for many early AIDS patients. Fearful that their apartments would decrease in value because of the large number of AIDS patients walking through the lobby, the board of a New York City cooperative apartment building unsuccessfully attempted to evict Sonnabend from his office.[43]

Fear had a particular impact in some hospitals. A staff member in a hospital especially hard-hit by the epidemic recalled:

> There was a lot of fear on everyone's part from the people that washed the walls to physicians to nurses to technicians to volunteers. Everyone read the paper, they heard the stories about food preparation, kissing and toilet seats. . . . In the beginning people were uneducated, very fearful. . . . the hospital buried its head in the sand. They did not start dealing with it soon enough. . . . In the beginning you would see transporters pushing AIDS patients through the hospital wearing gloves and gowns and masks so you definitely knew this poor individual was an AIDS patient. The horrible stories of nutrition people not putting the food in the patient's rooms but leaving it outside in the hall. That we did not have here because we educated [staff] and we had a policy that you would be fired if you refused to care for an AIDS patient.[44]

Some hospitals instituted a kind of internal quarantine by restricting patients to private rooms. This was done well into the 1980s—after the nature of transmission was clearly understood. This meant that precaution signs would be placed on the door of a patient's room indicating that he or she had an infectious disease.

One early GMHC volunteer viewed these responses as totally irrational even in light of the limited knowledge about the disease at the outset; in his opinion, people in health care institutions demonstrated

> not only a lack of leadership but an overtly hostile and phobic reaction. That is, in our finest institutions, I mean from Sloan Kettering to NYU . . . people were frightened to walk in the room. . . . People in those hospitals had dealt with tetanus, rabies, things that make AIDS pale by comparison. It didn't matter if it was airborne or not. Even if it was airborne we knew the precautions. There was absolutely no excuse except phobia. It was an irrational fear. . . . I could understand people being phobic . . . what surprised me was the hostility that was behind it and how flagrantly overt that hostility was and how sanctioned it was by the institutions. . . . It was OK for this to happen to those people. . . . The reaction was flagrantly irrational by any standard of medical practice.[45]

GMHC staff and volunteers responded to these problems in two ways. They trained health care professionals, and mediated a growing number of complaints. In 1985–1986, GMHC's ombudsman's office handled 485 cases; the number rose sharply to 1,240 two years later.[46]

In addition to the newness and uncertainty of the disease and the unresponsiveness and often neglect that early AIDS patients experienced, some features of the lives of gay men made the development of organized services particularly necessary. Although many received support from parents and siblings, others had strained or nonexistent relationships with families. An early GMHC volunteer recalled that "There were people who were alone, abandoned by their families, were too terrified to reach out to their families." For many, friends were their families and were often referred to in this way.[47] Some men lived at great distances from their families of origin and had come to New York because of the enormous difficulties of being a gay man in many parts of the country. Indeed, New York's gay community was filled with men who had left other parts of the country to take advantage of the anonymity, freedom, and sense of community. GMHC itself served as family. GMHC volunteer Barry Davidson noted, "It was like our own brother and sister and family we were taking care of. There was a lot of love between the staff and the volunteers. We were really family more than anything else."[48]

Many volunteers worked as buddies, visiting patients and doing practical chores. Called upon to do the kind of caregiving usually performed by women when a family member is ill, one early leader explained the willingness of GMHC's early volunteers to roll up their sleeves and do the dirty work involved in crisis intervention work: "They had also been kicked around enough in life having grown up gay."[49] It was difficult work since, "after working with two or three PWAs, . . . they were frightened. They were gay men and the illness brought up a lot of issues for them." Many of the early volunteers were fearful that they had AIDS, and others were concerned that the disease might be easily transmitted. Michael Quadland, a psychologist and early volunteer, recalled that he threw away the drinking glass that his first client used. Mark Senak, a volunteer attorney for GMHC, boiled the glass a client had used to drink wine.[50]

As survival time increased, many volunteers pointed out that they got more than they gave and found working with PWAs (Persons with AIDS) inspirational and transformative. A woman volunteer pointed out: "Before, I had lots of personal problems. I was often unhappy. . . . After I met people with AIDS, I saw that life must have value. Here are people who are trying so hard to live. They have everything wrong with them, and every part of their bodies is in pain. But they still want to live, even in pain. Seeing that changed me completely. Now I realize how meaningful and important life is. I'm growing up."[51]

Volunteers were doing the work of human service professionals with little background and training. Mitchell Cutler, a dealer in expensive art books, who designed the buddy program, recalled working "out of instinct and from my heart and what I thought was morally and ethically right."[52] Lay people worked alongside professionals, not always without differences and tensions, but instincts and professional knowledge were synthesized in creating services that responded to the needs of AIDS patients. Neither professionals nor lay volunteers were completely comfortable with this situation. Jed Mattes noted that many clients had complex lives that were sometimes "Gothic soap operas [with problems] bigger than what we could handle. . . . We were in a professional status and we weren't professionals. . . . But we couldn't really do what we wanted to do, which was to conquer this."[53] Ken Wein, the first director of clinical services, recalls that he was "kind of frightened. . . . We're talking about people with very serious and profound life crisis issues and they were working with paraprofessional volunteers."[54]

GMHC's rapid response and the ingenuity and commitment of its volunteers were a stark contrast to the lack of responsiveness of mainstream social service and public health organizations.[55] The rapid development of GMHC's services is testimony to its ability to attract a talented pool of staff and volunteers. The fact also reveals an enormous gap in our society's safety net. Social services tended to be organized for children, old people, and poor families, not for men in their thirties with acute and fatal diseases; and the public health system had not been very involved in preventing sexually transmitted diseases since the development of antibiotics. But the limited response was attitudinal, not just organizational. When I interviewed an executive in a major health agency in the city in the late fall of 1988, he candidly admitted that "AIDS wasn't a sexy item. AIDS was the kind of item where people most definitely didn't want to get too involved. They didn't want to get too close for fear that people would start to talk about who they were, what they were doing, why they were doing it."[56]

GMHC responded to the stigma of the illness as well as to its enormous uncertainty. For patients, their friends, and health and human service professionals, AIDS was stressful and frightening because it was not clear what needed to be done and because the risks of getting the disease were unknown. Physicians were baffled and unsure about how to treat patients. GMHC's volunteers played an important part in the development and diffusion of knowledge about AIDS patients. Once the knowledge base had been developed, GMHC's staff and volunteers established its Professional Education Program which trained health and human service professionals working in the city. Volunteers and social workers assisted clients in obtaining public benefits like Social Security Disability Insurance.

GMHC sponsored a number of fundraising events in 1982 and 1983 including a raffle and a cocktail party and auction at the home of Craig Claiborne, the *New York Times* food critic.[57] One year after the Showers, in April 1983, GMHC sold out Madison Square Garden for the Ringling Brother's Circus.[58] It was able to provide a $100,000 deposit by borrowing $1,000 from one hundred people.[59] The circus raised $300,000, double its goal, and the eighteen thousand people who filled Madison Square Garden were told that it was the "greatest gay event of all time." The conductor Leonard Bernstein led "The Star Spangled Banner" and Mayor Ed Koch gave a speech.[60] Along with nearly $300,000 from New York State and $25,000 from two New York City agencies, proceeds from the circus allowed GMHC to move to new quarters and to hire more staff. [61] Potential donors were told "we have instituted a very ambitious program of Patient Services—to help our friends and lovers who may be ill with AIDS. . . . We are proud of this work, and we hope that you are too. We are growing very quickly, as is, unfortunately this epidemic. . . . For us to continue this growth, we need your continued support. . . . We need your money and we need your support. Please help us help all of us."[62]

By then, the growing demand for services and the agency's greater complexity required more paid staff. The agency had organized four major educational forums, printed one-half million pieces of educational material, and trained eight teams of crisis intervention counselors. Popham told the people at the circus that "The need for our services continues to grow at such an alarming rate that we're dizzy and exhausted from trying to keep up with it. . . . We have created a gay Red Cross. Now we must professionalize it."[63]

At the end of 1983, there had been 514 AIDS deaths in New York City and GMHC's twelve staff and five hundred volunteers were engaged in a broad range of activities.[64] Described as "a sophisticated social-service organization with growing political power" by the *New York Times*, the organization found its sense of urgency and crisis unabated. GMHC'S second executive director, Rodger McFarlane, pointed out, "When persons with AIDS come to us, their lives are shattered and their heads are twisted. They've just been given the devastating news that they have a disease that's probably fatal with a stigma the size of Manhattan attached to it. . . . We're there primarily to handhold and troubleshoot and help these people get some control over their lives."[65] One year later, McFarlane pointed out that "The madness is relentless. They come in the door and across the telephone, and it's our task to manage the madness, not to be sucked into it."[66]

In the summer of 1985, Richard Dunne, a GMHC board member, became the agency's third executive director. Dunne had considerable background working in city government, and brought additional management expertise to GMHC. Growing public concern also meant that public funding was beginning to increase, and during Dunne's tenure, GMHC became a major social service agency, with an $11 million budget in 1989. Dunne resolved at the outset that, even though "government funding would double or triple on the city level, . . . we must continue to actively raise private funds, and must maintain our independence and integrity and not become overly dependent on government funding."[67] He was successful in this goal: the proportion of GMHC's income from public sources declined from one third in 1986 to twenty percent in 1989.[68] Private funds gave the agency autonomy. When Senator Jesse Helms claimed in 1987 that a GMHC video and its "safer sex commix" were "hardcore, pornographic, lustful [and] ugly," the agency was able to point out that the materials were not produced with public funds.[69]

Dunne wanted GMHC to increase its involvement in advocacy, "pressuring government agencies to fund research, improve health care delivery and patient services." To do this, he hired Tim Sweeney from the Lambda Legal Defense Fund as the full-time deputy director for policy.[70] The organizational culture and the mix of volunteers also began to change. A 1986 survey done by Philip Kayal found that 40 percent of GMHC volunteers had AIDS, were HIV positive, or suspected they had AIDS and 60 percent thought that they might need GMHC's services in the future. By the end of the 1980s, GMHC volunteers were much more diverse. Only about one in ten new volunteers were HIV positive and slightly more than half (54 percent) knew someone who was HIV positive or had AIDS. This also meant that four in ten did not have a close personal connection to the disease but became involved to join the AIDS community or to help the "gay family."[71]

GMHC's success and growth under Dunne's management was bittersweet. At the end of his tenure in 1989, he pointed out that "Most executives in my position would feel justifiably pleased. But when the reason for the expansion is AIDS, it's impossible to feel completely positive, because a part of you is always wishing that it weren't necessary."[72] The most visible evidence of the agency's growth was the opening of its first building, in the final quarter of 1988, an opening that symbolized the agency's permanence.[73] The board had decided that it was necessary to purchase a building to get the space it needed, because "whenever GMHC's real estate agent had found promising quarters, the landlord would learn the nature of the group and back out."[74] When they located a site in 1986, the broker handling the deal did not mention the name of the agency, to make sure that the sale went through.[75]

The new building gave the epidemic and the agency a greater permanence. Echoing Richard Dunne's bittersweet feelings about GMHC's growth, the board president, Joy Tomchin, pointed out, "Our new building has said to the world that we're here to stay. But we must not allow this image to impede us in our struggle for the speedy elimination of HIV infection."[76] Most volunteers, like most Americans, thought that the disease would be conquered quickly and the need for the agency would end. Board member James G. Pepper recalled that "Like most people in 1981–1982, I felt that AIDS would be rapidly crushed by the miracles of modern medicine. In 1986 I had to face the reality that organizations such as GMHC would have to provide services for a greater number of people that ever anticipated in the early days."[77] GMHC's ability to rely on volunteers reinforced the organization's sense that it was temporary, since an agency with unpaid staff could be dismantled when it was no longer needed.

But the epidemic was not ending soon and the number of cases was escalating. Three-and-a-half years after GMHC opened its new building on Twentieth Street, the building was again too small.[78] By then, GMHC was the center of a network of AIDS organizations in the city. Many consciously modeled themselves after GMHC. Others, like the PWA Coalition, took a different approach and were far more interested in empowering individuals to take charge of their lives. Together, the volunteers and staff in this expanding network of organizations began to see themselves as part of an AIDS community that defined its mission as "fighting" the epidemic and fighting for their lives.

Chapter 2

Fighting the Victim Label

Those of us crazy enough to publicly identify ourselves as having the most stigmatized disease of the century agreed that it felt strange to be treated like "celebrities" for having AIDS. Only in America, I thought, would it be necessary to make a career out of being sick in order to compel a more humane and appropriate government response.

—Michael Callen, *Surviving Aids* (New York: Harper Collins, 1990)

A 1984 article in the *Native* presented a chilling fantasy of the epidemic in 1987 and in 1988. Over two million people had been diagnosed with AIDS or AIDS-Related Complex. The epidemic had been declared a health emergency; there was mandatory testing of all health care workers, flight attendants, food handlers, and teachers. Gays were changing their identities and fleeing New York and San Francisco for smaller cities because they feared they would be placed in detention camps. Cremation was required for all AIDS deaths. The theater district had closed because of the large numbers of actors who had died of AIDS. An underground Homosexual Liberation Army ambushed religious leaders, killed three senators, and was at war with the U.S. government.[1]

Looking back, this scenario may seem exaggerated, but some elements were not inconceivable. Between 1983 and 1986, the complexity of the disease and the magnitude and the impact of the epidemic were becoming clearer. The sense of panic was growing. Although many Americans were compassionate, there was a great deal of indifference, some condemnation, and mostly a lot of fear. Several recommendations for reducing the spread of the disease—quarantine, tattooing people with AIDS, mandatory HIV testing, and case reporting—were viewed with alarm by an emerging AIDS community.[2] The fantasy of fighting the disease and also fighting an indifferent and potentially repressive society was also beginning to take hold. In the face of enormous uncertainty and panic, people with AIDS began to organize to fight the disease, and, in the process, they created an AIDS community based on a sense of shared risk, a source of social solidarity that is growing in importance in an increasingly technologically sophisticated global society.[3]

GMHC's founding marked the beginning of creating an AIDS community. Its volunteers refracted ideas from various helping professions to respond to the needs of people who were dying quickly. Within a short while, survival time began to increase, and people began to publicly identify themselves as persons with AIDS (PWAs). They faced two significant challenges—uncertainty about the disease, and the enormous stigma, both physical (since many PWAs had visible signs of having the disease in the form of skin lesions from Kaposi's Sarcoma) and psychological. PWAs began to meet in GMHC-sponsored support groups and in other groups, where they developed an AIDS culture. The AIDS culture operated as a collective action frame, a cognitive map that guided individuals living with AIDS, a framework that included what Indyk and Rier describe as grassroots AIDS knowledge.[4] The expertise GMHC drew upon was professional; it adapted ideas from the fields of social work, psychology, and psychiatry. The AIDS community also tapped another type of expertise, knowledge based on the experience of living with AIDS.

There were two key dimensions to the AIDS culture: an emphasis on interacting with other PWAs and becoming empowered; and reframing the disease as life-threatening but not immediately fatal. The emphasis on individual and communal self-determination and empowerment promoted a sense of shared identity and also served as a blueprint for collective action.[5] Clearly, the personal concerns that brought people into the support groups and other organizations in the AIDS community led to political action, which supports Paul Lichterman's observation that the search for individual fulfillment does not preclude communal and political action.[6]

Enormous uncertainty about the disease, combined with a sharp rise in the number of cases, contributed to growing concern in the society and a sense of panic in the gay community. In July 1982, 11 new cases were being diagnosed in the United States each week; this increased to nearly 170 cases each week in 1985. Government officials announced in 1985 that it was unlikely that effective medications would be available before 1990 or that the epidemic would be under control before 2000.[7] Costs were rising. Public funds for hospital care in New York City were between $51 million and $77 million in 1985, and the amount was expected to rise to $100 million the following year. The state comptroller estimated that the city would be spending about $500 million on AIDS in 1989.[8]

Americans became even more fearful after new routes of transmission were identified. Five thousand people a day were calling the federal government's month-old AIDS hotline in August 1983.[9] The identification of cases that were the result of blood transfusions or of hemophiliacs receiving HIV-infected blood products led to a concern about the safety of the blood supply. A 1983 article in the *Journal of the American Medical Association* suggested that AIDS might be transmitted in ways other than through sexual contact, drug use, or exposure to blood products—through routine household contact, a possibility not disproven until 1986.[10] The prospect of other as yet unknown routes of transmission contributed to the concern that the epidemic could spread to the so-called general population. In some instances, the responses were extreme, if not irrational.

Public attitudes and a number of events indicated that the *Native* scenario might not be so bizarre. Some of the fears were obviously irrational, since they persisted well after scientific evidence showed that they were groundless. From 28 percent who thought that AIDS was transmitted by sharing a drinking glass in 1983, the proportion rose to 47 percent in September 1985, when large numbers of Americans either thought it was "unsafe to associate with someone with AIDS" even if one did not have "intimate physical contact" (36 percent), or did not know whether this was safe (7 percent)."[11] One in five young American women interviewed in 1988 believed that HIV could be transmitted if a person donated blood or was bitten by an insect. [12]

From 1984 until 1987, the gay community directed enormous amounts of attention and resources to protect the civil liberties of people with AIDS. Northwest Airlines excluded people with AIDS, and later required that they present a medical certificate testifying that they were not infectious.[13] Legal issues abounded: evictions, job discrimination, and the need to establish eligibility for Social Security, SSI, and other public benefits. Staff in the federal Department of Justice noted that people with AIDS and "carriers" could be dismissed from their jobs since they were not covered by federal guidelines protecting disabled people from being dismissed arbitrarily.[14] Violence toward gay men increased—from 2,042 incidents nationally in 1985 to 4,946 the following year.[15] Numerous cases of discrimination were reported in New York City and in New York State; this accelerated in the second half of the 1980s when cases rose sharply, from 154 in 1983 and 1984, to over 900 by the end of 1987. Some incidents involved people who were *thought* to have AIDS, which in most cases meant gay men.[16] Public policy debates included serious discussion of measures like quarantine, mandatory screening and testing, contact tracing, and reporting the names of people who tested HIV positive. Conservative journalist William Buckley suggested in an Op Ed column in the *New York Times* that people with AIDS could be tattooed on their buttocks or arms to warn others that they were infected, a proposal he later retracted.[17]

When the New York City schools opened in September 1985, eleven thousand students stayed home on the first day because a child with AIDS would be attending a public school in the borough of Queens.[18] In Kokomo, Indiana, a teenage hemophiliac named Ryan White was told not to attend school, and received his schooling over the telephone for several months. When he returned to school under a court order, Ryan was taunted, the windows of his family's home were broken, their car tires were slashed, and store clerks refused to put change into his mother's hands.[19] The three Ray brothers, also hemophiliacs, had their home burned down in Florida. Although it was not clear why, an AIDS patient caught on fire in 1984 in one of the city's most prestigious hospitals.[20]

Some leaders and journalists contributed to the stigma and irrational response. Fundamentalist preacher Jerry Falwell pointed out that, by failing to take adequate public health precautions, President Reagan was to be blamed for "allowing this awful disease to break out among the innocent American public."[21] In the summer of 1986, about a fourth of Americans polled by the *Los Angeles Times* agreed that AIDS was "a punishment God has given homosexuals for the way they lived."[22]

For many in the gay community, these events served as the basis of enormous concern and alarm that there was an AIDS backlash. At the end of 1985, one third of Americans surveyed in a Gallup poll indicated that they had more negative feelings toward homosexuals, as a result of AIDS.[23] One long-term gay activist pointed out to me in 1990 that he had long thought that there might be a serious backlash against gays in the country, a kind of pogrom, but that "It would be done in some medical way." Tim Sweeney recalled, "It was a completely bleak time controlled by the radical right. My energy was spent trying to block the anti-gay campaign in the U.S. Congress . . . which had been sponsored by U.S. Senator Jesse Helms."[24] This was the setting in which growing numbers of people were learning that they were "immune deficient" or had AIDS. Looking at AIDS as a moral issue, not just a disease, heightened PWAs' guilt, self-blame, and stigma.[25] Some, especially gay men, turned to one another for support.

An anonymous interview with a "gay cancer" patient in the late summer of 1981 indicated that, already, people living with the disease were beginning to turn to one another for information and for support. He pointed out that "I've become very close with one of the other patients whose disease is more extensive. I really feel I understand what he's going through in a way that those who haven't been in this situation can't. Our communication has meant a lot to both of us. I'm sure it's going to have a positive influence on our getting well. Hope, the will to live, these are important aspects of the healing process. As more of us come together, the more positive that influence will be."[26]

The connection between these two patients was part of an important trend in American life, where increasing numbers of people were joining self-help groups, especially groups for people with specific diseases.[27] Even though some people viewed support groups as promoting introspection and narcissism, many such groups had a significant political aspect.[28] Health psychologists were also beginning to document what the anonymous gay cancer patent knew: that social support had a beneficial impact. People lived longer if they reached out to other people, particularly people with the same illness. Social isolation was toxic. The course of a person's illness was affected by social and psychological support and by changes in lifestyle, which were, in turn, very much influenced by being in contact with other people who could provide information and support.[29] Participation in self-help groups and in patient activism would prove enormously beneficial for individuals, and served as an important basis for communal empowerment.[30]

The stigma of the disease, combined with a lack of clarity about transmission, converged to promote social isolation and despair among many early AIDS patients. Bob Cecci, GMHC's ombudsman, recalled about those early years:

> Nobody knew what to advise us so we were advised about everything. Things that were ludicrous. Don't touch money. Don't go into restaurants. Don't go into grocery stores during the day when there are a lot of people in there. . . . Don't breathe the air—that was the big one. So I literally sat in my apartment for six months afraid to open the windows. Afraid that if I took a deep breath I would get pneumocystis. Afraid to really be around other PWAs.[31]

Another early PWA, Kenny Taub, went into seclusion after his diagnosis, since he "figured, what's the use?" Like other gay men diagnosed with AIDS, Taub tried to commit suicide, and woke up two days later feeling sorry that he hadn't died.[32] In the first several years, the stigma and social isolation, which made the groups important, also made it difficult to start them. Men were fearful of going out of their homes and being in a room with other people with

AIDS. The formation of these groups marks the beginning of a shift in the disease: they included men who were living with AIDS, not just those who were dying quickly. Men with KS were reluctant to be seen in public and, according to Luis Palacios, who ran the first group for men with KS, they had a lot of shame, confusion, helplessness, and "internalized toxicity," and were "confronting existential issues we seldom confront. Life is unfair, unjust, and that ultimately nothing saves you from the ultimate pain of death."[33]

Ideas that would later coalesce into an AIDS culture were developed in a number of different groups. The support groups were a lifeline: most people with AIDS were dying quickly and in the process were experiencing abandonment, stigma, and an enormous sense of isolation. Knowing they had a fatal illness, they simply did not know what they ought to do until they died, since some of them had periods of relatively good health interspersed with periods of serious illness. Participating in a group helped them to cope. Michael Callen, who joined one of GMHC's first support groups, recalled that "Most of us felt that some terrifying force had taken control of our lives. . . . We saw AIDS as yet another 'closet,' and took comfort in knowing that we were not alone. We shared our hopes, fears and anger as well as love, support, and practical tips on how to handle the stigma which was attached to a diagnosis of AIDS."[34]

In the summer of 1982, Callen formed Gay Men with AIDS (GMWA), a support group that met in his living room.[35] Ads in the *Native* solicited prospective members who were "immunosuppressed gay men who want to break the habit of promiscuous behavior . . . to support each other during the difficult transition from a promiscuous lifestyle to medically safer lifestyles."[36] At about the same time, Jim Fouratt started Wipe Out AIDS! The membership included "people that were sick, and people who were afraid of being sick, and people who were well but were concerned about people who were sick." Many of the speakers who came to the group urged its members that "Hope is realistic."[37] Callen described his experiences to members of the New York State congressional delegation in the spring of 1983:

> We talk about how we're going to buy food and pay rent when our savings run out . . . how we are going to earn enough money to live when some of us are too sick to work . . . how it feels to get fired from our jobs . . . the pain we feel when our lovers leave us out of fear of AIDS . . . the friends who have stopped calling . . . what it feels like when our families refuse to visit us in the hospital. . . . We share our sense of isolation—how it feels to watch doctors and nurses come and go wearing gowns, gloves, and masks. . . . Mostly, we talk about what it feels like to be treated like lepers who are treated as if we are morally, if not literally,

contagious. We try to share what hope there is and to help each other
live our lives one day at a time. What we talk about is survival.[38]

They also discussed doctors and treatment. Drawing on ideas from the
woman's health movement and the critique of the medical system offered by
writers like Ivan Illich,[39] the group urged people to be active health care consumers, not passive patients. Its announcements in the *Native* gave people the
tools to achieve this, citing articles published in medical journals, warning
people about questionable treatments, and urging them to be critical of the care
they were receiving, since "AIDS is a new syndrome and there are NO authorities. Clearly, much of what is being done is not working. . . . educate yourself
by going outside the gay press. Get as broad a view and as many different opinions as possible."[40]

Several members allowed themselves to be interviewed for newspapers
and on television. This took enormous courage. Having real people be interviewed—and named—put a face on AIDS, identifying actual persons with
the illness rather than allowing the disease to be only an abstract, statistical
reality. Phil Lanzaratta, diagnosed with KS in October 1981, was the first person to write about his experiences in the gay press, in a 1982 *Christopher Street*
article. He was also quoted in the *New York Times* and appeared on several
television talk shows in 1983.[41] David Summers was interviewed and photo-
graphed for a *New York Times* article, and was the subject of a Public Broad-
casting System documentary, "Hero of My Own Life." Crew members for NBC
walked out on a taping session with Summers because they were afraid to be
in the same room.[42] These efforts personalized the epidemic, making it real,
something that could happen to one's son or brother or friend.

The members of GMWA also began to participate in the city's nascent
AIDS community, which had expanded beyond GMHC to include the AIDS
Network, an organization that brought together people from a broad cross-section of gay and AIDS organizations. The AIDS Network's weekly meetings featured a count of the newly diagnosed AIDS cases, a sobering reminder of the
growing impact of the epidemic.[43] The AIDS Network was open and inclusive;
Callen and other members of GMWA began attending regularly and met staff
and volunteers from GMHC and from other gay organizations, and gay political leaders like Virginia Apuzzo and Hal Kooden. Funds from the AIDS Network allowed two members of GMWA, including Callen, to attend the Fifth
National Lesbian and Gay Health Conference in Denver in June 1983.[44]

The Denver conference marked a major turning point in the creation of a
national AIDS community, since it was the first time that a group of self-

identified people living with AIDS met to determine how to respond to the disease. Remarkably, they were able "to see beyond the hysteria of the moment" and develop the Denver Principles, which served as the ideology for the emerging national AIDS community.[45] The central principal had already been articulated by a PWA group in San Francisco, whose representatives brought a banner to the conference proclaiming that they were "FIGHTING FOR OUR LIVES." One by one, each member of the group announced the principles at the closing session of the conference. People who were there recalled this as a "key emotional catalyst for the conference" ; Callen noted that "There wasn't a dry eye in the house."[46]

The Denver Principles pointed out, "We condemn attempts to label us as 'victims,' which implies defeat, and we are only occasionally 'patients,' which implies passivity, helplessness, and dependence upon the care of others. We are 'people with AIDS.'" This was a forceful rejection of the commonly used term "AIDS victim." Callen reminisced about his initial reaction: "How California, I thought. But time has proven them right. . . . The difference between the descriptors *person with AIDS* and *AIDS victim* seem subtle until one watches oneself on reruns on TV. To see oneself on screen and have the words *AIDS victim* magically flash underneath has a very different feel about it than when the description *person with AIDS* appears."[47]

Although the mortality rate was still very high, the number of people who were alive after an AIDS diagnosis was just beginning to increase; there were 140 people living with AIDS in New York City at the end of 1982, a number that would increase more than ten times in the next three years, to 1,733.[48] These numbers did not include people who were being called immunosuppressed. The idea of being people, not victims, extended to the principle that people with AIDS ought to live satisfying sexual and emotional lives, had the right to quality medical care, had the right to privacy and confidentiality, and had the right "To die—and to LIVE—in dignity." At the same time, the Denver principles recommended that health care professionals should get in touch with their own feelings and treat people with AIDS "as whole people." Other principles were directed, more broadly, toward "all people;" they called for support "in our struggle against those who would fire us from our jobs, evict us from our homes, refuse to touch us, or separate us from our loved ones, our community, or our peers," and asked people not to "scapegoat people with AIDS, blame us for the epidemic, or generalize about our lifestyles."

A central theme was an emphasis on individual and communal empowerment. The Denver Principles noted that PWAs should "form caucuses to choose their own representatives, to deal with the media, to choose their own agenda, and to plan their own decisions," and to be vocal and active both in the political arena and in AIDS forums.

Callen and the other New Yorkers at the Health Conference returned to New York enthusiastic about forming Persons with AIDS—New York. Attracting about ninety members in its first month, the organization became mired in controversy over the issue of gay bathhouses. Members reviewed grant proposals for the Centers for Disease Control, and participated in GMHC's November 1983 conference organizing a workshop called "Safer Sex: A Presentation from People with AIDS."[49] Eventually, PWA—New York lost momentum, because, according to Callen, GMHC "strongly resisted the notion of a rabble-rousing group of PWAs" and as a result of "internal dissension, the deaths of many of the founders, and a generally inhospitable environment."[50] It is also likely that the potential for organizing was limited because the critical mass of people living with AIDS was still small.

In April, 1985, Callen and eight other PWAs—and one woman who was not a PWA—founded the PWA Coalition, "with a lot of faith and very little in the way of funds."[51] The by-laws noted what was especially distinctive about the PWA movement, that "People with AIDS *are* the experts on the subject of the epidemic."[52] Since empowerment was highly contingent on being informed, the group's *Newsline* would be a "forum for the expression of the diverse opinions of those with and affected by AIDS," to "encourage other PWAs to take control of their lives and plan an active role in whatever mode of treatment they choose to combat this illness."[53] The Coalition recognized the political dimension of its work, noting in its by-laws that "we are born of and inextricably bound to the historical struggle for rights—civil, feminist, lesbian and gay, disabled and human."[54] In addition to creating a blueprint for living with AIDS, the Coalition stressed that PWAs' experiential knowledge gave them enormous legitimacy in fighting the epidemic. The Coalition was founded as a reaction to GMHC, which they believed was not especially concerned about empowerment; and, in fact, PWAC members criticized GMHC, noting "that it is inconvenient, irritating, and time-consuming to let people take an active part when you are busy trying to control them."[55]

PWAC's members wanted to "break through the 'client vs. healthy volunteer' feeling [that] often seems to pervade GMHC" and improve the poor communication between clients and staff.[56] They were interested in working with GMHC as representatives of PWAs. In an article entitled, "So What Are PWAs/ PWARCs Anyway? Chopped Liver?" Coalition member Ken Meeks complained about a conference for service providers at which there were no PWAs on the program.[57] The desire for participation had a deeper source; in a second article,

Meeks explained that "This is 1986: if the gods of medical science can't give us the instant cure we desire, the gods of all professions had better prepare to include us in their plans."[58] GMHC acceded to the Coalition's request: Max Navarre soon joined GMHC's Quality Assurance Committee and its board.

PWA's first major project, the *Newsline*, a monthly newsletter created by and for PWAs, was the AIDS community's first regular source of written information that tied together this expanding community. The first *Newsline* was typed and duplicated on a copying machine. The original run of two hundred was quickly depleted and an additional four hundred copies were distributed.[59] Early issues included notices about free massages, a plumber willing to help PWAs, and "Oysters: A Raw Deal," a summary of a study published in the *Journal of the American Medical Association* that pointed out that raw oysters as well as raw fish and beef "can be deadly" for people with weakened immune systems.[60]

The *Newsline* filled an enormous need, and the number of readers grew rapidly. It appeared at a time of transition in the dissemination of information, just as computer databases, computerized bulletin boards, and email discussion lists were coming into existence. Even though it primarily focused on the AIDS community in New York, its readership was nationwide. In early 1986, the *Newsline* was posted on a computer bulletin board, the precursor of more elaborate systems of information dissemination that would occur after the expansion of the internet. A year later, it became possible to obtain selected Associated Press stories, Medline, and specialized AIDS information via computer.[61]

Circulation rose rapidly and fourteen thousand copies were printed in 1987.[62] The *Newsline* attracted numerous contributors. People shared their feelings and experiences, both positive and negative; announced meetings; discussed policies and programs; and offered information about treatment methods. The information was practical: tips on selecting a doctor; the benefits of diet, exercise, massage, and holistic approaches to health care; reasons to join a support group; reasons to be angry; and tips on grieving.[63] Articles offered hints about how to lengthen survival time, stressing the importance of diet and of alternative and holistic approaches to health. The publication's resource guide listed AIDS organizations and services available in the metropolitan area. The weekly "Living with AIDS" show, produced by GMHC in collaboration with PWAC, was another important source of information for the evolving AIDS community.[64]

The participatory nature of the *Newsline* was empowering. Each issue began with a disclaimer: the articles were for "information only and do not necessarily constitute an endorsement."[65] Articles were written by members of the Coalition but also by prisoners with AIDS, caregivers, and PWAs from all over the country. One caregiver commented that "GMHC gave me the bureaucratic cold shoulder because my lifemate hadn't been 'officially diagnosed' . . . *PWA Coalition Newsline* was my lifeline, my sole source of information and human contact with other living, vibrant gay human beings wresting with the implications of this vile epidemic and their own mortality."[66] With Callen, as editor, feeling that the readers were "sentient adults capable of sorting out what is useful from what is not," the magazine had a policy of printing everything submitted.[67] Even when having to be more selective, Callen tried to publish everything he could because "At heart, I'm a softy. I know I have published a lot of bad writing, but there were always reasons other than style to publish a piece. More than once I got a frantic call from an intensive care nurse saying that the last words spoken by a PWA before going on a respirator was a desire to see something he or she had written published in the *Newsline*."[68]

In addition to discussing mainstream medical findings, the *Newsline* published pieces expressing dissident views on the cause of AIDS. Although most experts agree that HIV, the human immunodeficiency virus, is the cause of AIDS, other explanations were suggested, including Dr. Jane Teas' idea that AIDS was caused by the African Swine Flu virus and that there was a connection between the disease and research taking place at a federal research laboratory on Plum Island, located off Long Island.[69] Some PWAs, like Callen, supported a multifactor thesis originally proposed by Joseph Sonnabend in a 1983 issue of the *Journal of the American Medical Association (JAMA),* which pointed out "that multiple factors provoke immune regulatory and surveillance defects in a subset of homosexual men. Recurrent cytomegalovirus (CMV) infections and immune responses to sperm are likely major causative factors of AIDS." The idea was expanded into the theory that AIDS was a consequence of the continued assault on gay men's immune systems by repeated bouts of sexually transmitted diseases.[70]

The *Newsline* supplemented informal channels of communication. In fact, the starting point for being empowered was to become involved with other PWAs. By the mid-1980s, there were more and more social opportunities. GMHC sponsored several recreational programs such as Friday night movies and weekly dinners. PWAC sponsored potluck dinners and singles teas, and opened the Living Room, a safe space for relaxing, support groups, and lunch.[71] In the winter of 1986–1987, PWAC offered an apartment sharing service, was serving between seventy-five and one hundred meals each week, presented Saturday night comedy films in a program called the "Laughter

Lab," and attracted a hundred people to the first of its monthly singles teas. One afternoon each week, Debra Provenzano taught PWAs how to use makeup to cover their KS lesions.[72] PWAC also sponsored support groups for people with ARC (AIDS-related complex) and for mothers of PWAs, and one that attracted three or four women with AIDS.[73] More and more people came to the support groups and to the Living Room: the mother's group doubled in size, the women's group grew to between ten to twenty members, and a Spanish-speaking group was attracting between eight and fifteen people each week.[74] In 1988, about eight hundred meals were served at the Living Room each month.[75]

PWAC founders like Navarre assured people about the importance of connecting with other people, since "no matter how you're feeling, you're not alone . . . lots of people have survived an AIDS diagnosis and are here to tell the story." Rather than being a death sentence, an AIDS diagnosis was an opportunity and an important turning point. Phil Lanzaratta reflected back about the initial reaction to the idea of living with AIDS: "In those days, if you suggested the possibility of survival, healthy caregivers would smile sadly, humor you, and hand you Kubler-Ross."[76] Early issues of the *Newsline* contained positive articles about survivors—how long they had had AIDS, various ailments they had overcome, and strategies they used to stay alive, including traditional and nontraditional forms of health care. These articles played an important role in reframing the illness at a time when doctors were just beginning to treat the opportunistic infections that affected people with AIDS. Thus, "We at the *Newsline* have decided that it's about time we balanced the books a little on the subject of survival."[77] Callen echoed these views in a speech to the American Public Health Association in 1986, seven years before his death. He pointed out that "AIDS is the moment-to-moment management of uncertainty. It's a roller coaster ride without a seat belt. . . . But if I can challenge one assumption about AIDS in this speech, it is the assumption that everyone dies from AIDS—that AIDS is an automatic death sentence—that AIDS has a 100 percent mortality rate. There are a handful of us—estimated variously at ten to eighteen percent—who happen to be quite alive more than three years after our diagnoses and who intend to be alive for many more years."[78]

Disclosing a diagnosis to friends and family was difficult, but for many people, once HIV testing was approved in 1985, learning of an HIV-positive diagnosis became a turning point. Many people believed that it gave them a new lease on life. One man told a reporter for the *Body Positive*, a magazine similar to the

Newsline, that "In some ways I was reborn the day I tested positive. The only life I know now is that of being positive and fighting or facing this virus. . . . Most of my friends now are HIV positive, or others who deal with HIV on a daily basis. It has taken everything I have to build a new life. I am thrilled with the new people who've entered my life these last years. I am glad to have taken what I first considered a death sentence and turned it into a more conscious and passionately lived life than before."[79]

An emphasis on self-determination developed early. By 1983, GMHC crisis intervention volunteers were being instructed, "Patients should . . . be encouraged to take as much of an active role in treatment as possible. . . . Patients should be encouraged to participate in as many social, recreational, leisure, and occupational pursuits as possible."[80] Being empowered lengthened people's lives. According to Callen, long-term survivors were "frisky, opinionated, educated," and many had thrown doctors or health care providers out of their hospital rooms.[81] Drawing on principles from the women's health movement, PWAs were told that

"Self-empowerment is about *YOU,* the individual human being, being *In Charge* (the Captain of the Team). It is about *YOU* being the final decision maker, consulting with who/whatever and following whichever path that *YOU* decide is the right one. It's not other people and certainly not institutions or laws/dogmas which need to be in control. (It is *YOU* picking up that scepter and bringing court to regal order."[82]

Perhaps the most critical reason for being in control was that PWAs needed to be active health care consumers: carefully selecting doctors, learning to be their own advocates when hospitalized, willing to question and challenge physicians, and actively seeking not only traditional but also alternative, as well as experimental and unapproved, treatment methods. PWAs were advised: "While you're talking, talk to your doctor. There is no such thing as a stupid question. . . . ASK THEM. If the answers that you receive do not satisfy you, say so. . . . It is your right and your responsibility to yourself to see to it that you understand what is being done to your body. If your doctor insists that a certain procedure is essential to your health, and you have qualms about it, get a second opinion. If getting another opinion makes you feel uncomfortable, *feel uncomfortable* and get another opinion."[83]

Like growing numbers of Americans, PWAs did whatever they could to improve their sense of well-being, combining conventional medical interventions with alternative and holistic treatment methods.[84] They joined support groups and engaged in other strategies, like watching comedy shows on television if they believed that having a positive frame of mind would lengthen their lives. The critical stance toward mainstream medical care began early in the epidemic. The members of Wipe Out AIDS! (later renamed Health Education AIDS Liaison, or HEAL) were interested in nontoxic and alternative therapies. Its members were concerned about the overly aggressive and possibly lethal methods used to treat AIDS, like chemotherapy, which suppresses people's immune functions.[85] Alternative healing strategies were especially attractive because "The magic bullet that we all eagerly await is, by all sober estimates, a long way off."[86] PWAs began to actively pursue alternative and holistic cures, including some that bordered on quackery, like using snake venom, algae, swamp water, and injections of hydrogen peroxide. The first issue of the *Newsline* contained announcements of yoga, meditation, and relaxation classes at the Metropolitan-Duane Church and of holistic health workshops for PWAs, including religious and psychic healing, as well as an article describing Lincoln Hospital's acupuncture clinic. Contributors to the *Newsline* discussed the benefits of absentee healing, acupuncture, metabolic therapy, homeopathy, massage, herbal remedies, vitamin therapies, self-hypnosis, yoga, Shiatsu, and mental imaging.

The use of a broad range of health and healing strategies is not unique to AIDS. Interest in nonmedical forms of healing has increased over the past two decades, as is evident in the wide popularity of books on alternative medicine. PWAs were another group of fatally ill patients willing to try untested treatments, and many of them asserted that they had a right to explore any treatment they wished.[87] In fact, in 1990 Americans made more visits (425 million) to providers of "unconventional therapy"—"interventions neither taught widely in U.S. medical schools nor generally available in U.S. hospitals"— than to all "mainstream primary care physicians" (388 million); when individuals face serious, life-threatening conditions, 83 percent combine alternative and mainstream treatments.[88]

Several other organizations concentrated on alternative treatments. Michael Hirsch, PWAC's first executive director, founded AIDS Action, which sold tapes, sponsored workshops with alternative health expert Louise Hay, and provided instruction in Reiki.[89] In early 1986, two PWAC members realized that a weekend workshop, Mastery of Acting "might lend itself to the needs of people with AIDS and ARC," and established the AIDS Mastery, a workshop that continued for more than a decade under the auspices of the Northern Lights Alternative.[90]

Being an active health care consumer was understood as central to individual empowerment, which in turn led to collective action. PWAC's members "soon came to the conclusion that we no longer wished to attend AIDS forums at which doctors, lawyers, social workers, insurance brokers, and politicians explained second-hand what it was like to have AIDS. We felt that we had a right to tell our own stories. . . . Our experiences were a reaffirmation of the feminist principle that the personal is indeed political.[91]

Besides espousing a philosophy of self-help—and hope—by providing information, PWAC members articulated the contours of empowerment for PWAs in ways that set the stage for them to become actively involved in social policy. In a history of the PWA self-empowerment movement, Callen recalled that the early groups mainly provided emotional support, because "we all had our hands full staying alive; it didn't occur to us to organize politically."[92] Their work had an impact on the formation of AIDS policy in many ways, including the inclusion of PWAs in conferences and on boards and advisory committees. People in the AIDS community fought for their own lives by becoming empowered; at the same time, they were also beginning to try to save other people's lives by providing a blueprint for reducing the transmission of the disease.

Chapter 3

The Invention of Safe Sex

Twenty years later, with condom ads running frequently on MTV, it seems like such a no-brainer: why would safe sex have to be invented, when it's just common sense to use condoms for protection against AIDS and other sexually transmitted infections?

—Richard Berkowitz

You must remember the urgency that we felt. I can't even begin to describe to you what I used to think could and might have happened had things been different. . . . Bill Buckley in those days was not apologetic about saying let's tattoo them. Pat Buchanan was not remotely afraid of saying this is God's wrath and punishment against these people, let them die. We were up against the wall in days. . . . The frightening part was trying to keep the sort of rational public health discussion and not let the underlying deep stigma of homophobia and addictophobia and racism and fear just sort of overwhelm us.

—Timothy Sweeney

Berkowitz's and Sweeney's words evoke a time of uncertainty and contention.[1] Soon after the first reports about "gay cancer," gay men, their doctors, and public health officials began to try to understand the connection between their lifestyle and the new disease. In a *New York Native* (hereafter, *Native*) article at the end of July 1981, Dr. Lawrence Mass asked "What is it about male homosexuals—or a subgroup of male homosexuals—that distinguishes their susceptibility to this disease?" He reviewed some theories that were being discussed: heredity, environmental factors, distinctive sexual practices, immune system depletion from repeated sexually transmitted diseases, and the use of amyl nitrates ("poppers") by nine out of ten reported cases. Mass's article concluded that "many feel that sexual frequency with a multiplicity of partners—what some would call promiscuity—is the single overriding risk factor for developing infections diseases and KS."[2]

This was the beginning of a quest to understand the transmission of the disease. Epidemiological information began to identify a number of factors associated with getting AIDS.[3] Public health officials, physicians, and gay men began to grapple with ways to prevent the transmission of whatever was causing the disease. The discussion of AIDS prevention took place in a highly politicized environment. The issues that needed to be confronted tapped into the very heart of gay identity, unleashed powerful emotions, and revealed the diversity of the gay community. Guidelines about how gay men might protect themselves, developed by gay health professionals and other leaders in the city's AIDS community, were adopted by large numbers of gay men who radically altered their behavior. Looking back nearly two decades after the changes began, David Nimmons observed that "we were saving each other's lives every night of the week."[4] The AIDS community's involvement in the invention of safe sex reveals another important dimension of the community's role in defining and influencing policies; it was actively engaged in the production of knowledge, not just in the interpretation of medical information.[5] The development of prevention policies also involved a major shift in the gay community's relationship to the state.

In the fall of 1981, the CDC initiated a national case control study comparing 50 men who had been diagnosed with the syndrome with a control group of 120 homosexual men who had been located through private physicians or through sexually transmitted disease (STD) clinics. Although designed to provide robust epidemiological data, the study's validity is probably questionable because many of the controls were in fact probably infected with HIV.[6] Preliminary findings, reported the following spring, confirmed what many gay men already suspected: many early cases were gay men with numerous sexual partners.[7] An earlier study, begun in New York in the spring of 1981, comparing twenty men with KS with forty controls, had reached a similar conclusion.[8] The identification of a cluster of AIDS cases provided evidence that the disease was sexually transmitted. CDC interviews with thirteen of the first nineteen AIDS cases in Los Angeles and Orange Counties documented that "nine of the 13 cases had direct sexual contact with another person who had or later developed AIDS"; one man in the cluster was linked to two patients with PCP through a healthy sexual partner, which made it likely that there were asymptomatic carriers.[9]

A new disease in their community was not a total surprise to many gay men since the incidence of sexually transmitted diseases had been increasing since the late 1960s. These diseases were not perceived as a serious threat, because they could be treated with antibiotics. Some gay physicians pointed out that their colleagues perhaps unwittingly contributed to this attitude; Dr. Dan William pointed out at an early AIDS conference that "Physicians caring for gay patients reinforced the concept that judicious promiscuity did not entail unacceptable health risks."[10] This view was not unique to the gay community. The public health system did not place great emphasis on preventing STDs. Indeed, according to Daniel Fox, "Public health officials . . . considered treatment a method of controlling venereal disease."[11]

Soon after the first AIDS reports, some doctors began to tell their gay patients to limit their sexual contacts.[12] Some were involved in the national gay health movement, a network of clinics and professional organizations that challenged the "prevailing heterosexist biases of medicine."[13] This movement also provided an infrastructure for the response to the epidemic, since existing organizations and networks of gay health professionals played a central role in providing care and developing innovative programs and policies.

The advice doctors gave, to restrict the number of sexual contacts, met significant resistance. When Dr. Alvin Friedman-Kien suggested at GMHC's first fundraising meeting that gay men ought to "cool it," the men asked "endless questions" and, according to Larry Kramer, some thought he "sounded like a born-again fundamentalist" who had no right to tell men to "stop having sex, on the basis of thirty cases."[14] The recommendation hit a raw nerve. An article by sociologist Marty Levine in GMHC's first newsletter, in the summer of 1982, described some of the changes in gay life. Levine pointed out that "The threat of disease and death erases more than a decade of gay pride. Internalized homophobia steps out of the closet as 'homosexuality' is blamed for the illness." To further illustrate the complexity of the response, he quoted one gay man as saying "I always knew being gay was wrong . . . I knew all the drugs and sleeping-around was sinful, and now it just might kill me."[15]

Larry Kramer took Friedman-Kien's recommendation seriously. Kramer had long been concerned with high levels of sexual activity in the gay community. As 1981 was ending, Kramer told the readers of the *Native* that "something we are doing is ticking off the time bomb that is causing the breakdown of immunity in certain bodies, and while it is true that we don't know what it is specifically, isn't it better to be cautious."[16] Kramer's March 1983 *Native* article "1,112 and Counting" pointed out that "Whatever is spreading is now spreading faster." Mincing no words, he exhorted his readers to change their behavior, and pointed out "I am sick of guys who moan that giving up careless sex until this blows over is worse than death. . . . Come with me guys, while I visit a few of our friends in Intensive Care at NYU. Notice the looks in their eyes, guys. They'd give up sex forever if you could promise them life."[17] There was vocal opposition to Kramer's views; one critic charged that "Kramer's ideology springs from a profound contempt for sex; this disdain enables him not only to condemn those who are sexually successful, but to devalue desire itself."[18]

Best known for his screenplay for the film version of D. H. Lawrence's *Women in Love*, Kramer became a controversial figure after the publication of his book, *Faggots*, was stridently critical of the sexual hedonism of gay life in Greenwich Village and on Fire Island.[19] The overwhelming majority of GMHC's board members disagreed with Kramer's position that GMHC ought to tell gay men to alter their sexual behavior; most believed that gay men had fought hard for their sexual freedom. Kramer's position endorsing abstinence especially pitted him against GMHC's president, Paul Popham. Several years later, Kramer recalled "Everyone sided with Paul."[20] The consensus was that the group should "educate without moralizing." Rather than "preaching," the "organization would present as many facets as possible . . . and allow everyone to make up their own mind."[21]

In June 1982, GMHC told the readers of the *Native*, "So much conjecture and unfounded rumor circulates among gay men that we feel there is a growing threat to our mental as well as physical health. We do not advocate taking any measures: each man must do what he feels is right for him. But we want you to know who is saying what, how the arguments stand, what is fact and what is fiction." GMHC provided cutting-edge information through its hotline and educational forums. Thinking back about these early forums, Michael Quadland remembers that we "told them everything we thought they ought to know" and what they might do and not do, including avoiding bathhouses and suggesting that they "get married and settle down."[22]

The first major discussion of prevention took place at the first National Lesbian and Gay Leadership Conference, in Dallas in August 1982. Representatives from gay political and health organizations, including GMHC, heard a keynote speech by Dr. James Curran, who headed the CDC's AIDS Task Force. He described the results of the CDC's case control study and led a workshop to develop guidelines for gay men's sexual behavior. One report of the conference noted that the group "came up with a directive that cautioned only against having sex with large numbers of anonymous contacts."[23]

The recommendation to reduce the number of partners raised vexing questions about the sexual behavior of some gay men. The term *promiscuity* was thought old-fashioned, judgmental, and moralistic, yet the issue had to be addressed.[24] As the issue of whether and what to tell gay men continued to be debated privately and in the gay press, there was growing empirical support for the strong connection between high levels of sexual activity and developing AIDS. PWAs Michael Callen and Richard Berkowitz confronted the issue head on, in an article in the *Native* called "We Know Who We Are: Gay Men Declare War on Promiscuity." They pointed out:

> Those of us who have lived a life of excessive promiscuity on the urban gay circuit . . . know who we are. We could continue to deny over-whelming evidence that the present health crisis is a direct result of the unprecedented promiscuity that has occurred since Stonewall, but such denial is killing us. . . . Every sexually active gay man knows that he is much more likely to pick up any of a variety of sexually transmitted disease today than he was five years ago. . . . There can be no equivocation. Promiscuity is a considerable health hazard. . . . This is not a moralistic judgment, but a clear statement of the devastating effect of repeated infections. . . . While a fatally disorganized gay leadership scrambles for a way to present promiscuity in a manner palatable to a generally unso-phisticated heterosexist world (and an understandably defensive gay community), gay men are dying unnecessarily. As individuals, we must care enough about ourselves to begin this re-evaluation: gay men are dying. As a community, we must initiate and control this process our-selves. Be assured that if we aren't willing to conduct it, others will do it for us. . . . The motto of promiscuous gay men has been, "So many men, so little time." In the '70s we worried about so many men; in the '80s we will have to worry about so little time. For us, the party that was the '70s is over.[25]

Their conclusion was echoed by Peter Seitzman, president of the New York Physicians for Human Rights, who was reluctant "to proclaim promiscu-ity immoral, but simply dangerous. Very dangerous right now—perhaps so dangerous that gay men might begin to completely revamp their sexual mores. Perhaps its time for good old-fashioned dating. . . . Perhaps it is time to use monogamy as a survival technique as well as in hopes of finding emotionally fulfilling involvement."[26] Seitzman distinguished his position from Callen and Berkowitz, noting that "They believe promiscuity is the cause, I believe promiscuity allows the spread."[27]

Some gay doctors, like Dan William, began recommending that men choose their "sexual partners from a small group who have all agreed to limit their different sexual contacts [and that this] will significantly improve one's chances of staying healthy."[28] This position was endorsed by the newly founded New York Chapter of the Physicians for Human Rights in July 1982.

Based on the available epidemiological evidence, AIDS seemed to be spread in the same ways as hepatitis B: sexually, through contaminated needles, or through blood transfusions. In the minds of some gay health professionals, this meant that, as with Russian roulette "the longer you play, the worse the odds become, and it's also possible to lose on the very first spin of the gun barrel."[29]

Sociologist Marty Levine questioned the recommendation to reduce sexual activity, in GMHC's second newsletter, noting:

> The pages of our periodicals continuously harangue us with the latest medical research. . . . All of this talk has produced a poisonous side effect. We are overcome by hysteria. . . . The panic originates in the widespread belief that clonedom—that is, drugs and fast sex—causes the diseases. While our doctors and journalists have been meticulous to inform us about the pitfalls of this notion . . . most gay men blindly accept the idea . . . [but] the clone lifestyle theory does not hold water. It is inadequate because it is based on correlational findings and fails to explain all cases, especially those among men who use no drugs . . . and who are sexually celibate.[30]

GMHC's second newsletter, published in January 1983, included a joint statement, by the New York Physicians for Human Rights and the New York City Department of Health, endorsing restraint. Admitting candidly, "We don't know yet what causes AIDS. Until we do: Cut down the number of different men you have sex with particularly with the men who also have many different partners."[31] CDC recommendations issued two months later repeated these ideas almost verbatim, noting that "Sexual contact should be avoided with persons known or suspected to have AIDS. Members of high risk groups should be aware that multiple sexual partners increase the probability of developing AIDS."[32] An October 1982 announcement in the *Native* noted that "current opinion points to something like a virus that may be transmitted sexually. THEREFORE: UNTIL WE KNOW BETTER, it makes sense that the fewer different people you come in sexual contact with the less chance this possibly contagious bug has to travel around. Have as much sex as you want—but with fewer people and with healthy people. If you don't know whether your partner is healthy—ask him directly to be honest with you."[33]

In addition to challenging a central feature of gay mens' lives, the development of AIDS prevention guidelines and policies required significant changes in the complex relationship among the gay community, health care professionals, and the state.[34] Jeffrey Levi provided an overview of the challenges that the gay community faced in the mid-1980s:

The medical profession has not welcomed gay practitioners or patients, and it has been only just over a decade since the American Psychiatric Association removed homosexuality from its list of mental disorders. The public health community has done little better. For example, the same Public Health Service that leads the federal government's fight against AIDS also enforces the legislative ban on gays entering the United States under immigration law . . . indeed, it is no accident that in many communities the first gay institution established is a gay health clinic because the existing medical and public health establishments are not serving the need.[35]

For many gay men, government had been—and still was—the enemy, since homosexual relations were illegal in many places. Police raids on gay bars were not a very distant memory. In the first several years of the epidemic, the Bowers v. Hardwick case was yet another reminder of gays' disadvantaged status. The case involved the arrest of two gay men in Georgia, where sodomy was illegal. In 1986, the Supreme Court affirmed the legality of Georgia's anti-sodomy statute, in the Bowers v. Hardwick case. The case had a chilling effect since some people believed that agents would begin entering people's bedrooms, which is what had happened when Bowers was originally arrested.[36]

This historic lack of trust and collaboration provided a challenge for government officials and for the gay community. Expanded state involvement in the name of public health was simply frightening to many. A group of community activists pointed out that "We must always remain aware of the political context in which AIDS research is occurring. We are inviting into our lives a government which does not recognize our fundamental rights to be free from discrimination on the job or in housing or our right to love whom we choose. . . . While it is clear that research into the causes of AIDS must proceed quickly, we cannot forget the long history in this country of the misuse of information gathered by governmental agencies."[37]

Wariness about dealing with government officials, especially scientists and physicians, was underscored in a *Native* review of *Bad Blood*, a study of the Tuskegee experiment. Written at a time when there was serious consideration of rejecting all gay men as blood donors, the author, Marty Levine, pointed out that "They say we have bad blood. Nearly forty years ago, they told some black men they had bad blood."[38] Drawing additional and more disturbing parallels, he noted:

> The Centers for Disease Control's actions . . . raise serious questions about its activities in AIDS. . . . We need to know if any of the present

AIDS researchers participated in the experiment. We know where one former member went. Dr. David Sencer is the Commissioner of Health in New York City. Sencer says now that under no circumstances would he condone similar (non)treatment of AIDS patients . . . [and] at his direction the Health Department voluntarily submits its AIDS-related projects for review by the Gay Men's Health Crisis Scientific Review Committee. . . . The parallel between the social positions of the two sets of players, however, also engenders concern. In both Tuskegee and AIDS, the socially franchised studied the socially disenfranchised. . . . Everyone I spoke to felt it is time to be more cautious. What happened in Macon County means we cannot blindly trust the Centers for Disease Control.[39]

By the time AIDS began, there had been some formal collaboration between the gay community and the state, dating back to the 1970s. Thousands of gay men, recruited through STD clinics, volunteered in clinical trials of a Hepatitis B vaccine.[40] But the distrust was significant. An influential group of gay community observers noted in the mid-1980s that the computerized files for this clinical trial had been retained and the CDC wanted to use them to determine how many of the men had developed AIDS. Instead, the New York Blood Center, which had participated in developing the vaccine, got a list of AIDS patients from the CDC and matched them with its files, an obvious breach of federal policies ensuring the protection of human subjects.[41]

Concern about a breach of confidentiality of the Hepatitus B data was not atypical. One long-term gay activist pointed out to me, in 1990, that he had long thought that there might be a serious backlash against gays in the country, a kind of pogrom, but that "It would be done in some medical way."[42] In fact, there was substantial public support for repressive public health measures. A Los Angeles Times poll conducted in 1985 found that 77 percent of Americans would support a law that made it a crime for homosexuals or other members of high-risk groups to donate blood, half supported quarantine of people with AIDS, 45 percent supported testing job applicants for AIDS, and 48 percent thought they would approve of "identity cards" for those HIV positive. More than one in eight approved of tattooing people with AIDS.[43]

In this context, a conference sponsored by a coalition of gay activists was called "AIDS: Should Panic + Prejudice = Policy." Two sessions introduced an analogy between AIDS and the Holocaust, an image later popularized by Larry Kramer. One session, called "Nazi Germany, 1933–1940: Lessons for Today," looked at the similarities between then-current "anti-gay" sentiment and the

"Nazi purges"; a second session was called "America's Concentration Camps: The Round-Up of Japanese Americans, 1941–1946: Lessons For Today."[44] Although suspicious about the government's role in researching AIDS—and some were suggesting that the disease was intentionally created by the government in research labs—the gay community recognized that it depended on government resources and expertise to understand the disease.

Jeffrey Levi observed in 1985, "Progressing from a basic goal of keeping government out of their lives, gays now seek ways to spur the government into saving lives and providing their share of needed services—while still fending off government intrusion into private affairs."[45] Even before the epidemic began, gay health professionals began to realize that there was a need to collaborate with public health officials.[46] Meanwhile, public health officials, like James Curran, also recognized the need to collaborate with community organizations. Curran consulted with gay organizations and AIDS groups throughout the country, including GMHC, and was the guest speaker at the first meeting of the New York Physicians for Human Rights, in early 1982.[47] Officials understood that guidelines imposed from above would meet resistance and they needed the community's cooperation.

In May 1983, Michael Callen and Richard Berkowitz, who described themselves as a slut and a hustler, coauthored and self-published a pamphlet called "How to Have Sex in an Epidemic," which outlined an approach they called "medically safe sex." They had worked closely with their doctor, Joseph Sonnabend, in formulating the guidelines. Recognizing that "Advice which focuses only on *numbers* and ignores ways to interrupt disease transmission is incomplete,"[48] they synthesized guidelines being offered by gay groups in San Francisco like the Sisters of Perpetual Indulgence (which encouraged men to use condoms), the Berkeley Gay Men's Health Collective, the National Coalition of Gay STD Services, the KS/AIDS Foundation in Houston, and the Bay Area Physicians for Human Rights (which recommended "AVOID THE DIRECT EXCHANGE OF BODILY FLUIDS"). [49]

Avoiding the stridency of their earlier *Native* article and the use of the highly charged term *promiscuity*, they noted that "Today in most large urban centers, what began as sexual freedom has become a tyranny of sexually transmitted diseases. . . . In the end, how you have sex is a matter of personal choice. But in the age of AIDS, it is important to realize that each one of us is now betting his life on what changes we do or do not make. . . . If we are to celebrate our gayness and get on with gay liberation, we must stay healthy. To stay healthy, we must realize that the issue isn't gayness or sex; the issue is simply disease."[50]

The brochure included suggestions about how men could screen prospective sexual partners by asking them about their sexual contacts and frequency of bathhouse attendance or by looking for external signs of illness like rashes and sores. It also recommended reducing drug and alcohol use so that one could stay in control, and discussed the relative risks of various sexual acts. The authors' ideas and the name "safe sex" caught on. One AIDS activist took it upon himself to paint "The AIDS epidemic isn't over. Use condoms" all over Lower Manhattan.[51]

GMHC began to publicize these ideas, producing pamphlets, doing outreach, and developing workshops. A fall 1983 conference, cosponsored with the Hunter College School of Social Work and the New York Physicians for Human Rights, featured a presentation on safe sex by Callen and Berkowitz and a workshop called "Sex and Intimacy: Looking for Love in All the Wrong Places."[52]

Volunteers set up information tables on the sidewalks of Greenwich Village and in other neighborhoods, noting, in a 1983 *Native* announcement, that "It's important that New Yorkers understand that this isn't a gay plague; gay New Yorkers need to know that sex can be healthy and fun." The outreach was not only directed to gay men, since "our tables provide answers for caring New Yorkers of all races, gay and straight, women and men, so we're not just looking for areas with a strong, visible gay community."[53] Early outreach workers faced hostility. Barry Davidson remembers that they were "physically assaulted" when they set up a table at 86th Street and Broadway since "They just didn't want to hear about it. That was stuff that belonged downtown with those queers."[54]

GMHC continued to provide information so that gay men could make their own decisions. In the late spring and the summer of 1984, advertisements in the *Native* entitled "Guidelines Save Lives," and "No Moralizing" pointed out that "We have to make some judgments—in editing, in deciding just what is risky—but they have to be judgments based on 'safe' versus 'unsafe' not 'good' versus 'bad.' We can provide information and recommend safe sex but ultimately only you can make moral and ethical decisions about your own life."[55]

An upbeat announcement in the spring of 1984 noted that "The fight against AIDS is four years old and, on many fronts, we're winning. We're winning by stopping disease. We have accurate guidelines on safer sex. Many gay men are protecting themselves."[56]

Two GMHC volunteers, Michael Shernoff and Luis Palacios-Jimenez, recognized that these changes had a host of emotional consequences. Ads and brochures provided guidelines, but they did not attend to the powerful emotions gay men were experiencing with the sickness and death of friends and lovers. Small group discussions were already taking place under the auspices of San Francisco's Stop AIDS Project. The level of panic and anxiety, though, was escalating. In the summer of 1983, *Newsweek* reported, "To be a male homosexual today is to be afraid of catching AIDS; since the incubation period can last as long as two years, many gays can only wonder whether some day soon their first symptoms will appear."[57] Rodger McFarlane recalled, "It was illogical to think that any of us were still uninfected."[58] Shernoff and Palacios designed safer-sex workshops because of what gay men were experiencing: "Uncertainty having to do with which sexual practices were low risk or how to change long-existing patterns of sexual behavior contributed to this anxiety. Many men were angry about AIDS and the changes necessary to protect themselves and their sexual partners. Some felt trapped into choosing celibacy and became resentful or depressed when faced with this choice. Others felt defiant and simply refused to practice safer sex, feeling that there was no sense in having sex if they could not do whatever they wanted."[59]

Shernoff and Palacios reasoned that there was a need to amplify and refine the information being distributed. They believed that the "safe sex" messages were overly negative, and that there was more to changing behavior than simply acquiring information.[60] The workshops could provide information, encourage men to change their behavior, but also remain positive about their sexuality. The goal was to eroticize safer sex, which involved using condoms while having satisfying sexual encounters.[61] Shernoff recalled, "Back then, many people were saying, 'Stop having sex.' . . . We wanted to say, 'Have sex safely.'" Although some view this approach as avoiding a discussion of multiple and sometimes anonymous sexual contacts in the name of being nonjudgmental, it is also possible to view the workshops as a realistic recognition of what would be heard.[62]

The workshops were an enormous success. A GMHC volunteer recalled that "all the Safe Sex forums were standing room only. All the gay men would come out on Saturday for these full-day forums." Reflecting back a dozen years later, Shernoff noted, "I am really astounded, because we did not conceive anything original. We took a little bit of sensate focus, a little bit of psychotherapy, and, in a very nonhomophobic way, talked to people about sex. But no one had ever thought to put it together like this before. . . . The community needed a place where they weren't going to be judged."[63] The workshops had much broader implications. A group facilitator remembered that "A lot of issues somehow presented themselves in the group. . . . A lot of the men were angry because they were either sick or they were going to get sick. . . . People were loaded with a whole lot of different emotions. . . . Some of them were very estranged from their families. They had just had a string of relationships they weren't satisfied with and they were worried about being sick. . . . We had a program to carry out . . . but what we didn't always anticipate was the real anger, the underlying anger that was to come with men who attended these programs."[64]

The combination of being better informed and the desire for self-preservation led to significant changes in sexual behavior in gay communities all over the country. More men were dating, monogamy was increasing, bathhouse attendance declined, and condoms were more widely used. [65] One study documented that gay men in New York sharply reduced the number of their sexual partners by 1984. Another reported that condom use had increased to 60 percent of sexual encounters in 1985 and that the amount of sex in public places declined by two-thirds.[66] There was a 40 percent reduction in sexually transmitted disease cases in the gay neighborhoods of Greenwich Village and Chelsea, a pattern found in other cities.[67]

Gay bathhouses were another dimension of gay life that needed to be addressed in the effort to fight AIDS. Since the bathhouses were places that specifically existed for sexual encounters, government officials and the AIDS community recognized the significance of altering the behavior taking place in them. This was another issue that provoked controversy and underscored enormous differences of opinion within the emerging AIDS community.

Decreasing attendance at gay bathhouses was part of a broader set of changes in gay men's sexual behavior and a response to exhortations like "Don't risk your life and the lives of your brothers."[68] Five of the city's fifteen bathhouses closed by the mid-1980s.[69] But some men continued to go to the baths. PWA–NY was the first group to address the issue. Its members produced and distributed safe sex posters but found that few owners cooperated, the posters were torn down, and they were criticized as inaccurate.[70] In late 1983, Roger Enlow, the director of the City's Office of Gay and Lesbian Health Concerns, chaired the first meeting of the Safer Sex Committee of New York, which attracted Callen, Berkowitz, representatives of GMHC, of Wipe Out AIDS, and of the Community Health Project, and public officials like Mel Rosen from the State AIDS Institute. Some members demanded the immediate closure of all bathhouses, while others insisted that there be no government intervention in people's lives. Bridging these differences, the Safer Sex Committee mounted a "Great Sex is Healthy Sex" campaign, developing brochures and posters and reaching out to bars and to bathhouses. The group proceeded cautiously, "to avoid a sudden, hysterical, negative community response." Within six months of their first meeting, they had contacted thirty-six establishments—bathhouses, backroom bars, movie theaters, and bookstores—and distributed more than two hundred posters and thirty-five thousand pamphlets. GMHC underwrote most of the cost and took over the responsibility for education in the baths.[71]

With a continued need to do something about the issue, several veterans of gay organizational life formed, in late 1984, the Coalition for Sexual Responsibility to reduce high-risk behavior by educating men who went to the baths and by persuading owners to make needed changes.[72] Coalition members believed that government closure could be the first step in reimposing sodomy laws, a concern not unfounded, in light of the fact that the Bowers case was still pending. Voluntary cooperation by owners was preferable to closing the baths, since, the members believed, the same behavior would take place elsewhere.[73] They drew up a set of guidelines dealing with lighting and hygiene and with the availability of brochures, posters, and condoms; and they inspected the baths to see if the owners were adhering to these principles.[74]

Callen had a different position. He believed that government inaction on bathhouse closure was enabling "suicidal, perhaps homicidal" activity to take place. Although closing the bathhouses would be a "political and civil liberties nightmare," he asked "do promiscuous urban gay American citizens have the right to commit suicide—to pursue happiness even if it kills them—free from state intervention. Perhaps. If a man is about to jump off the Brooklyn Bridge, should police physically restrain him? . . . The man jumping off the bridge should be restrained . . . he may live to jump again."[75] Callen also thought that the voluntary approach was not working, because few of the bathhouses had free condoms or displayed safe sex posters.[76]

In New York in the fall of 1985, city and state officials began to seriously consider closing gay bathhouses. The idea had been dormant for several years but had been hotly debated in several other cities. Mayoral candidate Diane McGrath made it a central issue in her campaign. It attracted attention because the number of new AIDS cases was rising sharply and health officials estimated that as many as one in ten adults in the city might be infected.[77] Public fears were at a high point, with the Queens school boycott and the death of Rock Hudson. The cover of *Life* magazine announced to Americans in July that "Now, No One Is Safe from AIDS,"[78] symptomatic of a growing concern that everyone was at risk. Public health officials throughout the country, including the city's health commissioner, David Sencer, did not support closure.[79] An epidemiologist on Sencer's staff estimated that closure would have a minor impact on HIV infections.[80]

About a month before the city's 1985 mayoral election, the State AIDS Advisory Council recommended that New York City adopt San Francisco's policy of regulating bathhouses, a policy that was adopted. The city could close establishments where risky sex was taking place; to remain open, bathhouses would have to comply with a set of guidelines concerning the distribution of condoms and educational materials, and to improve the lighting to discourage unsafe and anonymous sex. Several gay bathhouses and one establishment catering to heterosexuals were closed in December 1985 but most were able to reopen.[81] One and one-half years later, only four gay bathhouses were in business.[82]

Gay men began to fight for their lives by trying to figure out how they might reduce AIDS transmission without compromising their right to lead their lives as they chose. They achieved this by collaborating with health care professionals to develop new knowledge and, at the same time, devising new ways of dealing with public health officials. Although the issue of safe sex was much more than a matter of putting on a condom or closing the baths, these issues were complex because gay men needed to protect themselves yet maintain some central features of gay culture. As Americans began to recognize that the disease was not a "gay plague," and could potentially affect a broad cross-section of the population, the kinds of people involved in fighting AIDS became more varied. These people participated in groups that began in the gay community, like GMHC and PWAC, but were drawn to the issue for a host of other reasons. By the mid-1980s, the AIDS community began to expand.

Chapter 4

Fighting AIDS is Everyone's Business

AIDS is the focus of my life. The crisis of AIDS is not diminishing; it's getting worse. I am resolved to make people understand this fact with all the resources I have. Everyone must join in this fight.

—Judith Peabody

Peabody's passion and her commitment reflected a growing sense that fighting AIDS was not a task solely for the gay community.[1] GMHC's 1987–1988 Annual Report noted that "GMHC Volunteers come from all walks of life and from all communities for one purpose: to join in the fight against AIDS."[2] By then, the epidemic was expanding in terms of the numbers and types of people living with AIDS. The AIDS community was also becoming more diverse—not only people living with AIDS but also their family members, friends, and a host of others. The image of the epidemic as a gay plague was being replaced by another view, the idea that everyone was at risk. A 1986 article in *Newsweek,* called "Future Shock," told Americans that "AIDS is not a disease of homosexuals or intravenous-drug users alone: it threatens millions of sexually active Americans regardless of age, gender, race or place of residence."[3]

Members of the AIDS community recognized that framing the disease as affecting everyone would increase public support. In the mid-1980s, the AIDS community was expanding to include elite and grassroots support from a broader range of stakeholders, who enlisted members of their social networks to become volunteers and donors. In a context of growing concern and, in some respects, panic about the epidemic's future impact, the expansion of the AIDS community had two important consequences: it increased resources and it moved AIDS higher up on the political agenda.

Support from several groups outside the gay community amplified the AIDS community's growing influence. The first response came from the city's religious community, whose members were moved by a concern and compassion for people affected by AIDS and by its strong connection to two other emerging problems, homelessness and hunger. A second came from women, including some highly visible elite women. Many had friends and family members who were gay, and their names, their friends, and their reputations transformed AIDS from a largely gay issue to a fashionable charity.[4] A third source of support came from the foundation community. Individual policy entrepreneurs in local foundations promoted AIDS as a fundable issue; several large national foundations also moved the issue up on the public agenda, creating the impetus for local programs that served as a template for national policies.

During the early part of summer 1985, the film star Rock Hudson went to Paris to receive experimental treatment for "liver disease." Hudson had been a matinee idol in the 1950s and 1960s and, in an era when the homosexuality of well-known people was rarely known, his gayness was widely rumored but never made public, nor admitted by Hudson himself. At the end of July, a hospital spokesperson revealed that Hudson was being treated for AIDS. When Hudson died the following October, he was the first person many Americans, including President Reagan and his wife Nancy, knew who had had AIDS. Hudson's death put a face on the epidemic and, in the minds of those Americans who continued to doubt that Hudson had been gay, offered proof that anyone could get the disease.[5]

The diagnosis and death of Hudson is viewed as a turning point in public awareness, concern, and policy development. By the time his illness was revealed, nearly 12,000 Americans had been diagnosed with AIDS and the number of cases was doubling every ten months.[6] The largest number of cases was in New York City, where the number of adults diagnosed with AIDS reached 3,587, and nine in ten of them had died.[7] As the epidemic expanded, people motivated by a sense of compassion rooted in their religious traditions were the first outside the gay community to respond.

In 1983, a small group of people established the AIDS Resource Center (ARC) to respond to an emerging problem, the growing number of PWAs who needed help with housing. Some needed housing because their families, roommates, or lovers were fearful of being in contact with them; in a few cases, people were thrown out of their apartments. The problem was becoming especially obvious in the city's hospitals, where some patients could not be discharged because they had no place to live. A rapid and creative response was needed, since it was costly for people to remain in hospitals. GMHC's executive director, Mel Rosen, told a congressional subcommittee in August 1983 that, contrary to existing policies, "People with AIDS are being discharged from hospitals penniless and homeless." Some obtained welfare and were living in single room occupancy hotels (SROs), places that were "dirty, dangerous, and certainly not a place where a very sick person should live." Although city officials denied it, some PWAs were living in city-sponsored homeless shelters, huge cavernous places, usually in armories, that were dirty, crime- and drug-filled, and especially unhealthy places for people with weak immune systems.[8] Reverend Meade Bailey saw firsthand the problem of people remaining in hospitals, in his work as a chaplain at Belleview Hospital. Bailey brought together a diverse group of clergy, writers, journalists, local business people, and a gay porn star to deal with the problem by establishing a residence for people with AIDS.[9] Since this would take some time, they devised an interim strategy: helping people to pay their rent. The first year, they helped forty people and distributed thirty-thousand dollars.[10]

ARC volunteers and staff also rented apartments for people who might not otherwise qualify as tenants, creating a model they called scatter-site housing. Rather than try to help people to rent apartments, the organization signed leases for tenants who were not creditworthy and had a short life expectancy. ARC signed five leases in the spring of 1985 and was housing twenty-one people in September. By then, ARC was relying more heavily on public funds from the city's Human Resources Administration than on individual donations. The group was barely making a dent in the problem since there were four times as many people on its waiting list. There was enormous turnover; the first group of tenants died quickly, staying in their apartments for an average of four months.[11]

At the end of 1986, ARC opened Bailey House, a 44-bed residence that provided medical, recreational, and social services in a facility that was a hybrid between a shelter and a nursing home. The city purchased a former hotel and gave ARC a contract to manage it.[12] Bailey House was the prototype for an emerging housing form called supported housing, where support services were available on-site. There was enormous resistance to establishing community-based residences for people with AIDS. A prevailing attitude in many neighborhoods, NIMBY ("not in my backyard") blocked the placement of ten patients in a city-operated nursing home in Rockaway, Queens, and plans to use an empty convent on the Upper West Side of Manhattan as an AIDS residence.[13] Bailey House experienced less opposition; it was located in the former River Hotel, on the waterfront at the end of Christopher Street, the heart of the city's gay community. Another AIDS facility, a hospice operated by the Missionaries of Charity under the direction of the world-renowned Mother Teresa, was also being planned in a former rectory in Greenwich Village.[14]

The AIDS Resource Center was part of a "faith-based" response to the AIDS epidemic.[15] During the first several years of the epidemic, clergy ministered to the needs of the dying and the mourners.[16] Existing and new organizations mobilized to provide care for people living with AIDS, offering both corporal and spiritual acts of mercy. By 1991, there were 2,810 AIDS ministries throughout the nation.[17] Some clergy and members of religious congregations became involved with AIDS because of its strong links to two other important problems, homelessness and hunger. The faith-based response to the epidemic involved members of existing congregations, gay religious groups, and individuals influenced by spiritual concerns. Clergy and nuns working at hospitals with large numbers of AIDS patients, including St. Luke's, St. Vincent's, and Belleview, attended to the spiritual needs of patients. Drawing on Jewish and Christian traditions of compassion, they recognized their obligation to help these patients cope with the sickness and the death and the mourning. By 1985, Sister Patrice Murphy at St. Vincent's Hospital had worked with ninety AIDS patients. The issue was very personal for some clergy because they were gay or had AIDS.[18]

Religious traditions had a paradoxical impact on the social response to the epidemic: both a source of stigma and the basis of enormous concern and compassion. Some religious leaders used AIDS as an object lesson illustrating moral decline. Others preached compassion and emphasized the obligation to care for the sick and the dying. The condemnation continued into the 1990s, when the Rev. Billy Graham pointed out to a large crowd, "Is AIDS a judgment of God? I would not say for sure, but I think so," a statement he later retracted. The AIDS National Interfaith Network's annual report declared, in the early 1990s, "AIDS is *not* a punishment from God."[19]

The pronouncements of religious leaders framed the public debate. The position of the Catholic Church illustrates the complex role of faith, preaching compassion but not condoning homosexuality. At a 1983 conference at Lenox Hill Hospital, Terence Cardinal Cooke's opening benediction focused on the importance of "loving and caring." His successor, John Cardinal O'Connor, affirmed the church's belief in the "sinful and unnatural" nature of homosexuality; however, under O'Connor's watch, the Church expanded care for PWAs in hospitals and in nursing facilities.[20] An interfaith group of clergy called for the public not to judge people with AIDS, and to offer them compassion. The strongest and most consistent voice promoting tolerance was Rev. Paul Moore, Episcopal Bishop of New York, a member of the State AIDS Advisory Committee, who announced at a press conference in June 1983:

Never in recent history has an epidemic brought such fear to the people of New York . . . let it be strongly stated that AIDS is not God's vengeance upon the homosexual community. The God whom Jews and Christians worship is a loving merciful God who does not punish his children like a wrathful father. . . . Furthermore, whatever so-called sins may have been committed by persons with AIDS can in no way compare in seriousness to the social sins of our generation which have brought war and poverty upon millions of innocent people. We believe, on the contrary, that God has a special love for his children when they are suffering persecution such as has been brought upon the homosexual community over the years.[21]

Moore's moral authority reframed the discourse and influenced Governor Cuomo of New York to increase state funding.[22]

Individual congregations started special religious services to help people with AIDS to cope with the enormous stigma and pain of their illnesses and to give them hope.[23] Members of the Unitarian Church of All Souls on the Upper East Side formed an AIDS Task Force that sponsored a forum and raised money for several AIDS organizations including the PWA Coalition, which received two hundred dollars each month for the *Newsline*.[24] Several lesbian and gay congregations and gay religious groups (such as Dignity for Catholics, and Integrity for Episcopalians) established committees to help individuals and families and to host special services of hope and healing.[25] The Jewish Board of Family and Children's Services recruited volunteers and developed a host of social services. In the 1990s, a small organization called the Tzvi Aryeh Foundation began serving Orthodox Jews.[26] Two individuals who had clear visions about the need to respond to the epidemic developed programs that quickly became major service organizations: Momentum, founded by Peter Avitabile, an early GMHC volunteer, and God's Love We Deliver, founded by Ganga Stone.

Momentum started out as a dinner and yoga/massage/stress reduction workshop sponsored by GMHC at St. Peter's Church. It was initiated by Peter Avitable, a GMHC volunteer, who had been working with a network of religious groups in mid-Manhattan that provided food and shelter to 350 people.[27] Momentum's first dinner, in September 1985, attracted about thirty people.[28] GMHC advertised the program and referred the "guests," and St. Peter's provided money, space, and pastoral counseling. The costs were relatively low, about one thousand dollars each week in 1987, because the program was staffed by volunteers—including Avitable, who spent full time coordinating the program.[29] Avitabile was inspired by the Catholic Worker movement's commitment to hospitality, and saw the dinner program as the beginning of a much more extensive set of activities, including the development of a residence for PWAs.[30] Just as the leaders of the AIDS Resource Center wanted to create a home for PWAs and disagreed with the city's vision of the facility as primarily a shelter, Avitabile was interested in hospitality, not only food. He wanted to keep the dinners small and to use fine china. The program's supporters were religiously diverse; in 1987 it was "funded by a Jewish widower, inspired by an Episcopal priest, held in a Lutheran church, and attended by over 70 persons each week."[31]

The dinners were so successful and the demand was so great that Momentum was serving twice the number of people Avitabile thought it could accommodate, by the end of 1987. Rapid growth and financial support from the city and from the Robert Wood Johnson Foundation also changed the organization. The china was replaced with paper plates, the guests became more diverse, the program expanded to include drug counseling, and, by early 1989, Momentum was operating in eight congregations located in three boroughs.[32] The AIDS Resource Center and Momentum attracted a diverse group of stakeholders, many motivated by the groups' compassionate missions. The groups raised funds from individuals, foundations, and corporations, but most of their growth was the result of an increase in public funding.

Another faith-related organization, God's Love We Deliver, attracted large donations from individuals, especially from members of the city's economic, social, and political elite who began to identify themselves as part of the AIDS community. The story of the organization's founding has a mythic quality that contributed to its early success; numerous versions appeared in print, and staff were familiar with these varied versions.[33] In May 1985, Stone went to visit an AIDS patient named Richard who was living alone in a fifth-floor walk-up in Greenwich Village. By then, public entitlements and services had expanded; welfare payments covered his rent and medical insurance was paying for a nurse. Stone, a volunteer for the Cabrini Hospice, brought him a bag of groceries, which Richard threw on the floor. The contents were useless to him: he couldn't get out of bed and his nurse was not paid to cook his meals. Richard was hungry; he hadn't eaten in two days. Stone went to a local deli and bought him prepared food with her own money. Vowing that he would not be hungry for the rest of his life, she called seven friends listed in his phonebook, each of whom took responsibility to provide him with his meals one day of the week.

This encounter was the beginning of God's Love We Deliver, an organization founded as "a response, not an idea" to the "horrible hole in the thin safety net that our various public and private agencies put under people with AIDS."[34] With a friend, Jane Ellen Best, Stone got meals donated by several restaurants. Stone and Best envisioned a broader set of activities in the future. God's Love's incorporation papers indicated two objectives: meals and other "non-medical and non-nursing services to ill persons at their homes" and the creation of a hospice. At the beginning of 1987, the organizers were getting food from sixteen restaurants and had forty-five volunteers.[35]

As demand grew, Stone decided that the organization ought to prepare its own meals, and opened a kitchen in the basement of an Upper West Side church in August 1987. The agency expanded rapidly. From 30 lunches each weekday that fall and 130 meals in early 1989, God's Love expanded to serve 900 clients, who received both lunch and dinner each weekday, in the early part of 1990.[36]

God's Love We Deliver created an elaborate delivery system involving a network of volunteers who picked up meals at distribution sites in churches, community centers, and even one bar. The meals themselves were the mission: they were high quality and of high caloric content to help AIDS patients gain weight. The clarity and the uniqueness of the service, Stone's eclectic spirituality and interesting life history—and the totally noncontroversial nature of the mission—made the organization attractive to foundations and to elite donors. God's Love We Deliver expanded the range of services and the membership in the AIDS community, attracting large numbers of individual donors. Like GMHC, it raised funds and attracted support from the city's economic, social, and political elite, some of whom began to identify themselves with the AIDS community.

At the end of the 1980s, God's Love and GMHC were the city's largest AIDS service providers. Both organizations depended on a core group of gay supporters and a broad range of volunteers and donors, including several well-placed, wealthy women. For GMHC, the transition from a small grassroots gay organization to a major social service agency between 1985 and 1988 involved changes in lay and professional leadership and in organizational culture. Growing support for GMHC and God's Love We Deliver benefited other AIDS organizations, too, since the fight against AIDS was becoming "everyone's" issue.

Under the leadership of Nathan Kolodner, as president, and Richard Dunne, as executive director, GMHC attracted a broad range of donors and volunteers and became more formalized, aiming to become a "sensitive bureaucracy" that applied standard management methods, like strategic planning, to effectively respond to a crisis.[37] Kolodner, a successful art dealer whose work brought him into contact with wealthy clients, began volunteering for GMHC in 1983, and was instrumental in mounting an art auction for GMHC.[38] In contrast to earlier fundraising events, which mainly attracted gay men, the auction attracted a range of people. While continuing to rely on the generosity of gay men and women, GMHC expanded its support to other people with a personal connection to AIDS patients, and to others who thought AIDS an important social issue.

By 1986, a larger number of women started to become involved; the proportion of women volunteers at GMHC doubled from 16 percent in 1982 to 33 percent in 1990. Although many key volunteers were lesbians, the majority of women were heterosexual; only 4.3 percent of new volunteers in the late 1980s were lesbians.[39] Many of the women had gay sons, and others worked in industries with large numbers of gay men, like fashion.[40] Mothers of PWAs were also clients and volunteers; some began attending the PWA Coalition–sponsored Mother's Group, beginning in the summer of 1986.[41]

The involvement of straight women reframed and brought greater attention to the issue. *Glamour*, the popular women's magazine, profiled GMHC board member Barbara Grande LeVine, a successful model, who began volunteering in 1983 after deciding to go beyond the "gossip and self-absorption" around her and because she "identified with the rejection and isolation."[42] Two elite women, Judith Peabody and Joan Tisch, were especially newsworthy.

Peabody, a "Park Avenue Debutante" who married the scion of an old New England Brahmin family, was first profiled in a *New York Magazine* article, one year after she began to volunteer for GMHC in the fall of 1985. The article's photograph showed her sitting on a bench next to Michael Callen. She became the co-leader, then the leader, of a carepartners group. Peabody had a long history of direct community service and had been trained as a counselor. Her commitment to GMHC was based on a concern over the stigma, blame, and marginalization of AIDS patients, and the belief that "This is everybody's disease. We are all in a high-risk category no matter how well we live our lives."[43]

Joan Tisch became involved with GMHC in the mid-1980s. At first, she labored anonymously, working the switchboard, stuffing envelopes, and organizing files. Reflecting back on what it was like to move between the culture of the agency and her friends who only dimly understood the nature of her work, she recalled that one friend asked, "When you stay down there five or six hours, what do you do when you have to go to the bathroom?"[44] Nathan Kolodner, GMHC's president, noticed her name on a sign-in log and invited her to join the board. Tisch pointed out that Kolodner "never asked me to give money directly. I was going to be the credibility bridge between the downtown gay community and the uptown business community." Tisch strongly believed that she was making a difference: "For the first time in years of volunteering, I had become emotionally involved. I witnessed the signifying of wills of men younger than my children. I saw people with Kaposi's Sarcoma try in vain to hide lesions with makeup. I listened to cases of harassment at work or by landlords. . . . When failing health or burnout prevented people from returning to the volunteer ranks, I realized that these people had become my friends, and I missed them. And in missing them, I also was saddened by the terrible tragedy of this terrible disease."[45]

God's Love We Deliver also attracted elite women, like Blaine Trump, who "hailed a cab to the God's Love kitchen after reading a fundraising letter" and hosted a party in 1988 that raised more than forty thousand dollars.[46] In 1987, the organization's board included Roberta Flack, the well-known singer, the ballerina Heather Watts, and Patricia Caesar, a consultant to nonprofit organizations, who had been referred to the group by a program officer at the New York Community Trust. Caesar lent her considerable talents to the organization, guiding it to develop the infrastructure it needed to grow and to survive. When she stepped down as chair and became vice-chair in 1992, the organization's newsletter stated that her "knowledge and guidance have been priceless to us. . . . She has been available to answer questions and handle emergencies on week-ends, at night, or whenever we needed the benefit of her judgment. . . . Patricia taught us what staff positions were needed, and then made sure that the right people were hired. It is to her that the lion's share of the credit for the overall excellence and professionalism of this agency must go."[47]

As the range of stakeholders expanded, AIDS funding increased rapidly. First GMHC and then other groups in the AIDS community moved from relying on small contributions to hosting major fundraising events. Before GMHC, fundraising for gay communal efforts had been limited. In 1982 and 1983, GMHC's work was primarily supported by gay donors. In an effort to reduce reliance on government funding, the group took steps to expand the donor base. The response to the GMHC's first direct mail campaign was unprecedented in the gay community, attracting over $723,000 in 1987.[48] A fundraising letter from GMHC's president, Paul Popham, pointed out: "To me, New York City without the Gay Men's Health Crisis would be the most frightening city in the world. . . . We need your help because GMHC is funded largely by people like yourself. People who want to help, who want to feel the satisfaction of being involved—people who want to make a real difference. And unless I'm very wrong, you are one of those people."[49]

GMHC evolved, from being an organization created and supported by gay white men, into one of the city's most visible charities and a member of federated fundraising appeals like the United Way and the State Employees Federated Appeal. The increasingly varied group of volunteers expanded its donor base, recruiting their friends and acquaintances to attend fundraising events and to donate money to GMHC. GMHC's first AIDS Walk, in 1986, raised $708,000, and an art auction at Sotheby's raised $925,000. The second AIDS Walk raised more than double the amount, $1.6 million, and attracted 12,000 people.[50] GMHC's first Dance-A-Thon, in 1990, drew 6,200 participants; 82 percent had "Never before participated in a GMHC fundraiser and only 18 percent had previously done the GMHC AIDSWalk."[51]

By the late 1980s, a number of prominent families had become active supporters and major donors for AIDS organizations. The pattern of involvement is consistent with Francie Ostrower's observation that members of the city's philanthropic elite are active in organizations and do not restrict their involvement to just donating funds.[52] This style of participation was evident in these people's commitment to AIDS. Some AIDS fundraising events became mainstream upscale affairs chaired by well-known celebrities and philanthropists, like Edgar Bronfman, Brooke Astor, and Ann Getty, and honored influential and philanthropic people, like James Wolfensohn, the former chair of Carnegie Hall and future president of the World Bank. Wolfensohn's foundation, like the family foundations of several other donors, began to contribute substantial sums. Ganga Stone recalled that a check from the Rudin family arrived at an opportune moment, when her organization was in dire straits.[53] The Rudins, who had access to the power centers of the city and donated funds through several different foundations, lent enormous legitimacy to AIDS and attracted their friends and business associates to AIDS fundraising events. Ad hoc and permanent fundraising groups were established to raise money through special events, including Art Against AIDS, Dancing for Life, Red Hot, the Design Industries Foundation Fighting AIDS, and Broadway Cares/Equity Fight AIDS. A 1985 recording of "That's What Friends Are For" by Dionne Warwick, Elton John, Gladys Knight, and Stevie Wonder raised more than a million dollars for AIDS organizations over four years.[54]

In 1985, GMHC cosponsored the largest single fundraising event until that time, with the AIDS Medical Foundation. Called "The Best of the Best," it was a gala performance with well-known singers and ballet dancers, held at the Metropolitan Opera. It too raised more than one million dollars.[55] The AIDS Medical Foundation was founded in 1983 by Dr. Joseph Sonnabend and Dr. Mathilde Krim, an interferon researcher at Sloan-Kettering Medical Center.

Krim had strong ties to wealthy and influential people through her husband, an executive in a major media company. She became involved in AIDS because she was "incensed" about the indifference to the young men who were dying, and because "My parents were passive anti-Semites. . . . They didn't believe the rumors coming out of Germany about what Hitler was doing to the Jews."[56] Krim's work had a profound impact on both the AIDS funding economy and the political opportunity structure. She became an icon, the "socialite scientist" who was also an AIDS activist willing to speak out on behalf of what she recognized as a social crisis.[57]

Krim recruited a large and prestigious advisory board for the AIDS Medical Foundation, including AIDS researchers, scientists such as Jonas Salk, scholars, businessmen, celebrities like Paul Newman and Tony Randall, and Rosalyn Carter, wife of the former president.[58] Yet, despite Krim's contacts and the support of those willing to lend their name to the effort, the initial fundraising efforts were relatively disappointing: $183,000 in the first year, double that amount the following year.[59] In 1985, the efforts began to take off: a benefit called "Comic Relief" raised half a million dollars. Recognizing the need for a national effort to raise funds for research, Krim merged the AMF into a California group called the American Foundation for AIDS Research, or AmFar, in late 1985.[60]

Krim became the co-chair of AmFar, with Elizabeth Taylor, the movie star and friend of Rock Hudson, whose estate served as a major source of AmFar's original funds. Yet another heterosexual woman who gave a "face" to those affected by AIDS, Taylor appealed for public and private funds, noting how her life had been "diminished by the deaths of beloved friends who have died of AIDS."[61]

Fundraising events had interlocking functions. They promoted awareness, served as a way to recruit influential donors with access to the corridors of power, and, at the same time, refocused the issue from a disease affecting gays to one of concern to the society as a whole. Krim told a *Newsweek* reporter in 1987 that "We had to have credibility; we had to be seen as a mainstream group and not a gay organization." In fact, Krim repeatedly told reporters, "Viruses do not discriminate on the basis of sexual preference. I think that it is a fluke that AIDS started in the gay community."

Growing awareness and support also mobilized another elite group, the "foundation community." Although foundations supply a relatively small share of private funds for nonprofit organizations, they play a role that far outweighs their economic impact. Contributing ten percent of nongovernmental support to nonprofit organizations, and greatly overshadowed by public funding, private foundations are important through setting the policy agenda, developing innovative solutions, and providing expertise, legitimacy, and investment capital for new organizations. Small grants to fledgling organizations enabled some of the city's new AIDS organizations to hire their first staff member and obtain their first government grant. Family foundations were especially critical in GMHC's growth, and allowed it to achieve autonomy in carrying out the prevention work that government was unwilling to support because of contested aspects of HIV prevention. Large national foundations, like the Robert Wood Johnson Foundation, developed models for services and policy. In short, foundations, as individual organizations and as an overarching institutional entity, gave AIDS greater visibility and legitimacy.

Initially, AIDS was of little interest to foundations, because of the small number of cases, the stigma associated with the modes of transmission, and the fact that many foundations and charities, even those with a particular interest in health care, would not support "single disease" organizations. During the 1980s and early 1990s, foundations reduced their support for health issues, from 25 percent to about 18 percent in 1992.[62] In the very early days of the epidemic, it was also not clear how foundations ought to respond. The president of the Charles A. Dana Foundation noted in 1986 that "It was relatively easy to identify some of the emerging problems, but it was very unclear how and where a grantmaker could make [an] . . . appropriate response."[63]

As with the mass media, where coverage was contingent on journalists' having a personal connection to the story,[64] foundations became interested in AIDS when they had a concerned staff member who lobbied to have the issue placed on the foundation's list of funding priorities. Some gay staff members were in a difficult position, since directing attention to AIDS might lead to a loss of privacy about their sexual orientation.[65] In some cases, such as the New York Community Trust and the MONY Foundation, the policy entrepreneurs were women who either had a friend with the disease or recognized the importance of the problem.

Foundations have different styles and strategies. Some foundations are interested in responding to new policy issues, while others are committed to supporting ongoing enterprises. In contrast to individual donors, whose support is based on an individual decision to write a check, foundations move slowly, since their funding practices are more formalized and they rely on written proposals from prospective grantees (in contrast to the more diffuse and informal decision making of individual donors). Foundations can only support organizations that have obtained a nonprofit status. As a group, they prefer to support organizations that will utilize funds responsibly and ensure they have an impact. In the first several years of the epidemic, there was little demand for AIDS funding by foundations, for there were few new organizations seeking foundation funds; foundations did not begin to fund AIDS projects until new AIDS organizations were established or existing organizations became involved in the epidemic.

The first AIDS grants in New York City, totaling $166,000, were given out in 1983 by two local funders, the New York Community Trust and the United Hospital Fund. The grants were for medical research, and for a volunteer program at Roosevelt Hospital. Grants to organizations in New York comprised the bulk of the $216,000 in foundation funding given out to organizations all over the country that year. Funding to organizations in New York City declined to about $86,000 in 1984 but, in response to the rise in number of cases and to growing public awareness, increased ten-fold during 1985 and continued to rise sharply, reaching $3.9 million in 1986, $9.4 million in 1987, and $15.4 million in 1988. By the end of 1987, fifty foundations had given AIDS grants to organizations located in New York City.[66]

In a context of increasing public concern but continuing lack of leadership by the federal government, the Robert Wood Johnson Foundation—the nation's largest health care funder—announced a four-year grant program, at the beginning of 1986, called the AIDS Health Services Program. Funds were targeted toward the twenty-one metropolitan areas with the largest numbers of AIDS cases, particularly the three metropolitan areas with the largest number of cases, Los Angeles, New York, and San Francisco. The total amount of $17.2 million was remarkable, considering that support by foundations had totaled $1.3 million between 1983 and 1985. The Robert Wood Johnson Foundation's request for proposals noted that the number of AIDS cases would double during 1986, and that the anticipated inpatient costs for someone with AIDS, estimated at $147,000 per person (an amount that may have been overstated), could be reduced by developing outpatient services and community-based care, a model developed in San Francisco.[67] With a small grant from the Fund for the City of New York, the Gay Men's Health Crisis coordinated the development of a successful grant proposal to the Foundation. The $972,275 award to a nonprofit fiscal conduit of the New York State Department of Health provided an infusion of funds to a handful of local organizations, both public and nonprofit, including GMHC and the AIDS Resource Center.

The announcement of the AIDS Health Services Program was a turning point and gave AIDS greater visibility and legitimacy as a national health policy issue. Previously, foundation staff members faced significant barriers to selling AIDS to their foundations, but the support of the Robert Wood Johnson foundation made AIDS more fundable.[68] More and more foundations, both local and national, began to include AIDS as a funding priority. The Ford Foundation sponsored a major research project documenting the limited amount of AIDS funding, and initiated the National Community AIDS Partnership (NCAP), a network of local funding mechanisms designed to raise support from foundations and individuals.[69]

Ford and other foundations also supported two other activities intended to increase foundation funding and to frame policies. Beginning in 1985, representatives from seven foundations started to meet informally to identify strategies to increase foundations' support of AIDS. Two organizations resulted from these informal meetings. One, Funders Concerned about AIDS, an affinity group of foundations, was to educate foundations and document the strategic role foundations play in supporting research, prevention, and services. A second organization, the Citizen's Commission on AIDS, established as a temporary organization that was to map out AIDS policy in the New York region, was sponsored by a consortium of fourteen foundations and other private funders "to stimulate private-sector leadership in responding to AIDS as a health care, social, and economic crisis at a time when there was relatively little public perception of the dimensions and long-term implications of the HIV epidemic." Its elite members were a broad cross-section intended to represent the city's racial and ethnic groups; through its meetings, press releases, and policy papers, it refocused discourse on the epidemic.[70]

By the late 1980s, the growing political influence of the gay community combined with broader membership in the AIDS community—people motivated by strong religious convictions, women (especially elite women), and foundation staff members—such that AIDS became a fight with a much broader base of support. More people were concerned about the issue, and donated their time, money, expertise, and political influence. They reframed the disease and the epidemic as affecting *everyone*. Although this view was not altogether correct, since some people were at higher risk than others, conceptualizing the epidemic in this way, and giving it greater salience, was not only valuable but necessary, because the epidemic was indeed changing in two significant ways: the numbers of cases was rising exponentially, and its face was changing.

Part II

A Changing Epidemic

Chapter 5

The Changing Face of AIDS

People talk about the changing face of AIDS. But it was there from the beginning. It was just not being identified.

—Miguelina Maldonado,
  Executive Director,
  Hispanic AIDS Forum

We're years behind in minority neighborhoods. We are still just trying to raise consciousness that AIDS is our problem. There's just not been the urgency that there was in the gay community.

—Roberto Soto,
  President,
  Hispanic AIDS Forum

It was clear that the government, the state, was not making a response to the AIDS epidemic. And a lot of us were very upset about it. And most of us who were upset about it were ex-addicts working in the treatment system or for the state. . . . And what we saw was that they were going on with business as usual and we had this AIDS epidemic on our hands. And gay men had come together and formed an organization and drug addicts were doing nothing.

—Edith Springer, ADAPT volunteer

In the mid-1980s, policymakers and journalists referred to the "changing face of AIDS" to describe a major shift in the epidemic.[1] Called Gay-Related Immune Deficiency or GRID during the first year, the epidemiological construct of the epidemic as a "gay plague, and then, in the middle of the decade, as a disease affecting everyone, were both facile oversimplifications.[2] More cases were being diagnosed among drug addicts who injected drugs (IDUs), women and children, African Americans and Hispanics, and outside of Manhattan.

The face of the epidemic was not changing; rather, our understanding was beginning to match the reality. The epidemic affected a diverse group from the very beginning, but many cases were not recognized as AIDS. Media coverage focused on gay men and interesting but relatively unusual cases like white women infected through blood transfusions, Alison Gertz (infected in a one-night stand with a bisexual man), and Kimberly Bergalis (one of a number of patients infected by a dentist in Florida). Although Gertz and Bergalis used their notoriety to increase public interest, the message of these cases was that everyone was at risk.[3] Even though this was theoretically true, the levels of risk varied considerably; the media images detracted from our understanding that the future of the epidemic was in the country's inner city ghettos, not in suburbia or on Park Avenue.

The overall growth in the number of cases, especially among people of color, women, and IDUs, and a change in the geography of the epidemic posed significant challenges to existing AIDS organizations. The future growth was alarming. The first estimate, which was later halved, was that there were four hundred thousand HIV-positive people in New York City.[4] Organizations anchored in the gay community did not have the capacity or, some thought, the cultural competence to serve such a growing and more diverse population. There was a need for organizations created specifically by and for people of color, for people infected through drug use, and for people still actively using drugs.

In contrast to the gay community, which mobilized quickly and tapped significant numbers of volunteers and donors, there was limited voluntarism in response to the changing face of AIDS. The people concerned about AIDS in African American and Latino communities faced enormous obstacles.[5] Local politicians did not provide much leadership. New AIDS organizations did have modest success raising private funds and recruiting substantial numbers of volunteers, but their growth, beginning toward the end of the 1980s, depended on the expansion of public funding.[6] Government agencies also played a more critical role in designing the fight against AIDS in these communities, providing personnel who volunteered time, designed programs, and developed new knowledge. Once funding began to increase, additional AIDS organizations were established and non-AIDS organizations began to compete with them for funds. A similar pattern occurred for women, with a large number of relatively small organizations developing. By the end of the 1980s, there was a large number of nonprofit organizations involved in fighting AIDS in the city.

An article in the 28 August 1981 issue of the *MMWR* documented the first case of immune deficiency in a woman. The following December, a description of eleven men with PCP revealed that six had histories of substance abuse.[7] The numbers of IDUs, women, and nonwhites diagnosed with AIDS began to increase in New York City: 139 IDUs and 64 women before April 1983. Nearly half of all AIDS cases in the city during that time were nonwhite: one quarter were African Americans, 19 percent were Hispanics, and 3 percent were Haitians.[8] By 1987, a similar pattern occurred nationwide. The number of cases per million was far higher (764) for African American men than for white men (291); the differential was even more striking for women: nine cases per million for whites and 105 for African Americans, with the rate slightly lower for Hispanic men (730) and women (73).[9]

The high concentration of the first AIDS cases in the gay ghettos of Chelsea and the West Village gave the epidemic a sense of urgency in these neighborhoods. This was not duplicated in Harlem, the Bronx, or Central Brooklyn. By the end of 1983, just under half of AIDS cases—49.5 percent—were in Manhattan. The second largest number were in Brooklyn (14 percent), the city's largest borough. A smaller proportion (11 percent) but a higher incidence were in the Bronx, and 7.5 percent were in Queens.[10] Clearly, the toll of sickness and deaths was expanding outside the boundaries of the city's gay ghettos.

Within boroughs, cases were more concentrated in some neighborhoods than in others. Rates of HIV infection were highest in the Bronx, especially in the South Bronx. Ernest Drucker of Montefiore Hospital estimated that one in five men between the ages of 25 and 45 living in the South Bronx were infected with HIV. HIV infection rates at one of the area's major hospitals, Bronx-Lebanon, indicated how serious AIDS would be in the future: between 5 and 10 percent of all women giving birth in the hospital, 14 to 25 percent of emergency room patients, and one quarter of all non-AIDS admissions were HIV-positive.[11] Among clients entering drug treatment, there were striking variations, with the highest proportion HIV-positive in Brooklyn (37 percent) and the Bronx (30 percent) but substantial proportions in Queens (19 percent) and in the counties surrounding New York City (21 percent).[12]

The changing face of the epidemic was also apparent in the growing number of drug addicts in the city being diagnosed with AIDS. The cases of "junkie pneumonia" in the late 1970s were the tip of the iceberg. The proportion of HIV-positive drug addicts rose sharply from 29 percent in 1979 to 52 percent in 1982.[13] There was a significant undercount of the number of drug addicts dying of AIDS during the first several years of the epidemic. The number of drug-related deaths in New York rose from 263 in 1978 to 1,091 in 1986; since most of these cases (80 percent) had AIDS-like symptoms, the researchers estimated that 2,520 AIDS deaths had been attributed to other causes.[14] Despite this undercount, a substantial number of people who were past and current

IDUs were diagnosed with AIDS. By mid-April 1983, 139 people, or one in five of the city's AIDS cases, were traced to drug use.[15] At the end of 1984, nearly one third of the city's AIDS cases were IDUs.[16]

This was an alarming change. There were an estimated 200,000 drug addicts in the city, a large proportion of the 1.1 to 1.3 million IV drug users in the country.[17] Injecting drug users, most of whom were men, could infect their female sex partners, who, in turn, would transmit the disease to their fetuses. In fact, 80 percent of women with AIDS were in the prime childbearing years.[18]

As with drug addicts, large numbers of the early cases among women went undetected. A study conducted in an emergency room in a public hospital in the Bronx revealed larger proportions of women than men who were sero-positive but not diagnosed as having AIDS.[19] In addition, the original surveil-lance definition of the disease excluded symptoms and infections that were unique to women. Given these facts, it is striking that, in 1984, one in ten AIDS cases in New York City and 7 percent nationally were woman. Six women were diagnosed with AIDS in 1981, 302 in 1984.[20] In 1985, AIDS became the second leading cause of death in New York City for women between the ages of 30 and 34.[21] The occurrence of AIDS in women became a particular concern because they were the source of infection for nearly all children who developed AIDS.

The five major AIDS organizations in the city—GMHC, PWAC, God's Love We Deliver, the AIDS Resource Center, and Momentum—altered their pro-grams and modified their organizational cultures in response to changes in the kinds of people who were living with AIDS. At the same time, they continued to be responsive to the gay community, which provided them with money and with volunteers.[22] Many of the staff, volunteers, and clients in these organiza-tions bridged race, class, and ethnic differences to develop strong connections, sometimes viewing PWAs who were different from themselves as "family."[23] But the lifestyle and cultural differences between gay men and people infected through drug use were sometimes unbridgeable. Existing organizations were transformed, and people in black and Latino communities stressed the need for their own organizations.

Despite a name that firmly linked it to the gay community, GMHC attracted a broad range of clients, including, in the early years, street people, who bene-fited from GMHC's open door policy: people could drop in and get help. Staff estimated in 1983 that 35 percent of its clients had a history of injecting drugs; this was twice the proportion of such cases in the city at the time. By 1986, 30 percent of GMHC's clients were black or Hispanic, and when GMHC volunteers began to do AIDS prevention work in gay bathhouses, they went to the Mount Morris Baths in Harlem.[24] GMHC also provided important leadership in policies and services for women, establishing support groups and developing legal services for women, drafting "Safer Sex Guidelines for Women," and assigning buddies to work with children, which led to the development of a Child Life program.[25] Despite its commitment to serving anyone who needed help, and despite the active involvement of women, African American, and Hispanic staff and volunteers, GMHC was criticized for being insensitive to minorities and to women, a description that one long-term African American staff member deemed an "urban legend."[26]

Other organizations added to or modified their programs. The PWA Coalition sponsored support groups for women, for mothers, and for gay men of color, collaborated with African American organizations to recruit writers for the *Newsline,* and started a Spanish language magazine called *SIDAhora.*[27] Momentum expanded to eight congregations in three different boroughs, began serving a more diverse group of guests, including homeless people and families, and ensured that clients could receive substance abuse counseling.[28] God's Love increased its geographic scope; it recruited volunteers from community groups located in the new neighborhoods it was serving, like the Addicts Rehabilitation Center in Harlem, and had more meals delivered by paid van drivers once the logistics of relying on meals delivered by volunteers became too difficult. In 1988, Ganga Stone told the organizations' supporters and clients, "There is no way to generalize about who we are. We are young and old, straight and gay, black and white, political and apolitical, religious and otherwise. . . . We care deeply about the people we feed. They are our brothers and sisters, sons and daughters, friends, husbands and wives."[29]

The changing population altered the organizational culture of some groups. Momentum developed a set of behavioral guidelines for guests and volunteers that suggested a host of problems at the dinners, including clients borrowing money, using drugs, stealing, and being physically or verbally abusive.[30] By the time the AIDS Resource Center's Bailey House opened, more of its residents were street people than originally envisioned, and there were tensions and conflicts. A Harvard University case study reported that "Most of the staff members at Bailey House came to the job full of empathy for their clients but were caught off-guard by what they encountered: a difficult group of people, many of whom were drug addicted and some of whom stole things, dealt drugs from the facility, and operated prostitution businesses in their bedrooms."[31]

The word on the street was that the staff were "naive beyond belief" and the agency hired substance abuse counselors and created a strict set of rules that banned overnight visitors, drug use, and drug dealing. Residents were evicted if they violated these rules.[32] Some of the same problems confronted the PWA Coalition's Living Room, where tensions were so great that a gay man thought that a drug deal was taking place when one man gave another an aspirin.[33] A newspaper article in the early 1990s indicated that gay clients at GMHC's recreation program were uncomfortable mingling with drug users who sometimes heckled them and called them faggots.[34]

Several years after the epidemic began, it became apparent that there was a need for new community-based organizations. Existing organizations were growing rapidly but were still unable to keep up with the demand. New, grassroots groups would have community support and would be more effective, having a better understanding of the needs in their particular communities. Like GMHC, they could attract money and volunteers. New York State began a slow process of developing a coordinated network of groups. The state legislature established an AIDS Institute (AI) in 1983 to fund scientific research and coordinate the development of the GMHC service model throughout the state, including "a hot line, crisis intervention counseling, home care, and legal services."[35] In the fall of 1983, the AI issued a request for proposals to establish seven Community Services Programs (CSPs) in different regions of the state plus one for New York City (GMHC was funded for this) and another for the Haitian community.[36]

The plan was intended to create a coordinated system of care. Calls to the state-sponsored hotline would be directed to each CSP. Like GMHC, the CSPs would rely on volunteers. In addition, they would also be "catalysts for service coordination, developing referral linkages for clients with health and human services."[37] The task was not easy; the groups were given relatively modest support to carry out a broad portfolio. In 1986, the state allocated $1.9 million to create task forces in Brooklyn, Queens, and the Bronx and later established task forces in Upper Manhattan (1988), Staten Island (1989), and Lower Manhattan (1990). Part of the difficulty of establishing the programs was the limited interest in many communities, especially minority communities. Staff in the AI had to work hard to get groups to apply. Rosen admitted that "Sometimes when people from minority communities hear the words AIDS, they just don't want to be involved, and we have taken a lot of heat for not doing enough programs with minority communities."[38]

The first nonwhite community to respond was the Haitian community. A group of professionals and community leaders started the Haitian Coalition on AIDS in 1983. The incidence of AIDS was high among Haitians during the first several years of the epidemic; the Haitian Coalition was formed to challenge the CDC's designation of Haitians as a high-risk group, and the fact that they were banned from donating blood. The Haitian Coalition remained small; it concentrated on advocacy and received little financial support because of the enormous stigma of the disease in the Haitian community. It did, however, achieve its two major objectives: Haitians were eliminated as a risk category in 1985, and, after a major demonstration in 1990, the ban on their blood donations ended in 1990.[39]

GMHC tried to promote interest in AIDS among minorities at a public forum cosponsored with the Ad Hoc Committee of Black Gay Activists, and the organization attracted a number of minority volunteers. [40] There was limited leadership from black and Hispanic elected officials, who, when they did consider the issue, focused on the impact of the epidemic on women and children.[41] Hispanic politicians were also cautious. When the Bronx Borough President Fernando Ferrer wrote in a weekly newspaper column that Hispanic women ought to cooperate with a Department of Health study about their knowledge, attitudes, and sexual practices, he received angry letters and phone calls. With enormous candor, he told a *New York Times* reporter in 1989 that "Elected officials are in a tougher position because, when you talk about speaking forthrightly, especially in the context of our culture and connectedness with religion, you're asking for trouble."[42]

Three new organizations, the Hispanic AIDS Forum, the Minority Task Force, and the Association for Drug Abuse and Treatment, were established in the fall of 1985. Each had the possibility of becoming the central organization for their communities, just as GMHC was for the gay community. In reality, each grew slowly, because of limited community support, a lack of public funds, and growing competition.

The Hispanic AIDS Forum (HAF) was organized by a member of the Mayor's Task Force on AIDS who convened a group of human service professionals to enlist support from community leaders, to disseminate information about the disease, and to become involved in planning services. Despite the fact that Spanish was the city's second language, the health department was still in the process of developing AIDS prevention material in Spanish and hiring bilingual staff; because the material was a direct translation from English to Spanish and had not been tested in the Hispanic community, the members of HAF were concerned that it would not be culturally appropriate. At its second meeting, the group's members agreed that the organization "must formally demand that all materials distributed by official governmental agencies be pretested in the Hispanic community." They were also concerned about getting "a fair share of any revenues" directed toward AIDS.[43]

At the same time, representatives of several organizations, including the Association of Puerto Rican Executive Directors, the Chinatown Planning Council, and the Department of Psychiatry at Harlem Hospital Center, were planning a major conference on minorities and AIDS.[44] Sponsored by the Council of Churches of the City of New York, the conference was held on the same day the *New York Times* announced that the proportion of AIDS cases among blacks was double their proportion in the population.[45] After the conference, a group of gay men in Harlem formed the Minority Task Force on AIDS (MTFA).

Having two groups, HAF and the MTFA, seemed inefficient, especially because the MTFA was intended to serve all minorities in the city. Potential funders encouraged them to merge. A HAF founder recalled that "Basically, what we were told is why is it necessary to have two organizations that are going to address the needs of minorities and AIDS in New York City. Isn't one organization enough? We have limited resources."[46] A foundation executive whom both groups approached remembered thinking, "Can't you people work together?"[47] HAF's founders did not want to merge because "Our experience in the past with so-called minority organizations was that most of them were controlled by African Americans and the agenda would be set by African Americans, and the needs of our communities are very diverse. And although we have common issues and common problems, we also have very diverse needs and different ways of dealing with problems and issues . . . in the area of HIV prevention and education, that culture played a critical role and that we had to develop our own organizations to address the needs of our community."[48]

HAF and the MTFA both grew slowly. AIDS was highly stigmatized because of its association with homosexuality and drug use. For individual African American and Hispanic men, the concept of being gay was not salient and, in fact, statistical reports and policy statements began to make reference to "men who have sex with men." It was also not uncommon for men to define themselves as bisexual even when their sexual contacts were exclusively with other men.

For gay men living in Harlem and in other neighborhoods, the epidemic did not have the same sense of urgency as it did for gay white men living downtown. The social networks of minority men who were homosexual did not intersect with gay white men's networks; further, they did not identify with the downtown gay white community since, as AIDS educator George Bellinger Jr., observed "We black gay men have been male first, black second, gay whenever."[49] An ethnographic study of gay men in Harlem noted that they distanced themselves from AIDS and saw it as a disease affecting drug addicts, and that "the gay men who have died or are ill all had or have social and sexual connections with the mainstream gay community downtown or with gay friends and sex partners in other areas of the city that have been affected by the epidemic"[50] African American gay men occupied a complex position in their communities. As a group, many led highly closeted lives. They were an integral and often important part of their families, since they provided economic support and assistance, especially to aging parents. Some were pillars of their communities. Mindy Thompson Fullilove and Robert Fullilove point out that homosexuality was openly condemned in black churches but at the same time "homosexuals are accorded a special status . . . they provide the creative energy necessary to African American religious experience . . . responsible for creating the music and other emotional moments that bring worshipers closer to God."[51]

The slow response of African American communities has complex roots. A poll conducted in the fall of 1985 found that many more African Americans (71 percent) than whites (48 percent) agreed that "AIDS was the most serious medical problem facing the country."[52] The message that African Americans were at risk was blunted by a lack of trust and the belief that AIDS was a government conspiracy. Much of this distrust was linked to the federal government's support for the Tuskegee experiment, which had become well known by the early 1980s.[53] The parallels to AIDS were disturbing. Here was a new and mysterious illness that was being linked to black people and to Africa. Numerous critics, including reputable scientists, were questioning its origins, and some suggested that AIDS was originally produced in a government laboratory to kill off undesirables like gay people and drug addicts.[54] A 1988 Nation of Islam publication likened AIDS to genocide and the idea was discussed in the mainstream media on television programs like Tony Brown's Journal, and in widely read magazines like Essence.[55] Polls indicated that some, although not a majority, of African Americans shared these suspicions. A New York Times/WCBS-TV poll conducted in New York City in 1990 found that one in ten African Americans agreed that HIV was purposely created in a laboratory to infect black people. Another 19 percent agreed that this might be true, compared to 91 percent of whites who thought that the idea was certainly not true. Two thirds of blacks thought that drugs are permitted to be easily available in poor black neighborhoods to harm people. One quarter agreed that "the Government deliberately makes sure that drugs are easily available in poor neighborhoods in order to harm black people," and an additional 35 percent noted this might possibly be true.[56] Another survey, conducted in the early 1990s, found that one fifth of African Americans believed that the government was using AIDS to kill off minority groups and 43 percent believed that doctors and scientists were not revealing all that needed to be known about the disease.[57]

For Hispanics, the barriers to community mobilization were also considerable. Hispanic culture condemned homosexuality and emphasized the importance of keeping intimate details private. This was especially true concerning discussions of sex and sexuality, which meant that "it's indiscreet to bring up the whole topic."[58] Hispanic families covered up diagnoses and attributed illness and deaths to other diseases like leukemia.[59] Homosexuality was not just a source of stigma for an individual but a source of shame for an entire family.[60] HAF needed to mobilize a geographically dispersed and closeted group of men who, like African American men, did not necessarily define themselves as gay.[61] A lack of candor about homosexuality occurred among HAF's founders. All of the men on the board were gay, but one member recalled that this "was not discussed at all. . . . Issues about homosexuals were discussed as if they were someone else's issues." In fact, one founder who died of AIDS kept the other members "in the dark" about his illness.[62]

HAF faced considerable obstacles to adopting safer sex practices. Barriers to condom use were enormous not only because between 85 and 90 percent of Hispanics in the city were Catholic, but also because condoms were associated "with prostitution and uncleanliness."[63] Prevention programs needed to be tailored to Latino culture, which emphasized machismo (male pride) for men and marianismo for women. Since "a good woman is always ready for her man and should not exhibit comfort with sexuality issues or ease with the sex act itself," the process of negotiating condom use had some distinctive features for Hispanic women.[64] There were also important considerations in teaching men who had sex with men. The request that a partner use a condom was interpreted as implying that he was promiscuous.[65] Hispanic gay men were geographically dispersed, with one definable community in Jackson Heights in Queens. HAF, along with GMHC and the AIDS Center of Queens, did HIV prevention in gay bars and clubs in Jackson Heights, using a performance format in neighborhood bars that was developed by the Fundacion SIDA of Puerto Rico.[66]

Both the MTFA and HAF depended on funding from foundations, corporations, and the state because their communities offered limited financial support, and relatively few volunteers stepped forward. The MTFA expected to have a similar experience to GMHC's: once people in the community became educated, they would tap into strong traditions of self help and informal assistance, and volunteer and donate money.[67] This did not occur; the group attracted a small number of volunteers and obtained private funds primarily from foundations.[68] The organization attracted a significant amount of foundation funding in its first several years, but this source dried up relatively soon because of financial and organizational problems.

The MTFA also faced another important dilemma: many community leaders lent support to a second organization, the Black Leadership Commission on AIDS (BLCA), founded in 1987. Initially sponsored by the Urban League, BLCA's membership included a cross-section of the city's religious, political, and economic elite: politicians, college professors, clergy, and professionals.[69] It also attracted significant funding from foundations and provided technical assistance so that community organizations could obtain funds for AIDS programs.[70]

It took several more years, until the late 1980s and early 1990s, for African American elected officials and organizations like the NAACP and the Urban League to make AIDS a priority.[71] There was a sharp spike in media coverage and awareness following the 1991 announcement by the basketball star Magic Johnson that he was HIV-positive.[72] Toward the end of the 1990s, when blacks were estimated to account for 57 percent of new infections, the U.S. Department of Health and Human Services and the Congressional Black Caucus announced a $156 million initiative to fight AIDS in minority communities.[73]

In contrast to the MTFA, HAF's founders expected to get little community support, and they concentrated on advocacy and community education. Members spoke to a broad range of groups, including hotel employees fearful of changing sheets and cleaning bathrooms. They encountered enormous indifference; one member recalled going to a tenant's association meeting where two people showed up. HAF's founders undertook the task of ending the silence since, according to one founder, AIDS "wasn't spoken about too much by Hispanic elected and appointed officials. . . . We were the only ones out there raising the issue about HIV and AIDS in the Latino community. The impact hadn't taken hold yet; people were still in a mindset because of the way that the epidemic was defined in the beginning—that this was not our issue, this was not our disease."[74] The group framed AIDS as a community-wide concern, not an issue solely associated with gay men or substance abuse, noting "the whole community is at risk," an idea that resonated in Hispanic culture, which stresses the importance of the family and the community.[75]

There was limited leadership from other institutional sources. African American and Hispanic newspapers did not cover the AIDS story during the early years of the epidemic.[76] Churches and other religious institutions responded slowly. Most Hispanics in the city were Catholic, and the Catholic church was firmly opposed to the use of condoms. African American churches did not serve as a locus of mobilization, either. Although many accounts focus

on the institutional indifference rooted in the stigma toward both homosexuality and drug abuse, focus groups with African American clergy in New
York, conducted by Mindy and Robert Fullilove, revealed that, even though
both were concerns, "It was homosexuality, however, which seemed to be the
greatest stumbling block."[77] With limited institutional support, few individual
donations, and a lack of support from politicians, the MTFA and the Hispanic
AIDS Forum each operated on a shoestring during most of the 1980s.

The association of the epidemic with drug addiction had complex consequences for community mobilization. The early years of the epidemic were also a
time of growing concern about drug use.[78] It was difficult to generate interest
in an epidemic affecting drug users, because they were viewed as a major
source of community problems, and drug addicts victimized people to support
their drug habits.[79] In a seminal essay that explores key reasons why African
American communities were reluctant to "own" AIDS, Harlon Dalton points
out that "For us, drug abuse is a curse far worse than you can imagine. Addicts
prey on our neighborhoods, sell drugs to our children, steal our possessions,
and rob us of hope. We despise them. We despise them because they hurt us
and because they are us. They are a constant reminder of how close we are to
the edge. And 'they' are 'us' literally as well as figuratively; they are our sons
and daughters, our sisters and brothers."[80]

A similar ambivalence characterized Hispanic communities. In the mid-
1980s, several Hispanic neighborhoods had high crime levels, much of the
crime related to the drug trade. One early HAF leader pointed out that "there
was the whole notion that it [AIDS] promoted the stereotype that there was a
lot of drug use among Latinos, and nobody wanted to say that out loud. And
no politician or community leader, including the heads of agencies, wanted to
be associated with that message, because they felt that they would get criticism."[81] AIDS was only one of a number of issues in Hispanic communities
and owning AIDS meant admitting to the existence of a problem both painful
and a source of status anxiety, as it was in African American communities. It
is not surprising, then, that HAF and the MTFA did not focus much attention
on the link between AIDS and drug addiction. Another group, the Association
for Drug Abuse Prevention and Treatment (ADAPT), was established to
respond to this issue.

In late October of 1985, two dozen people attended a meeting to consider the
growing numbers of IDUs being diagnosed with AIDS. A series of recently

released studies indicated that a large proportion of current and former drug addicts were HIV-positive.[82] The meeting was initiated by staff in the Division of Substance Abuse Services (DSAS), the state agency that funded drug treatment programs. In spite of the fears and concerns about AIDS among staff and clients in drug treatment programs in the state, little was being done.[83] The meeting included drug counselors and social workers, representatives from the city's Department of Health, two social scientists who studied drug use, a physician, and a Legal Services lawyer. Many of them were personally affected as former drug addicts.[84] The group decided to revive an organization some had once belonged to, called the Association for Drug Abuse Treatment and Treatment (ADAPT).

The State AIDS Institute was planning to fund community education and case management for minorities, especially for drug users.[85] ADAPT and DSAS could be partners in fighting AIDS among drug addicts. DSAS was beginning to send out vans to do street outreach with homeless people and was developing posters to warn people about AIDS. ADAPT's volunteers could do the advocacy, innovation, and risk taking that were difficult for staff working in a public agency.

DSAS staff thought that that "ADAPT will become the prototype for a national model" just as GMHC had.[86] ADAPT emulated GMHC in several ways. The organizers developed innovative methods of fighting AIDS among active drug users and recruited an active critical mass of volunteers, most of them former addicts. Volunteers and staff played an important role in the creation and the diffusion of knowledge about how to reduce HIV transmission among active drug injectors (IDUs). ADAPT volunteers and staff trained staff of AIDS organizations throughout the country to adopt its methods.

The eleven committees formed at the group's second meeting were testimony to the complexity of what needed to be done.[87] The organizers acted quickly to expand membership, sending letters to staff and to clients in substance abuse treatment programs noting that "Our members include recovered and recovering substance abusers who are clinic administrators, social workers, client activists, housewives, the unemployed, a physician, and an attorney. However, YOU DON'T HAVE TO BE AN EX-ADDICT TO JOIN ADAPT."[88]

They had an elaborate set of plans including a speakers bureau, public service announcements, brochures and flyers, a buddy program, and a hotline, as well as professional education for health care and drug treatment staff. Two activities gained momentum: visiting prisoners in the city jail on Riker's Island, and street outreach with active drug injectors.

AIDS posed enormous challenges to correctional facilities, creating panic in prisons and in jails among guards and prisoners. Drug use was high; 85 percent of six hundred people arrested in New York in 1986 tested positive for "hard drugs," including 20 percent who had been using heroin.[89] One ADAPT member, Frank Tardalo, contacted officials at Riker's and enlisted a small group of volunteers to visit prisoners and teach them about HIV prevention.[90] The needs were far greater than they anticipated, since the conditions were horrible and prisoners with AIDS were "housed in practically the oldest and worst building on the island . . . [in] a cell block that was totally neglected, infected with rodents and infestation, . . . [with] no adequate heating during the winter and . . . no air conditioning during the summer. . . . The men were locked in their cells at night without adequate pain medication. The medical services were poor. The guards were scared.[91]

The prisoners mounted two hunger strikes, in June and October of 1986. The eight regular volunteers from ADAPT served as liaisons to the prisoners' families during the second strike, and one initiated a lawsuit challenging the conditions. These efforts led to some important changes, including a new infirmary, access to methadone, better medical staff, and improved medical care in city hospitals.[92]

A second set of activities, street outreach to active drug injectors, became the organization's major and best-known program, and allowed it to grow and to hire staff. In San Francisco and in Baltimore, also, groups were doing outreach with IDUs, a set of people who had been disconnected from the social service and public health systems.[93] Like the GMHC and Safer Sex Brigade volunteers who stood on streetcorners and went into the bars and the baths, ADAPT volunteers were trying to help drug addicts to do more effectively what many were already attempting: to save their lives by changing their drug-using behavior (see chapter 9). These volunteers took it upon themselves—without any funding or support—"to work with people to prevent them from getting sick"[94] There were scattered precedents for doing outreach with active drug injectors. Beginning their work on streetcorners, ADAPT volunteers began to do outreach in the "shooting galleries" where people purchased drugs; borrowed, shared, or "rented" injection equipment; and prepared and injected drugs. One outreach worker recalled that "a lot of people said we were doing a terrible thing, we were encouraging people to use drugs. We were enabling. But we felt we were doing the right thing. We saw it just like sexual risk reduction. GMHC didn't tell people not to have sex. They told them how to have safer sex. We weren't going to tell people not to use drugs, we were going to tell them how to avoid HIV. That was our goal."[95]

These outreach workers had two distinct objectives: to get people into treatment, and to teach them how to protect themselves—since, the workers realized, many addicts were not ready for treatment and the number of treatment slots was limited. Distributing copies of a brochure called the *Mainline Message*, ADAPT volunteers advised drug users to buy and keep their own injection equipment, warned them that used needles were being repackaged to appear new, and encouraged addicts to boil their needles or to clean them with alcohol or bleach.[96] One outreach volunteer thought back about the messages being conveyed and pointed out that "They were not according to the principles of health education. They were scary. There were tombstones. They were made by drug addicts."[97] Building on the fear of addicts, which was very real, the flyers reminded people that AIDS was "for keeps" and that carelessness would lead to death. But the volunteers were not just out to scare people; they wanted to provide them with tangible ways to prevent themselves from becoming infected or infecting other people. Like GMHC volunteers, who were "making it up" as they went along, ADAPT volunteers developed bleach kits: plastic ziplock bags with brochures, condoms, bottle caps used as cookers to prepare drugs, and cotton and bleach for cleaning needles and syringes.

The idea of ex-addicts fighting AIDS attracted attention. TV, radio, and news articles described ADAPT's street outreach especially its work in shooting galleries.[98] News stories described addicts telling outreach workers how they wanted to get off the streets and into treatment and stop wasting their lives. Former addicts were doing the kind of work that the average person could not. A description of an early outreach effort in Williamsburg noted that Tardalo's "street-wise savvy granted him free reign in the neighborhood."[99] An article in *Fortune* pointed out how Edith Springer "and other reformed addicts make the rounds of sleazy shooting galleries where as many as 100 addicts a day share a few sets of injection paraphernalia."[100] Many of the articles focused on ADAPT's president, Yolanda Serrano, who had not been an addict. Hailed as one of *Ms. Magazine's* women of the year in 1989, she was described as the "Avon lady to the dark side of society" who fearlessly stepped over crack vials and entered abandoned buildings to announce to those in the shooting galleries, "I have condoms. I have bleach."[101]

But the volunteers' enthusiasm and creativity were not enough to meet the enormous challenges of teaching prevention to the great number of drug addicts in the city. Although news accounts point to the group's large membership, 40 volunteers involved in an outreach effort in East Harlem, 100 active members in 1987, and 250 in 1989 and 1990, the names of two or perhaps three dozen active members appear again and again in the organizations' records.[102]

Members realized fairly quickly that they would have "serious problems" if they did not obtain funding. A grant application to the New York Foundation in 1986 noted that "The danger to ADAPT's voluntary leadership and membership from over-extension, stress, conflict, and 'burnout' is very real."[103]

The active members kept the group afloat, donating time and money. Its first and only fundraising event, a dance in a Manhattan club in the summer of 1986, netted only $4,500, far less than the $12,000 they expected to raise. A $24,000 grant from the New York Foundation allowed ADAPT to hire a coordinator and pay some of its expenses, and technical assistance from the Community Service Society allowed the organization to actively pursue funding from the city and the state.[104] The AI turned down ADAPT's application to coordinate services in Brooklyn, but the group succeeded in getting its first large contract, with the City Department of Health (DOH) to conduct "educational services to intravenous drug users, past/recovering intravenous drug users, and their sexual partners." The request for proposals (RFP) for this contract targeted seven "communities at high risk for intravenous drug use" and specified that applicants must have "previous experience in delivering services to the above-named target populations," which meant that there was not much competition, since ADAPT was the only organization doing this work. The initial timetable was ambitious, with a 30 June 1986 application deadline and funding to begin 1 August.[105] Although ADAPT was invited to negotiate a contract for $176,635 at the end of the summer of 1986, the approval process was slow, and the first installment of $15,000 did not arrive until the following June. In the interim, ADAPT used up most of its cash reserves and got a bank loan.[106]

Public funding quickly transformed ADAPT. The staff grew from one person to twelve by the end of 1987 and to thirty in 1989. The need for their services was so great that the DOH was ready to double the amount in a second contract even before it disbursed the funds for the first contract. Relying almost exclusively on public funds, ADAPT's income increased from $263,118 in 1988 to nearly $1.7 million in 1991. However, numerous internal problems, including the dominance of a relatively inexperienced albeit charismatic executive director and the departure of many volunteer leaders, led to a series of financial crises, a slow decline, and the agency's closure in 2005.

Despite efforts to create a coherent and coordinated system, the network of nonprofit organizations, hospitals, and government agencies involved in AIDS activities grew exponentially; a total of 166 new AIDS organizations were established in New York City by 1998. These organizations had a broad range of objectives. Some were involved in the arts; others provided services, were advocacy groups, or conducted scientific research. The number of organizations with broader purposes engaged in some type of AIDS-related activity was far larger. A study conducted by the Health Systems Agency estimated that there were approximately 400 AIDS service providers. My own estimate, based on extensive data collection, was that there were 554 organizations involved in AIDS-related work. By the end of the 1980s, a number of community-based Hispanic organizations were providing AIDS prevention and services. Nicholas Freudenberg and his collaborators documented the organizational response in two Hispanic communities, Washington Heights in Upper Manhattan and the Hunts Point section of the Bronx, in the late 1980s. More than half of the 47 groups they surveyed had some type of AIDS prevention activity, a remarkable figure in light of the few resources and enormous stigma. Most often, the groups had conferences or workshops to inform staff and clients. Some sponsored discussion groups for women and for teens, and trained staff to do HIV prevention and counseling. [107]

The sharp rise in AIDS-related funding, mainly public funding, contributed to this expansion. New York City spent $47.4 million of its funds for AIDS in 1986. Much of this went for hospital care. Total costs increased nearly four times, to $181.6 million in 1989.[108] A city Office of Management and Budget calculation of total funding (including city, state, federal and foundation funds) on AIDS in New York City, totaled $465 million in 1990 and $600 million in 1991.[109] Funds from New York State also rose sharply. The New York State AIDS Institute's budget was $5.25 million in 1983–1984. Five years later, its allocation was $30.4 million.[110]

The rapid and highly decentralized growth of AIDS organizations and services especially characterized services for women and for children. In 1993, the State AIDS Institute funded forty women's programs. One of the earliest efforts was the work of Dr. Joyce Wallace, who later founded the Foundation for Research on Sexually Transmitted Diseases (FROST'D). Wallace was one of the first physicians to recognize AIDS in women, and she began to do outreach and AIDS education with sex workers.[111] Beginning in 1986, the city's Department of Health started a support group for women referred by the city's AIDS hotline.[112]

Efforts to develop community-based groups were spearheaded by professional women. Beginning in 1986, members of the Women and AIDS Project began meeting regularly. The group's two leaders were staff members in state agencies, the Division for Women and the Division of Substance Abuse Services.[113] They organized a legislative hearing and initiated the Women and

AIDS Resource Network (WARN) in 1987, the first organization in the country that focused on women and AIDS. WARN attracted significant private funding: $262,000 from a dozen foundations and public charities between 1987 and 1990.[114] Noting that "AIDS disproportionately affects women with the least resources able to bear it," the group's founders recognized that many women with AIDS are not only PWAs but also caregivers for partners and children with AIDS. Initially, WARN was envisioned as a clearinghouse providing information, helping women to obtain access to services, assembling "a pool of expert professionals," conducting surveys, and influencing public policy.[115] By 1992, the organization became a multipurpose service organization offering telephone reassurance, case management, support groups, and information and referral. Continuing to receive support from various foundations, it became more dependent on public funds, which comprised 89 percent of its funding in 1992, its last year.[116]

The network of services for women and children expanded by the early 1990s. Large numbers of women and children living with AIDS needed income, housing, and psychological support as families confronted a highly stigmatized illness and the future prospect of the death of one or both parents.[117] Initially focusing on women as individuals, a host of new and existing organizations began to serve families affected by HIV. With the drug addiction, illness, and death of women with HIV, their HIV-positive and HIV-negative children needed foster care and long-term custody plans. Most children in families affected by AIDS were HIV-negative and would survive their parents and their HIV-positive siblings. Besides the psychological impact of the loss of a parent, the children who would get AIDS were a particularly vulnerable population because "a parent's illness from AIDS is just one piece of a chaotic puzzle of divorce and separation, drug addiction, incarceration, mental illness, domestic violence, and poverty."[118] For these children, especially the adolescents, anticipating and becoming orphaned were enormously traumatic. A study of AIDS families in New York revealed that "Adolescents informed of their parent's illness were more likely to engage in unprotected sex, substance use, and be emotionally distressed."[119]

AIDS organizations like GMHC, God's Love We Deliver, HAF, MTFA, and ADAPT, served women and their children. Life Force in Brooklyn (founded in 1989) and Health Force in the Bronx (founded in 1990) trained peer educators, many of them HIV-positive, to do outreach and education.[120] A Women and AIDS Working Group, under the auspices of the Manhattan Borough president, planned Iris House, an organization designed to provide family services in one location, and the Family Center was established in 1992 by former staff from the city's Human Resources Administration to serve families affected by HIV.[121]

Numerous non-AIDS organizations sponsored support groups, provided services, and did prevention education. The prevention program sponsored by Women in Crisis involved community education. Its staff members distributed condoms and did informal education in places, like beauty parlors and nail salons and other sites where women gathered and could speak freely and openly.[122] As survival time increased, women and children living with AIDS were able to receive support and mental health services from organizations like the Community Consultation Center, the Ackerman Institute for Family Therapy, and the Lower East Side Family Union. In 1987, staff at Beth Israel Medical Center started the Well Children in AIDS Families Project, helping children to understand what was happening to their parents, to deal with their own feelings, to learn how to cope with talking to people in their family and their community, and to talk about their feelings about losing a parent.[123] Several church groups sponsored women's centers.[124] Child welfare and home care agencies, like Self Help and the Visiting Nurse Service, provided foster care and homemaking services.[125]

As the 1980s were nearing an end, policymakers, journalists, and people in the AIDS community came to realize that the epidemic was not simply a medical event, but a total social event involving a broad range of social, psychological, economic, political, and cultural forces. The changing face of the epidemic was obvious. What was becoming more apparent was that the future was even more grim. The number of cases was increasing, future costs were alarming, and it was becoming more evident that AIDS was a disease of the underclass enmeshed in a host of social ills that needed to be addressed. An evaluation of New York's state-funded programs serving women pointed out that "The women had a wide range of service needs that went beyond problems with HIV. Women mentioned legal problems, difficulties with substance use, the burden of discussing HIV with their children, adolescent children who were facing their own crises, housing issues, transportation for appointments, and problems receiving entitlements."[126]

The clients were changing and so were their needs. It took the perception of an impending crisis for the federal government to expand its commitment to the epidemic.

Chapter 6

The "New Calcutta"

It's not in their face like the knife or the eviction notice. . . .
AIDS is a plague for people who are already plagued.

—Ernest Drucker

Ten major policy reports, released between May 1988 and July 1989, described the myriad implications of the changing face of AIDS.[1] They summarized the work of a number of elite groups including the Presidential Commission on the HIV Epidemic, the President's Commission on AIDS, and panels organized by the National Academy of Sciences, New York State, New York City, and major foundations.[2] The task forces and commissions gave the issue enormous visibility and legitimacy, because their members represented a broad cross-section of Americans who were impartial and became impassioned about the epidemic. Admiral James Watkins, the politically conservative former U.S. Chief of Naval Operations, took over an initially beleaguered Presidential Commission on the HIV Epidemic that was criticized for its lack of expertise. Watkins, a deeply religious Catholic who was described as having a "blend of pragmatism and compassion," noted that his past work was a piece of cake compared to trying to understand the epidemic.[3] Dr. David Rogers, a professor of medicine at Cornell University Medical School, also played an important role in drawing attention to AIDS, as head of the New York City Mayor's Task Force on AIDS and the New York State AIDS Advisory Council and co-chair of the President's Commission on AIDS.[4] The groups not only informed elected officials; they promoted public awareness and concern. Several months after the President's Commission on HIV report was released, a majority of Americans agreed that AIDS was the nation's most serious social problem.[5]

The reports mapped out a broad range of policy proposals—medical care, prescription drug development, vaccine development, drug treatment, prevention, and public health measures—and estimated future costs. Several, like that of the President's Commission on the HIV Epidemic, pointed out that the epidemic was "occurring disproportionately within the underclass, the largely minority population of the inner city poor."[6] It was becoming clear that the epidemic was strongly associated with several other important social problems—drug use, crime, domestic violence and homelessness—that exposed holes in the society's social safety net. More PWAs were living in neighborhoods with high rates of crime, unemployment, welfare use, teen pregnancy, violence, and shorter life expectancy. AIDS was a disaster for some communities; it was both a cause of disaster and a symptom of a broader set of social ills.

These two qualities—the association of the epidemic with the underclass and the sense of disaster—greatly contributed to rapid growth in funding and, in 1990, the passage of two important pieces of legislation, the Ryan White Comprehensive AIDS Resource Act (CARE Act) and the National Affordable Housing Act. These acts earmarked significant federal funds to fight the epidemic in the hardest hit cities and states. A third act passed that year, the Americans with Disabilities Act, provided important civil liberties protection for people living with AIDS.

The passage of the Ryan White and the National Affordable Housing Acts were a turning point in another way. The allocation of federal funds was evidence that federal officials and members of Congress recognized that local government funding, volunteers, and private dollars were inadequate. This was a sharp turn away from the Reagan administration's strong commitment to devolution and privatization. As nonprofit and government organizations looked to the future, it became apparent that the voluntary sector had significant limits. The neighborhoods that were becoming the most affected by the epidemic were areas with limited social capital and little access to private funds. A rise in funding was not needed only to respond to the epidemic; it was necessary to ensure the economic health of American cities.[7]

The epidemic was well under way when these plans were released; more than 100,000 people had been diagnosed with AIDS. The belated planning was evidence of a combination of a slow government response and an early lack of clarity about the epidemic. It took several years to begin to understand who was affected, how many people were infected, what kinds of health and social services were needed, and how much they would cost.[8] New York State's first comprehensive plan, in 1989, noted that planning had been difficult because the full dimensions of the geography and demography of the epidemic had not been clear.[9] Nationwide estimates of people infected with HIV rose rapidly from 200,000 in 1984 to between 1 and 1.5 million in the middle of 1986.[10]

The reports synthesized a growing body of research on the complex nature and impact of the epidemic. The outlook was grim. The report issued by the Presidential Commission on the HIV Epidemic raised public awareness and mapped a broad range of national policies needed to address "the full course of HIV infection rather than concentrating on later stages of the disease." This represented a major shift in the way the disease was framed: it had become clear that early intervention in HIV illness slowed the course of the disease. This meant that people living with HIV, not just those with AIDS, would need help. The expansion in the numbers of people with HIV illness, the longer life expectancies involved, and the growing availability of expensive but life-sustaining medications meant that future costs would skyrocket.[11]

Reports on New York City and New York State underscored the need for more federal funding but endorsed the existing "third way" approach, characterized by public-private partnerships between the nonprofit sector and all levels of government.[12] The New York City AIDS Task Force report projected fifty thousand AIDS cases by 1993. If true, this would more than double the demand for hospital beds, require ten times as many new nursing home beds and five times the number of housing units, and cost the city one billion dollars each year for hospital care alone.[13] The planning document for the New York City AIDS Fund, the local affiliate of a nationwide effort by the Ford Foundation to increase private funding, pointed out that "the care needs growing out of HIV infection and AIDS are placed on already overburdened and inadequate health care and social service systems, and most agree that these systems will not be adequate to meet the growing needs."[14] New York State's strategic plan pointed out that "New York State must reshape and rearm its response, combining the strengths of all levels of government and bridging the gap between public and private sector efforts."[15] Similarly, the New York City's Interagency Task Force on AIDS report observed that "It will take the combined resources of City, State, and federal agencies and the full participation by the voluntary and private sectors to confront the epidemic here."[16]

The future costs were striking. But what made the epidemic especially alarming was its connection to other problems. One report, "The Crisis in AIDS Care," developed by the Citizen's Commission on AIDS, had a particular impact on New York's civic leaders. The report pointed out that the number of diagnosed cases and deaths—about 18,900 in the metropolitan area—was the tip of the iceberg. There were between 30,000 and 50,000 people with symptoms of HIV illness, and another 130,000 to 170,000 who were HIV-positive but asymptomatic. Annual costs would spiral to $1.2 billion in 1990–1991 and to $1.9 billion three years later. At a press conference, John E. Jacob, the Commission's co-chair and the president of the National Urban League, pointed out that "we are all at risk. Some directly from the virus, others who will not be able to get into overcrowded hospitals, and many others because businesses—facing a city gripped by plague-like conditions in subways, terminals, and streets—will leave for a less daunting environment. It is not inevitable, but it is a realistic scenario if we fail to act now."[17]

A *New York Times* article on the press conference, called "AIDS Drives Jobs Away," quoted other commission members. John Zuccotti, former head of the city's planning commission and a partner in a prominent law firm, pointed out, "In locational decisions, more and more I hear people saying: 'What is happening with New York's health care? Are we going to be stepping over bodies, like Calcutta?'" J. Richard Munro, the chairman of Time, Inc., noted that people would "think twice" about moving to New York if there were no hospital beds.[18]

Several weeks later, the Citizen's Commission and the New York City AIDS Task Force organized a meeting of the city's civic and business elite, the kinds of leaders that influence policy decisions in large cities.[19] One participant, Felix Rohatyn, the investment banker who had taken a leadership role in responding to the city's near-bankrupcy in the 1970s, told a reporter that AIDS was even more serious than the city's fiscal crisis. Lewis Rudin and Preston Robert Tisch, whose families actively supported GMHC and God's Love We Deliver, pointed out that they were particularly concerned about the epidemic because friends had waited for several days in hospital emergency rooms before they could be admitted.[20] Like the founders of the Howard Associations in the South, who organized services in yellow fever epidemics in the nineteenth century to ensure that their cities were favorable places to conduct business, these business leaders were alarmed.[21] They urged the city, the state, the federal government, and the private sector to devote more funds to the epidemic. The backlog in the city's hospitals was symptomatic of a host of urban problems that affected the city's business climate and, in turn, its viability as a global city.

The Citizen's Commission's report outlined the strong links among crime, homelessness, drug use, and AIDS. Drug use was "ravaging" the city and was often described as a plague that contributed to a host of social problems. Between 1977 and 1989, drug arrests more than quadrupled (to 90,000), the number of prisoners in city jails rose from 7,000 to 19,000, and nearly 1,900 people were murdered.[22] A boy born in Harlem had a shorter life expectancy than a boy born in Bangladesh. Almost one in ten babies born in Harlem went directly into the city's foster care system.[23] There were nearly 9,000 more reports of child abuse (55,160) during the first nine months of 1988 than in all of 1987.[24] There were obvious signs of disorder all over the city: graffiti on almost every subway car, the sound of gunshots in neighborhoods with high rates of drug use, high levels of welfare use, and homeless people sleeping in the streets and in the city's bus and train terminals.[25] (In some neighborhoods, like my own on the Upper West Side of Manhattan, nearly every car had a "No Radio" sign to warn off thieves.)

Some drug users were addicted to heroin, but a growing number, particularly women, used a form of cocaine known as crack, the focus of a growing concern about drug use.[26] Crack had the advantage of being smoked rather than injected. The rise in drug use among women was having important consequences for HIV transmission and for the foster care system. In contrast to the users of other addictive drugs, an estimated 60 percent of crack users were women.[27] Many traded drugs for sex, which greatly increased their risk of getting HIV. The beginning of the crack epidemic coincided with a 30 percent increase in the number of abused or neglected children between 1985 and 1986.[28] A U.S. General Accounting Office study of New York City, Philadelphia, and Los Angeles found that although half of children entering foster care had at least one drug-abusing parent in 1986, this was true for more than 75 percent in 1991. During the same time, the proportion of newborns in foster care with prenatal drug exposure doubled from 29.5 percent to 62 percent.[29]

Six weeks after the Citizen's Commission's report, New Yorkers were shocked by the brutal rape of a young woman in Central Park by a group of teenagers. The attack was part of a nightlong rampage involving robberies and attacks—a "burst of random assaults" called *wilding*. Like an earlier case in 1984, when a frightened subway rider named Bernard Goetz shot four teenagers who tried to rob him, the attack stirred up New Yorkers' fear that the city was coming apart.[30] Journalists picked up on an idea being debated by scholars that there was an underclass in the nation's cities associated with these problems. Harkening back to nineteenth-century images of cities overrun by the "dangerous classes," a perception that had sparked local elites to support charities to reduce disorder,[31] the Central Park jogger case was another reminder of the need for an infusion of federal funds to fight AIDS and to deal with homelessness, crime, and drug addiction to ensure the city's fiscal health, growth, and stability.

As 1989 drew to a close, Kenneth Lipper, an investment banker and former deputy mayor, pointed out in the *New York Times Magazine* that New York was "sliding slowly into decline." Lifelong New Yorkers were thinking about leaving the city because their children were being mugged and harassed by drug dealers. Working-class neighborhoods had become "war zones" where police were hard pressed to intervene in drug dealing. Like *Bonfire of the Vanities*, a novel published in 1987, Lipper observed that even the upper class, whose apartment buildings were guarded by doormen and who could afford to avoid the city's dirty and dangerous subways, were not immune to this disorder and might also flee. This could further erode the city's tax base, where 180,000 households were paying half of the city's personal income tax and 1,000 of the city's 350,000 businesses were paying half of its business taxes. A tipping point might be reached where the city would lose its economic backbone. Indeed, 60 percent of New Yorkers polled in 1990 did not expect to be living there in five years.[32]

Although the sense of danger and disorder were pervasive, the "causal stories" on the epidemic's impact on the city concentrated on how hospitals were being affected.[33] The danger signs were not new. In 1985, Dr. Stephen Caiazza told a City Council hearing that "Hospital bed availability in New York is presently marginal. . . . It is now routine for me and my colleagues to wait days before finding a bed for a seriously ill patient."[34] Dr. Michael Lange, a physician at St. Luke's–Roosevelt, noted that "The whole system is falling apart."[35]

AIDS strained a hospital system already undergoing major changes. Foreign nurses were being recruited to deal with a nursing shortage.[36] Health care costs were skyrocketing, and cost containment strategies were being put in place. Between 1980 and 1985, eighteen hundred hospital beds in New York City were eliminated to reduce costs.[37] The payment methods for hospitals also changed. In the past, there had been a fee-for-service system, where hospitals billed insurance companies and were reimbursed for specific costs. This was replaced by a diagnostic-related-group (DRG) system where hospitals received a predetermined flat rate for each admission, based on the person's illness. This change was intended to discourage unnecessary tests and treatment, but it meant that hospitals could lose money on patients.[38]

Early estimates of the cost of treating AIDS patients documented that the disease was relatively expensive. These estimates, which may have overestimated the real costs, were used by politicians and hospital administrators to claim that AIDS had the potential of bankrupting the hospital system. Drawing on the findings of a CDC study that the average hospital costs for treating each AIDS patient was $147,000,[39] city officials pointed out that public hospitals were receiving $300 less per day than it cost to care for each AIDS patient.[40]

Public officials and health planners looked to San Francisco as a model of care. Early studies of AIDS care documented that San Francisco spent much less on each hospitalization ($27,571) than did Boston ($41,500) and New York ($55,700), because the average hospital stay was twelve days in San Francisco compared to twenty-one in New York.[41] This difference was attributed to San Francisco's integrated system of outpatient services, a "continuum of care" that included inpatient care in San Francisco General Hospital and an array of outpatient support services delivered by nonprofit organizations that relied on public funds and an "army" of volunteers.[42] Health planners began to realize that adopting the San Francisco model throughout the nation would reduce costs. New York State, the Robert Wood Johnson Foundation (in 1985), and the federal government (in 1986) provided funding and administrative support to adopt San Francisco's methods.

The AIDS Institute's CSPs and the designation of some voluntary hospitals as AIDS Centers were part of this strategy. AIDS Centers would receive higher reimbursement, and their case managers would coordinate inpatient and outpatient care. The goal was to get patients out of hospitals more quickly and "to increase access to essential services with emphasis on the use of home care and community based support services through individual patient case management and comprehensive discharge planning services . . . the AIDS Centers concept is based on a continuum of care model and designed to meet and/or arrange for all levels of care and needed services required by the AIDS patient."[43]

The AIDS Center policy was announced in late 1985, and ten voluntary hospitals in the city were enrolled as AIDS Centers by the spring of 1988.[44] Reducing the amount of time patients spent in hospitals by providing an integrated system of outpatient care was a formidable task in a disjointed and complex human-service delivery system.

New York City also received funds from the Robert Wood Johnson Foundation's AIDS Health Services Program, making the city one of eleven communities in the United States to receive these funds.[45] The foundation's legitimacy and strong links to government policymakers served as a wedge to begin obtaining federal funds to support AIDS services. In 1986, Congress voted $16 million for AIDS Service Demonstration Projects in four cities. By 1989, the effort expanded to twenty-five metropolitan areas and to nearly $50 million in funds.[46]

In New York, a combination of Robert Wood Johnson and federal funds (from the Health Services and Resources Administration, or HRSA, of the Department of Health and Human Services) went to Health Services Incorporated, a nonprofit fiscal conduit for the state's Department of Health.[47] Public agencies, including the New York City Human Resources Administration and the Department of Mental Health, Mental Retardation, and Alcoholism Services, also benefited from these funds.[48]

The effort to create a coordinated continuum of care was subverted by conflicts between various community-based organizations.[49] The idea of adapting the San Francisco model to New York was also difficult because the magnitude of the epidemic and the nature of the health care systems were quite different in the two cities. On any given day, there were ten times as many AIDS patients in New York City hospitals. While San Francisco General provided inpatient and outpatient care for half of that city's AIDS patients, no one hospital in New York had either the capacity or the desire to handle such a large share of the city's AIDS patients. Differences in the financial burden in 1986 were significant: the city of San Francisco spent $11.5 million of its own funds on AIDS while New York City spent between $42 million and $56 million. [50]

In retrospect, shorter patient stays in San Francisco occurred not only because of the system of care. They also resulted from significant differences between the kinds of people with HIV in the two cities. Only 1.2 percent of diagnosed AIDS cases in San Francisco through 1986 were drug users, compared to over 29 percent in New York.[51] And AIDS patients in San Francisco General Hospital may have had shorter hospital stays because a smaller proportion of them (31 percent) than of patients in New York (63 percent) were diagnosed with *Pneumocystis cariini* pneumonia, an illness that required relatively longer hospital stays.[52]

Hospital gridlock in New York City became more serious. In October 1987, thirty-four of the city's forty-six voluntary hospitals and all eleven public hospitals had 90 percent or more of their beds filled. People remained in emergency rooms for hours and sometimes days. Beds were put in hallways.[53] This situation was unprecedented and, by 1988, numerous observers were pointing out that the system was facing collapse.[54] In January, 1989, 950 people were in emergency rooms waiting for beds.[55] The problem was more serious in some hospitals than in others. In 1987 at Bellevue, the city's largest public hospital, more than 60 percent of AIDS patients who were ready for discharge were unable to leave because of a lack of housing.[56]

The problem of hospital gridlock was of greater magnitude in New York City, but it was occurring in a number of cities. Citizens, local leaders, and national policymakers began to realize that the triple epidemics of AIDS, homelessness, and drug use were affecting social institutions, especially hospitals, all over the country. It was becoming clear that, in contrast to the idea that everyone was at risk of AIDS, the epidemic was linked to an urban crisis that was most apparent in New York but evident in other cities, as globalization and deindustrialization "hollowed out" numerous urban centers.[57] Some social scientists saw many urban problems as associated with a growing underclass that was becoming more concentrated in certain neighborhoods.[58] Members of the underclass were isolated from mainstream values, had tenuous links to the job market, and lived lives where violence, drug use, crime victimization, and involvement with the criminal justice system were all too familiar.[59] AIDS had become another dimension of this pattern. The idea of an underclass dovetailed with a rightward turn in American politics and a shift away from the liberal policies of the sixties. Even though advocates for the homeless portrayed them as simply people who were victims of a housing shortage, it was becoming clear to these social scientists that a large number had an array of personal problems, including substance abuse and mental illness.[60]

The links among HIV, drug use, and disadvantage were especially apparent for women. Many women with HIV had been sexually abused as children and bore the scars of unhappy childhoods and of the drug abuse and drift of young adulthood.[61] Joyce Wallace estimated that many of the sex workers she served were enormously unhappy: 80 percent had children but only one in ten lived with any of them. Also, "Most of them [the women] lived in foster care or in homes where they weren't wanted or loved. Almost all the women admit to us that they were sexually abused as children."[62] Anitra Pivnick's study of methadone maintenance clients and of participants in a center for women with AIDS revealed that becoming HIV-positive was layered on top of earlier losses. Only 37 percent of the women she interviewed had lived continuously with all of their childrenm and 63 percent had at one point lost custody of at least one child for five months or more. Motherhood was important to them. Having a child was life-affirming since, in Pivnick's words, "children are perceived as their mother's lifesavers, the ones who can deliver them from uncontrolled drug use, prostitution, depression, poverty, homelessness, hopelessness, and death. A child can provide a constructive focus in a woman's life. . . . For HIV infected, drug-using women, the meanings represented in becoming a mother include compensation, regeneration, redemption, and the symbolic reclamation of losses accrued over a lifetime."[63]

A study of women in one HIV prevention program revealed that 68 percent of a sample of women with AIDS had a relative or close friend who had been killed, 47 percent had been the victim of a sexual assault, 51 percent had had a relative or close friend die of a drug overdose, and 19 percent had been in foster care or a group home.[64]

Some markers of being part of the underclass—teenage and single parenthood, lack of skills, and tenuous connections to the labor market—were more concentrated in some neighborhoods than in others. Two new strategies for dealing with these problems were emerging. Rather than replacing the slums, the policy of the 1950s and the 1960s, one strategy stressed neighborhood development and revitalization. Perhaps it was not poverty itself, but concentrated poverty in areas that lacked social and economic capital, that needed to be attacked. In another strategy change, social services were expanding and, according to observers like Lawrence Mead, social policy toward the poor was becoming more paternalistic: "Programs . . . help the needy but also require that they meet certain behavioral requirements, which the programs enforce through close supervision."[65] One dimension of this change was the reliance on case managers who coordinated access to services for PWAs; another was the emphasis on work as the nation moved toward a major transformation of its public assistance system in 1996.

In December 1989, Senator Edward Kennedy sponsored four days of hearings on the nation's health care system. Beginning in the Bronx, and moving to Los Angeles, the Senate Labor and Human Resources Committee also visited Maplewood, Missouri, and Sparta, Georgia. Kennedy pointed out that the hearings illustrated "the Nation's health care system is the fastest growing failing business in America." The hearings documented "a crisis in the delivery of essential health services more serious than at any time since the enactment of Medicare in 1965. And all of these critical problems are compounded by AIDS and drugs."[66] The epidemic was affecting some areas far more than others. Representative James Scheuer told a House Budget Committee hearing on "Hospitals in Crisis" that 20 percent of hospitals in the U.S. were treating 80 percent of all AIDS patients and 5 percent were treating half of them.[67]

There was growing momentum for some kind of "disaster relief." This approach, to target funds to areas hit hard by the epidemic, was an expansion of the program already being funded by HRSA, where support was directed to a handful of localities rather than to all cities. The problems linked to AIDS were found in numerous U.S. cities, not just in New York. Mayor Koch's claim in 1986, that the federal government had been indifferent to the epidemic because it mainly affected New York and San Francisco, was no longer true.

AIDS was perceived as a disaster in many large cities.[68] In fact, a *Washington Post* article pointed out in 1988 that many cities were looking "more and more like Calcutta." Between 1970 and 1990, the proportion of births in which the mother was unmarried more than doubled (from 11 percent to 28 percent) and the number of serious crimes rose from 8.1 million to 14.5 million.[69] An article in *The Nation*, "Thousands May Die in the Streets," pointed out that "New York City is the most extreme example of the emerging crisis, but the convergence of AIDS and homelessness is becoming increasingly evident around the country."[70] Substantial numbers of homeless shelter residents in Miami and Chicago tested HIV-positive. There were homeless people with AIDS and with tuberculosis in Richmond, Virginia, Dallas, Texas, and Birmingham, Alabama. Hospitals in Miami, Florida, and Fort Worth, Texas, were also experiencing strain.[71] The situation was so acute in public hospitals throughout the country that the National Association of Public Hospitals convened an emergency meeting, in March 1989, to discuss the issue. Patients in New York City emergency rooms were waiting up to three days for a bed. The waits were shorter but still distressing in other cities: eighteen hours in Los Angeles and twelve hours in Miami. One evening, five of the nine emergency rooms in Denver stopped accepting patients because all of their beds were filled.[72] Hospitals were not only caring for people who were ill, but becoming "catch-all neighborhood social-service agencies," serving as entry points to a human service system for people who did not know where else to go.[73]

Like the New Yorkers growing weary of panhandlers in the city's transportation terminals and subways, people in other cities were experiencing compassion fatigue and becoming insensitive and even negative about many social problems. The number of those who believed that people were homeless because of "circumstances beyond their control" decreased. People were less willing to give money to panhandlers, and begging was banned in the New York City subways.[74]

These concerns were amplified in an April 1990 report by the U.S. Conference of Mayors, "The Impact of AIDS Upon America's Cities." It discussed the best-known cities "hardest hit by AIDS," New York and San Francisco, but also Boston, Houston, Philadelphia, and Dallas. Homelessness, drug use, and AIDS had a huge impact on the nation's hospitals, the report noted, but it also pointed to the growing numbers of people who were uninsured. It called for federal funding because "local governments are increasingly unable to respond effectively to the health care needs of their citizenry."[75]

The epidemic began several months after President Ronald Reagan's inauguration. Reagan was committed to reducing federal spending and devolving power and responsibility to states and cities. The administration's logic was that, as the federal government did less, states and cities and the private sector would do more. The gay men in New York and in other cities who created organizations to care for the sick and the dying seemed proof that the voluntary sector could respond adequately. This conclusion had tragic implications for the AIDS epidemic and the nation's cities. By the mid-1980s, it was apparent that the voluntary sector was *not* adequate. In inner city neighborhoods, in particular, the mobilization of volunteers and the expansion of private funding was not taking place. AIDS organizations in inner city neighborhoods attracted relatively small numbers of volunteers, and the people they attracted were clients with limited job skills, histories of substance abuse, and low levels of self esteem.[76] Public funds were critical; city and state government funds were proving inadequate.

The cost of caring for people with AIDS began to rise sharply at the end of the 1980s. The President's Commission on the HIV Epidemic estimated that $380 million was spent for hospital care in 1985 and that medical care costs would rise to $8.1 billion in 1991.[77] The perception of AIDS as a crisis out of control was becoming widespread. Efforts to adopt the San Francisco model in New York City expanded services but did not resolve the problem.

In 1989, when AIDS services in the city cost nearly $700 million, news reports were describing a complex and disconnected system with numerous gaps and inconsistencies.[78] Nonprofits like GMHC were experiencing enormous strain. The agency was serving nearly three thousand clients in 1990, and the number of new clients requesting services each month was rising. GMHC realized that it would not be able to handle this growth and decided to limit the number of new clients it accepted. Its experience was not unique. The demand for services outstripped the capacity of many nonprofit AIDS organizations in the city.[79] A lack of funds also hampered city agencies like the Human Resources Administration. Its Division of AIDS Services, the entry point for receiving Welfare, Food Stamps, and Medicaid, was so overwhelmed that applicants waited for months and sometimes died before they received services, a situation that some traced to weak management, not merely limited funds.[80]

All these events suggested that federal funds were crucial. But an additional focusing event made the need for federal intervention even more critical—the fact that San Francisco's system of care was at the breaking point. In the summer of 1989, the Acting Executive Director of the San Francisco AIDS Foundation told a congressional hearing that the San Francisco model "is a marvelous model, and it is crumbling." A task force concluded, in early 1990, that "the San Francisco model is near collapse" from the burnout, "battle fatigue," and deaths of past volunteers, and an inadequate supply of new volunteers. (In fact, the actual reliance on volunteers may have been exaggerated since many needed services were always provided by paid staff.)[81] At this juncture, the National Commission on AIDS, a second national commission created in the summer of 1989, urged Congress to take action and provide disaster relief for AIDS services.[82]

In March 1990, Senators Edward Kennedy, a liberal from Massachusetts, and Orrin Hatch, a conservative from Utah introduced the Comprehensive AIDS Resource Emergency (CARE) Act. The Act had four titles, providing funds for cities with more than two thousand AIDS cases; to states, based partly on the number of diagnosed cases; for support for early intervention for people at risk or infected with HIV; and for women, children, and families.[83] As the bill moved through Congress, Kennedy pointed out that "There is a national crisis out there and without this, there is a very real chance the public health system in many parts of the country will collapse."[84] The idea of framing funding for AIDS as emergency or disaster relief dated back at least five years, to when Representative Ted Weiss of Manhattan wrote to his constituents, "when a community is damaged by a hurricane or flood, a wide range of Federal assistance is available. . . . I believe the same federal commitment should apply when a public health emergency such as encephalitis, legionnaire's disease, rabies, or acquired immune deficiency syndrome (AIDS) arises."[85]

The broad support, rapid passage and nearly unanimous vote for the Kennedy-Hatch bill, renamed the Ryan White CARE Act, can be traced to two factors. The first, discussed most often, was the growing political sophistication of the AIDS community and the support it garnered from the National Organizations Responding to AIDS, a temporary coalition of 125 organizations that was convened by the AIDS Action Council and included AIDS and gay organizations, professional organizations including the National Association of Social Workers and the American Medical Association, service providers like the American Red Cross, and groups like the National Parent-Teacher's Association and the National Council on La Raza. Some of these groups had already collaborated in lobbying for the Americans with Disabilities Act, which was passed earlier that summer. In addition to lobbying for the legislation, many of the participants in NORA, including the policy director of the AIDS Action Council, were involved in drafting the CARE Act.[86]

Less often discussed, but of perhaps greater importance, was the second factor, the fact that AIDS was part of a host of urban problems. Both the rhetoric—and the reality that AIDS was part of a national crisis accounts for the rapid growth in AIDS funding and the passage of the CARE Act. Designed to "provide emergency assistance to localities that are disproportionately affected by the Human Immunodeficiency Virus epidemic and to make direct financial assistance available to States to provide for the development, organization, coordination, and operation of more effective and cost efficient systems for the delivery of essential services," the Act authorized a major infusion of funds that would transform AIDS services nationally. A second bill, passed several months later, authorized funding to house PWAs. This measure was also designed to reduce hospital and institutional care.[87]

Even though the CARE Act was specifically focused on one disease, the testimony and debate focused on issues other than AIDS. Witness after witness, many of them high-profile personalities like film actors Elizabeth Taylor, a founder of AmFar, and Paul Michael Glazer, whose wife had AIDS, drew attention to the idea that the bill would save the nation's health care system from disaster.[88] Senator Kennedy noted that the crisis of health care institutions was "not the only cause of these problems. But it is adding to the stress that is leading toward a total breakdown of our health care system."[89] A content analysis of the debate found that the idea that "AIDS is spreading and must be contained" was only mentioned seven times. Much more common in the discourse were comments concerned that "AIDS is a crisis in cities and states," mentioned thirty-six times, or that "AIDS is creating a health care crisis," mentioned twenty-nine times. The discussion did not focus on the kinds of people most affected: gay men (mentioned fourteen times), and IDUs (mentioned nineteen times); many more comments were made about children, who comprised only 2 percent of the affected population but were mentioned in 41 percent of the comments.[90] Naming the bill for Ryan White, the hemophiliac who was subject to enormous discrimination and a source of shame for Americans, testified to the belief held by nine in ten Americans, "Regardless of who has AIDS, they deserve our compassion."[91]

The CARE Act provided cities and states with significant funds to expand services for people living with HIV. Fifteen cities received funds during the first year. The number of cities rose sharply, to 26 by 1995 and to 51 in 2001. Funding also increased rapidly, from $220 million in fiscal year 1991, a quarter of what was authorized in the original bill, to more than $2.0 billion in 2003. The funds were widely distributed in New York City, but some risk groups and neighborhoods were singled out for higher levels of assistance.[92] The CARE Act underwrote the cost of various services, especially medical care, for people living with HIV and AIDS (PLWHA). Some of the benefits provided under the Act's range of benefits—medical care, payment for prescriptions and dental care—were not available to other low income people or even, in the case of prescription coverage, for people of modest means.

This was only the second time in American history that a particular disease had been singled out in public policy. In 1972, Congress extended Medicare coverage to people with End-Stage Renal Disease (ESRD). This was the result of a long policy debate carried out sotto voce by medical professionals, elected officials, and a small but critical mass of advocates. The number of patients who originally benefited was small but the number of patients with ESRD, and the costs, have increased.[93]

The last word in the CARE Act's name, "emergency," is especially important. The Bush administration opposed the bill because, like the ESRD legislation, it had a "narrow, disease-specific approach."[94] Framing the bill as an emergency response is part of an important trend in contemporary social policy, since, according to political scientists Michael Lipsky and Steven Rathgeb Smith, issues like homelessness, hunger, runaway youth, and violence against women have also been framed in this way. While clearly a way to respond to an emerging problem, such a frame has other important implications including "temporarily deflecting attention from more deeply probing solutions, substantially surrendering control over admission to client rolls, and a degree of inequity in policy delivery."[95] Emergency legislation creates the sense that a policy is temporary, and, in the case of the CARE Act, meant that services and benefits were being given to a particular group rather than being offered universally. The CARE Act addressed two serious social problems: the growing numbers of Americans lacking health insurance, and the rising cost of prescription drugs. The Ryan White Act responded to these problems on a temporary basis, creating a mechanism so that states could finance care for people with HIV. Evaluations demonstrated that CARE Act funds were critical in providing access to medical care and prescription drugs by the kinds of people more and more affected by the epidemic—women, children, African Americans, and Latinos. Equally important in terms of its original objective, the funding contributed to a decline in hospital stays.[96]

The sense of social disorder was less salient at the end of the 1990s. Some neighborhoods, like parts of the South Bronx, which had had their housing supply reduced through arson and abandonment during the 1970s, were nearly rebuilt through a combination of federal, state, and private funds. Harlem, the best known black ghetto in the nation, became an empowerment zone attracting new merchants and new residents, beginning a process of gentrification.[97] Other neighborhoods, like Washington Heights, were stabilized and revitalized. The process of "saving cities" by saving neighborhoods involved a combination of policies spearheaded by foundations and by government, and implemented by nonprofit organizations and by the private sector—reducing crime, homelessness, and substance abuse, as well as welfare reform and reducing the concentration of an urban underclass viewed as central to these problems. Teen pregnancy rates declined, crime and drug use were down, the number of inmates in state prisons experienced a small decline, and the number of children in foster care began to decrease.[98] There was also a decline in "concentrated poverty." And the percentage of urban poor who lived in census tracts where more than 40 percent of the residents were poor declined from 17 percent in the 1980's to 12 percent in 2000.[99] The strategy that was used, public-private partnerships, or a "third way" between laissez faire capitalism and state socialism, envisioned a different role for the state, especially for the federal government. Indeed, funding from Washington to major cities like New York began to take a different form. More funds went to individuals, like housing vouchers and payments to landlords and service providers, rather than as grants to local governments.[100] Local governments played a key role in determining how funds were to be spent, a role they played under Title I of the Ryan White Act, HOPWA, and CDC funding where local planning councils determined priorities and distributed funds to the nonprofit organizations that were the major service providers.

The growing sense of disorder in the nation's cities clearly had an influence on AIDS policy. But, at the same time, the effective lobbying and activism of the AIDS community, and its alliances with a broad range of people who became concerned about the issue and drew attention to the epidemic, moved the issue higher up on the public agenda. Members of the AIDS community, once relative outsiders, came to the table to influence the direction of AIDS policy.

Part III

Saving Lives

Chapter 7

Our Place at the Table

This is not politics as usual.
This is our lives.

—David Rothenberg

I think we learned a lot about sort of finding our place. Instead of being the outsider and being hidden, we said "Take your place at the table. Come into society."

—Timothy Sweeney

The AIDS community was in fact becoming a force.[1] Federal funding for AIDS increased substantially by the end of the decade, and critics began to claim that AIDS was overfunded in contrast to other diseases, like cancer and heart disease, that affected larger numbers of people. This situation was attributed to the AIDS community's growing influence. A *Time* magazine article called "The AIDS Political Machine" pointed out that "By using Washington connections, media savvy, and even civil disobedience, the AIDS movement may have become the most effective disease lobby in the history of medicine."[2] The idea that the AIDS movement so dominated AIDS policymaking is not necessarily supported by recent scholarship on the impact of social movements and political organizations. Three literature reviews all concluded that, although political organizations—advocacy organizations, interest groups, and social movements—have an impact on social policy, the nature and the extent of their influence is unclear. There is a need to develop a better understanding of how political organizations, public opinion, and political opportunities individually and together influence public policy.[3]

This chapter considers the evolution and the structure of the AIDS community's political activities. It describes how a broad coalition of organizations and individual actors influenced HIV policies, and how people with AIDS fought for their lives in myriad ways. First gay men and then other people in the AIDS community raised money for scientific research, cared for the dying, taught the living to protect themselves, aggressively tried alternative medicine and new treatments, created organizations, and developed new ideas about services and prevention. Members of the AIDS community also challenged unresponsive economic, social, and political institutions by mounting litigation, appearing at public hearings, doing policy research, lobbying, and protesting.

Some people were outsiders and demonstrated in the streets; others were insiders and took their place at metaphorical tables in various centers of corporate, government, and nonprofit power. Members of the AIDS community were keenly aware of these distinctions and of the benefits of combining these methods: insider strategies like citizen advocacy, persuasion, public information, and lobbying; and outsider methods like political protest, civil disobedience, and strident and sometimes offensive political rhetoric.[4] Reflecting back on the impact of the AIDS community in 1997, Tim Sweeney pointed out that it "utilized an arsenal of tactics to foster change—we pushed the media, we lobbied the legislators, and we rallied in the streets."[5]

Often, insiders and outsiders—activists and advocates—were the same people playing varied roles either sequentially or simultaneously. Traditional categories used to understand organizations and policy development—activists, advocates, volunteers, staff, and bureaucrats—were not salient. Activists moved into positions in government; government employees and scientific researchers were also advocates and activists using their positions and their legitimacy to press for policies. Government officials and scientists were important allies serving as institutional activists. Some activists became government officials, and government officials and scientists were simultaneously activists using their scientific findings to reinforce the interests of the AIDS community. Many outsiders were, in fact, employed by AIDS organizations and combined being insiders and outsiders. John Moore, a researcher at New York University, pointed out, "It's possible for scientists to be activists, possible for activists to be scientists." Nilsa Gutierrez, the medical director of the New York AIDS Institute, pointed out at a New York State AIDS Institute conference in 1993 that "We are civil servants and we are activists."[6] To categorize people then as either activists and advocates, or bureaucrats, politicians, or members of a social movement (or as insiders or outsiders), greatly oversimplifies the nature of the AIDS community, as does the image of an AIDS political machine.

The gay communities that were first affected by the epidemic are a post–World War II phenomenon; they had become more visible after the Stonewall riot in 1969, when a police raid on a gay bar in Greenwich Village sparked off a two-day riot that marked the beginning of the gay liberation movement. After Stonewall, gay communities began to develop institutions such as local newspapers, community centers, health centers, and political, lobbying, and advocacy groups. A national magazine, the *Advocate*, served as an important communication link among local communities. There were also several national organizations, including two particularly important groups, the National Gay Task Force and the Lambda Legal Defense Fund, located in New York.

In contrast to San Francisco, where the gay community mobilized quickly and was visible and politically vocal, the gay movement was fairly weak in New York.[7] Gay political and service organizations had relatively few members, modest budgets, and few full-time staff. The National Gay Task Force, founded in 1973, had ten thousand members and a fifty-thousand-dollar budget in 1983.[8] The Lambda Legal Defense Fund, also founded in 1973, had a staff of four and a yearly budget of approximately two hundred thousand dollars during the first several years of the epidemic. There were only two lobbyists representing the gay community in Washington in 1982, and the number of openly gay elected officials could be counted on less than one hand.[9]

AIDS mobilized gay men who had been unconcerned about gay politics, and revitalized some veteran activists who, according to Cindy Patton, had become "burned out, discouraged, cynical."[10] The dense and interlocking social networks in New York's gay community were a natural locus for mobilization. By the time the epidemic passed its first anniversary, some observers thought that they had "never seen the gay community so together on anything."[11] GMHC's founders had not been involved in gay political activity before AIDS. Even Larry Kramer, who became an activist, wrote in GMHC's second newsletter that "There is one thing we must not allow AIDS to become, and that is a political issue among ourselves. It's not. It's a health issue for us."[12] GMHC volunteers were originally more concerned about funding medical research and helping friends and lovers than with influencing the political process, because of the enormous antipathy between many gay men and the state. There was a preference for autonomous organizations, since government meant arrests, raids on gay bars, and intrusions into men's lives. AIDS changed that.

Many of the early AIDS cases, at least those known to the founders of GMHC, were "clones," which was "a lifestyle that was prevalent in New York, [with a] hypermasculine look" that rejected "the prevailing cultural definition of homosexuals as failed men" and whose adherents' social lives involved "cruising, tricking, and partying." Marty Levine, who studied this scene, believed that GMHC's founders were "Essentially . . . a cohort of men who, while they benefited from gay liberation, never participated in gay liberation. . . . These gay men were in many ways the A-crowd in the clone scene within the gay community. And they perceived themselves and were perceived within that world as an elite."[13]

People's lives were transformed because of the epidemic, and previously uninvolved people became politicized. Many people changed jobs and even changed careers to fight AIDS full-time. Mel Rosen, GMHC's first executive director, left a large social service agency and began volunteering for GMHC because, "When I saw those men in the hospital, the same men I had seen walking down Christopher Street, the same men I had seen in the discos, it was 'there but for the grace of God'—it could have been me lying in that hospital bed."[14] Paul Popham, GMHC's first president, was originally unwilling to have himself be publicly identified, and admitted that he found gay politics "distasteful." The deaths of his friends, combined with discrimination and the fact that "nobody cared," led him to conclude that "silence was a luxury I couldn't afford."[15] As the organization evolved, GMHC attracted several politically active members, like Leonard Bloom, a former deputy health commissioner, who joined the board in 1983 and headed its government relations committee.[16]

AIDS had a paradoxical impact on gay political organizations, diverting energy from other issues, like civil rights, but also attracting money and members in response to a combination of AIDS backlash, discrimination, and increased violence. Ron Najman, of the National Gay Task Force, pointed out that "Every time the Rev. Jerry Falwell opens his mouth, more people come out of the closet."[17] The National Gay Task Force's budget rose to $700,000 in 1987, and donations to the Human Rights Campaign Fund's doubled between 1984 and 1986, when it reached $1.5 million.[18] The most vivid evidence of the growing willingness of gay men and women to come out of the closet and publicly support the gay movement was the October 1987 March on Washington. In contrast to an earlier march in 1979, which attracted between 25,000 and 100,000 people, the 1987 march drew between 200,000 (National Park Service estimate) and 500,000 people. Between 1983 and 1986, gay organizations and AIDS organizations began to take their place at the table, meeting with elected officials and government bureaucrats.[19] Jeff Levi, the executive director of the National Gay and Lesbian Task Force, pointed out in 1986 that "AIDS has totally transformed the way the gay political movement does business. Three years ago, the kind of access and influence we have now would have been unthinkable."[20]

The development of AIDS advocacy organizations in New York City dates back to July 1982, when a small group called the AIDS Network began meeting every week. In addition to recognizing the need to coordinate activities, the group was a response to the possibility that gay men and Haitians might be told not to donate blood. This was the first of a number of privacy and civil liberties issues that were an enormous threat to the gay community. The AIDS Network included representatives from GMHC, people who had been involved in the gay health movement, and veterans of gay and lesbian politics—like Dr. Hal Kooden, a psychologist influential in ending the American Psychological Association's designation of homosexuality as a disease. Virginia Apuzzo became the group's leader. Apuzzo believed that the proposed procedure, where gay men would voluntarily refrain from donating blood, was problematic. Many people donated blood at work, and Apuzzo was concerned that if a person did not volunteer to donate blood, this might be interpreted to mean that he was gay or had AIDS, which could result in stigmatization and discrimination. The Red Cross was beginning to discourage gay men, Haitian immigrants, and other people in high-risk groups from donating blood. The National Hemophilia Foundation, representing a group infected through the pooling of blood in the manufacture of a clotting factor, called for "Serious efforts . . . to exclude donors that might transmit AIDS," including "identification by direct questioning of individuals who belong to groups at high risk of AIDS."[21]

The AIDS Network expanded to include representatives from the New York Blood Center, Gay Men with AIDS, and the St. Mark's Clinic.[22] It became both the voice of, and a clearinghouse for, the city's AIDS community.[23] Apuzzo, the newly appointed executive director of the National Gay Task Force, had an insider's view of government and a willingness to work within the political system to demand a response. Tim Sweeney recalled that she "understood government and politics better than anybody that I saw in the early days of HIV and AIDS."[24] In spring 1983, she and a number of community activists had two meetings with editors of the *New York Times* to persuade them to expand coverage of the lesbian and gay community and of AIDS.[25]

In early March 1983, the AIDS Network sent a letter to Mayor Edward Koch requesting a meeting and offering several recommendations.[26] On March 9, Koch announced the formation of an Office of Gay and Lesbian Health Concerns in the New York City Department of Health and appointed an AIDS Network member, Roger Enlow, as director.[27] In late April, Koch, Enlow, the health commissioner, and the head of the Human Resources Administration met with ten representatives of the AIDS Network. Koch agreed to some of the points this meeting raised, declaring a "state of concern" about AIDS and affirming a commitment to press for federal funding for research, but, according to the *Native*, he did not agree to issues that would involve significant funding, like housing or donating a city-owned building for AIDS organizations.[28]

AIDS organizations began to promote citizen advocacy and strategies to promote awareness. In 1983, the AIDS Network and GMHC were both distributing preprinted postcards to mail to public officials.[29] Individual artists used their work to call attention to the epidemic and, in the late 1980s, Art Against AIDS developed a yearly "Day without Art" on December 1, World AIDS Day, shrouding statues and covering up works of art produced by people who had died of AIDS to demonstrate the extent of loss.[30] The AIDS quilt, which consisted of thousands of standard-size pieces, each the size of a grave, put a face on the epidemic, emphasizing the distinctive qualities of each person who had died. The quilt was already the size of two football fields when it was displayed in Washington, D.C., during the 1987 March on Washington.[31] The quilt's creator recognized its political impact when he called his biography *Stitching a Revolution*.[32] The best known icon of the epidemic was the red ribbon, invented in 1991. Worn by millions of people, including celebrities on nationally broadcast programs like the Oscars and the Emmys, the ribbon was featured on a postal stamp issued at the end of 1993.[33]

Citizen advocacy—marching, letter writing, wearing a red ribbon, and participating in events to increase public awareness—complemented behind-the-scenes meeting and lobbying. This work was, as I have noted, sometimes reinforced by institutional advocates working within the system. Active and intense lobbying was critical in the establishment of the State AIDS Institute. GMHC and the New York State Lesbian and Gay Lobby coordinated the efforts of several local gay groups and lobbied key legislators to establish and to press for continued funding for the AIDS Institute despite Governor Cuomo's opposition.

In spring 1983, the federal Social Security Administration determined that people with AIDS were eligible for disability benefits.[34] This was the result of a joint effort by GMHC, the National Gay Task Force, and the chief of staff for U.S. Representative Ted Weiss from Manhattan.[35] That August, officials in the Department of Health and Human Services (HHS) announced that they would request $40 million for AIDS research in 1984, $22.1 million more than originally planned. This decision followed meetings between representatives of the AIDS community and federal officials, and Congressional testimony by Apuzzo and Callen at a hearing on the weak federal response to the epidemic. The first such meeting was held at the White House, an important symbolic gesture. At a second meeting, between HHS officials and representatives from the NGTF, GMHC, and the San Francisco KS Foundation, Apuzzo asserted the necessity of "adding resources to rhetoric."[36]

Efforts were made to coordinate and to increase national AIDS advocacy, with the founding of the Federation of AIDS-Related Organizations (FARO) at the 1983 Gay Health Conference, the conference where the Denver Principles were developed. FARO would be a "single voice" for the AIDS community, speaking on behalf of its thirty-eight founding member organizations. Although all but one of these were gay groups, FARO was intended to broaden organizational support since it was an AIDS organization, rather than a gay organization.[37] FARO hired a lobbyist with extensive experience in health policy, who pointed out, "We cast it as a public health issue to give it the broadest appeal. . . . I'm not running away from the fact that this is a gay issue. . . . But I have to make the cross-section to the rest of the health lobby in town."[38] GMHC donated forty thousand dollars to FARO in 1983, but the group still foundered because of limited financial support.[39] A successor group, the AIDS Action Council, was established in 1986. AIDS Action, in turn, convened a broader coalition to operate as an issue network. This group, the National Organization Responding to AIDS (NORA), played a prominent role in numerous policies, including designing and lobbying on behalf of the CARE Act. NORA included 150 groups, only 4 of them gay organizations. The creation of NORA was consistent with a major trend in interest group politics in the United States, where coalitions focused on an issue, rather than individual organizations, have become critical in policymaking.[40]

Joint advocacy on the city and state levels began in 1986, when fifty organizations, including the PWA Coalition, the Gay and Lesbian Independent Democrats, the Hispanic AIDS Forum, and the Minority Task Force, advocated for an increase in funding for AIDS education. GMHC began to develop a more permanent coalition to influence funding priorities, convening the Committee on AIDS Funding (CAF). The CAF became autonomous, but GMHC provided staffing until it became part of the statewide New York AIDS Coalition (NYAC) in 1988. With its own staff and start-up funding from five foundations, NYAC is the major local AIDS advocacy organization in 2005.[41]

GMHC was an active participant and financial supporter of these coalitions. Within the first several years of its existence, GMHC became a hybrid organization, combining services to clients with political advocacy. GMHC itself developed policy recommendations, used insider tactics, and promoted citizen advocacy. Reminding readers of the *Native* that "Pressure Works," GMHC announced plans in mid-1984 to "step up its lobbying efforts" since "We have to fight harder than ever because we are still fighting for our lives."[42] GMHC formed alliances with gay organizations and other AIDS organizations, and temporary alliances with groups like the American Civil Liberties Union and the disability rights movement. The existence of independent coalitions that GMHC supported, like NYAC and AIDS Action, also meant that GMHC did not always need to act.

With the appointment of Tim Sweeney as the deputy director for policy in 1986, GMHC began to develop its own public policy department and professionalized its advocacy work. It hired a lobbying firm in Albany in 1987, testified to various commissions, task forces, and working groups, and met with legislators and public officials.[43] When New York City's health commissioner proposed mandatory name reporting of people with HIV in 1989, GMHC sent out an "action alert" that resulted in eight hundred calls or letters, and the proposal was dropped. During that year, GMHC and other local organizations defeated "over two dozen pieces of regressive AIDS legislation."[44] GMHC's ombudsman's office and its legal services department challenged AIDS discrimination. The number of complaints against health care providers rose dramatically from 485 in 1985–1986 to 1,240 two years later.[45] GMHC collaborated with the Lambda Legal Defense Fund on lawsuits, such as fighting the eviction of Dr. Joseph Sonnabend from his office, and launched a successful lawsuit challenging the federal ban on funding for AIDS prevention material that promoted homosexual activity.[46]

Two days after GMHC's successful circus benefit at Madison Square Garden, candlelight marches were held in New York, San Francisco, Houston, and Chicago. The May 1 march in New York involved between six thousand and nine thousand people, who walked from Sheridan Square in the heart of the city's gay community to the federal building. This was the beginning of visible public advocacy by the AIDS community. The march had several objectives: it mourned the dead, raised public awareness, called for more federal funding, and urged the Social Security Administration to designate AIDS a disability. The march, which preceded the Denver Conference, led many to realize that they were part of a community. Roger Enlow noted, "For the longest time I thought I was alone, but now I know I'm not."[47]

This was the first large public display of concern in the city, but it was not the first demonstration. Several weeks before, less than twenty people, including Larry Kramer, demonstrated at a conference on AIDS at Lenox Hill Hospital.[48] For the next several years, demonstrations and marches were relatively infrequent. There were other candlelight vigils, commemorations of people who had died of AIDS at the annual Gay Pride parades, a march in Washington (to request funding) that attracted fifteen hundred people in October 1983, and a "peaceful demonstration" organized by Rapid AIDS Mobilization during 1985 Gay Pride week (at which about two hundred people gathered at the Federal Building in Manhattan to display "anger and disgust at the lack of government action on AIDS").[49]

As the death toll mounted and signs of indifference and a conservative backlash increased, there was a growing sense that insider methods were inadequate. One critic noted that "The time for candlelight vigils mourning the deaths of our lovers and friends is over . . . it's time to wipe away the tears, clear our throats, and strike back at those who scapegoat, propose quarantine, and try to disenfranchise us. It's time to stop asking for help, and instead *demand* it, to make public health officials accountable for inaction and improper action."[50]

Negative media coverage of the bathhouse issue sparked the concerns of the eight gay activists who met to establish an organization, modeled on the Anti-Defamation League, to "monitor how homosexuals were portrayed, in the press and by the government." Six hundred people came to the first meeting of the Gay and Lesbian Alliance against Discrimination (GLAAD) in November 1985. Film critic Vito Russo, a former officer of the Gay Activists Alliance, told the crowd, "The AIDS epidemic is being used by right-wing fanatics and yellow journalists to create a witch-hunt mentality against lesbians and gays in this city."[51] Five days later, GLAAD mounted its first demonstration, outside a two-day City Council hearing on whether to close the bathhouses (approved) and on whether to bar teachers, students, and staff "who are victims or carriers of the AIDS virus" (not approved). About one hundred demonstrators carried signs proclaiming "1935—Juden Verboten, 1985—Homosexuals Verboten." David Summers, a member of the PWA Coalition, allegedly pushed and punched a policeman after unsuccessfully trying to enter the hearing room; Summers was the first person arrested at an AIDS demonstration in the city.[52] A second demonstration, at the *New York Post*, protested that the paper "whips up hysteria and defames us in a manner that no self-respecting community should have to bear."[53]

The following June, GLAAD organized a major demonstration in response to the Supreme Court decision to uphold Georgia's sodomy law in the Bowers v. Hardwick case. This was an enormous setback to the cause of gay rights. Despite GLAAD's efforts to keep the demonstration peaceful, some participants channeled their frustration and anger, stopping traffic for five-and-a-half hours. A subsequent demonstration, on July 4, attracted 1,200 people according to the police, between 3,000 and 6,000 people according to the organizers.[54] At about the same time, the Coalition for the AIDS Housing Crisis, a group concerned about the problem of homelessness, held a candlelight vigil in front of Gracie Mansion and demonstrated outside a fundraising dinner that Mayor Koch was attending.

Soon afterward, a group of GLAAD members formed the Lavender Hill Mob to concentrate on outsider tactics while GLAAD used an insider strategy.[55] GLAAD met with editors and writers at the *New York Times* to increase coverage of gay and lesbian issues, and, along with GMHC, persuaded William Buckley to withdraw his recommendation to tattoo everyone infected with "the AIDS virus."[56] The Lavender Hill Mob included former members of the Gay Activists Alliance (GAA); they employed a protest strategy used by the GAA called a "zap." This was a way that a small number of demonstrators could gain attention and have an impact; participants would gain access to an event, often by "dressing and acting the part of usual participants," and directly confront a person, target, or audience at an appropriate moment.[57] Boston's *Gay Community News* reported that the Mob had a "vocal role . . . using "costumes, leaflets, testimony, and disruption" to disrupt a CDC Conference on HIV Antibody Testing. Mob members called the conference "a hoax and a cover-up for government inaction," and labeled the CDC a "Center for Detention Camps . . . under the control of Mormons and bigoted right-wing conservatives"; two members dressed themselves as gay inmates in Nazi concentration camps, with pink triangles, and they heckled the CDC official who spoke at the closing session. In a workshop on confidentiality, one Mob member disrupted the discussion, noting "Don't tell me it's not possible to be rounded up. You did it with the Japanese in World War II and you will do it again as you want to."[58]

After the conference ended, a Mob member disrupted a news briefing with representatives of the Lambda Legal Defense Fund and the National Gay Task Force, proclaiming "You're completely out of touch with our anger, with what the gay community really wants. What you're doing today is just perpetuating this farce."[59]

Much of the rhetoric, the methods, and the emotions that fueled the work of the Mob—the Holocaust metaphor, the actions, the zaps, and the anger were carried over to ACT UP, founded one month after the CDC conference.

On 10 March 1987, Larry Kramer was a last-minute substitute lecturer at the Lesbian and Gay Community Center. Kramer had left GMHC after not being selected as one of the group's representatives at the AIDS Network's meeting with the mayor. Kramer began his speech by reminding the audience that it had been almost four years since the publication of his article "1,112 and Counting" in the *New York Native,* an article that exhorted gay men to change their sexual behavior and for the gay community to wake up and face the reality of the epidemic. Telling the audience that "We have not even begun to live through the true horror," he told the people in the room to stand up and told them:

> At the rate we are going . . . two thirds of this room could be dead in less than five years. . . . If what you're hearing doesn't rouse you to anger, fury, rage, and action, gay men will have no future here on earth. How long does it take before you get angry and fight back? . . .
>
> Did you notice what got the most attention at the recent CDC conference in Atlanta? It was a bunch called the Lavender Hill Mob. They got more attention than anything else at that meeting. They protested. They yelled and screamed and demanded and were blissfully rude to all those arrogant epidemiologists who are running our lives. . . .
>
> We can no longer afford to operate in separate and individual cocoons. . . . Every one of us here is capable of doing something. . . . We have to go after the FDA—fast. That means coordinated protests, pickets, arrests.[60]

During the discussion period, he singled out GMHC's Tim Sweeney and asked him, "What are you going to do about this, Mr. Sweeney? You're the great person . . . I had such hopes for you."[61] The *Native* reported that "An abundance of anger and frustration was vented, primarily at the American government for its lack of commitment to ending the life-threatening situation."[62] Kramer's earlier call for direct action, at the conference at Lenox Hill in 1983, had a small turnout. Four years later, the political climate was radically different—there was also a greater promise of government responsiveness—and emotions in the gay community had shifted.

Just as the founders of the PWA Coalition reframed AIDS as an illness that one could live with, the people who joined ACT UP responded to changes in the nature of the disease. With the introduction and greater use of the HIV test and the availability of AZT and other treatments that prolonged people's lives, people were living longer.[63] Keeping people alive meant that they might live long enough for a cure. In 1987, this did not seem impossibly far away. The optimism about the capabilities of medicine were enormous. The approval of new drugs also hinted at something else: AZT was not a newly discovered drug but had literally been sitting on a shelf with no clear use since the 1960s.[64] AZT's approval provided hope, and generated frustration. In a classic example of relative deprivation, where the promise of a cure heightened the sense of desperation since the drug's appearance made it seem a cure was closer, the

AIDS community moved to another level of mobilization, building upon the sporadic direct action tactics of the Mob and other ad hoc groups.

Two nights after Kramer's lecture, 350 people came to the first meeting of a group that became the AIDS Coalition to Unleash Power, or ACT UP."[65] Sweeney cofacilitated the first few meetings, until the group's natural leadership emerged. GMHC supported Sweeney's involvement and gave the group its first five thousand dollars.[66] ACT UP's major focus was to hasten a cure for AIDS by having promising drugs released rapidly, but the members also had other concerns. The new organization developed a set of operating principles that gave it a number of unique qualities. ACT UP's stationery pointing out "No more business as usual!" had two meanings—the organization's intention to influence the public agenda, and its own operation. Meetings were open, and people were eligible to vote after coming to two meetings. It was a highly participatory and totally democratic "collectivist organization" with no elected leadership and, initially, no paid staff.[67] The only structure consisted of co-facilitators who ran meetings, an unpaid elected officer who took care of routine matters, and workgroups, affinity groups, and committees that focused on specific issues. The bulk of the work was done by committees and affinity groups, including media, outreach, prison issues, treatment and data, and women's issues. As the agenda broadened, the number of subgroups expanded. Gilbert Elbaz, who did an ethnographic study of the group, described it as "a confluence of different social movements" whose members brought organizational skills from other organizations.[68]

ACT UP's first demonstration, a Wall Street sit-in on March 24, was organized under the banner of the AIDS Network, since the new group was still unnamed. Media attention was carefully orchestrated. The day before, an Op Ed article by Larry Kramer in the *New York Times* explained that "the FDA constitutes the single most incomprehensible bottleneck in American bureaucratic history—one that is actually prolonging this roll call of death."[69] A flyer proclaiming "No More Business as Usual!" outlined a series of demands: approval of several promising drugs, "massive public education," prohibiting discrimination, and the "immediate establishment of a coordinated, comprehensive, and compassionate national policy on AIDS" since "nobody is in charge."[70] The demonstration attracted six hundred people; nineteen were arrested for blocking traffic after they lay down on the street. The demonstration featured an effigy of FDA director Dr. Frank Young, and demonstrators chanted "Ronald Reagan, your son is gay! Put him in charge of the FDA." About the choice of the target and the rhetoric, Kramer pointed out that "our complaint isn't really with the stock market. We want the media."[71] The demonstration was successful: the evening news on the three major networks covered the story; a photograph appeared in the *New York Times*; and the next day's Donohue show featured footage of the demonstration.[72]

Attendance at ACT UP–New York's Monday night meetings rose quickly, and the group moved to a much larger space, Cooper Union's Great Hall. The meetings were described as joyous. One reporter recalled that there was "much laughter, spontaneous bursts of changing, and kissing. And weeping: when friends died, no one gave a thought to keeping a stiff upper lip."[73] There was a palpable sense of shared anger channeled toward the common goal of ending the epidemic. The meetings also offered the chance for new friendships and sexual liaisons. In the midst of ongoing deaths and the impending deaths of many members, meetings were a place to affirm life. Participation was goal oriented but also identity creating and identity affirming, an example of what sociologists call a "new social movement," an organization with a middle-class membership concerned with identity politics.[74]

Although some people went to socialize and the meetings were sometimes fun, the topics reflected the epidemic's complexity and utter seriousness. For the first several months, the demonstrations primarily focused on issues related to access to treatment and the need for a cure. ACT UP–New York's agenda expanded and the movement became national. The day after the 1987 March on Washington, two hundred AIDS activists met to plan a week of protest. The meeting was organized by ACT UP–New York and nine other groups, including the Minority AIDS Task Force, Citizens for Medical Justice, Mothers of People with AIDS, and the Lavender Hill Mob. The meeting led to the formation of ACT NOW (AIDS Coalition to Network, Organize, and Win) which adopted a nine-point AIDS Action Pledge calling for "massive" funding, a comprehensive AIDS education program, centrally coordinated AIDS research, public accountability, a "fully funded national Health care program," and "A worldwide, culturally sensitive funding program." The coalition opposed quarantine, mandatory testing, discrimination, and funding reductions. By spring 1988, more than three hundred organizations were part of ACT NOW and the group mounted nine days of protest. Each day focused on a specific issue, such as women, prisoners, people of color, substance abuse, homophobia, health care, the global impact of AIDS, and new treatments.[75]

ACT UP's rapid growth represented the channeling of powerful emotions that had been building for several years—anger and disappointment, yet hope that a cure would be identified. Vito Russo, the film critic who was also a founding member of ACT UP, described the group's formation as spontaneous combustion fueled by "The explosion of people's pent-up frustrations about AIDS, their anger, their [outrage] that their friends were dying." One member of the AIDS community told a reporter that he was "getting tired of candlelight vigils when, in fact, blow torches may be necessary."[76]

By the late 1980s, more people in the AIDS community were turning their desire for empowerment and control into public expressions of anger.[77] In the early years of the epidemic, some gay men expressed their desperation by committing suicide. The suicide rate declined with the introduction of promising treatments and recognition of the positive benefits of empowerment.[78] Although there is no scientific evidence that the decline in suicide was associated with the rise in anger, it is clear that anger rather than despair became a dominant emotion in the AIDS community.

Anger was widespread; perhaps, as Douglas Crimp pointed out, it was "the one emotion it seems OK to feel."[79] When fifty-three gay men in New York who had been diagnosed with AIDS for at least three years were interviewed in 1990, the researchers concluded that, considering that this "group of polite cooperative men who complied with a lengthy interview not designed for their benefit, who were willing to talk to strangers about personal matters in a study they had not volunteered to be in . . . it was the more remarkable to discover that three-quarters of the men felt very angry, most of them a great deal of the time."[80] Nearly two-thirds of the members of a direct action group interviewed in San Francisco in 1990 indicated that their major motivation was "To channel the anger I feel at this disease and the response of the government to it." In contrast, volunteers in an AIDS service organization did not express the same degree of anger.[81]

Anger was viewed as life sustaining.[82] An early GMHC volunteer pointed out in 1986 that "most of the very politically active, angry people with AIDS in New York are still alive."[83] Rather than mourn the deaths of friends, lovers, and family members, some AIDS activists, like ACT UP's Peter Staley, believed that "If you stop to spend a lot of time on mourning, you'll lose the war. We prefer to skip the mourning stage and go straight to anger."[84] Public expressions of anger were directed toward politicians, the government, scientists, drug companies, and "anyone who we think isn't doing everything they can."[85]

Death imagery pervaded many of the group's actions and its culture, especially the idea that people with AIDS were being 'murdered.' At a 1988 rally, Vito Russo proclaimed, "If I'm dying of anything it's from homophobia. If I'm dying from anything it's from racism. If I'm dying from anything it's from red tape. . . . If I'm dying from anything I'm dying from Ronald Reagan. If I'm dying from anything I'm dying from the sensationalism of newspapers and magazines and television shows which are interested in me as a human interest story as long as I'm willing to be a helpless victim but not if I'm fighting for my life."[86]

By the end of its first year, ACT UP–New York had mounted twenty-seven actions—one every two weeks.[87] The choice of targets and strategies illustrated how clever the group could be. They were comic, dramatic, and outrageous, and combined civil disobedience with street theater. ACT UP's second demonstration took place at the city's main post office, on Eighth Avenue and 34th Street, on April 15, the deadline for mailing tax payments.[88] On 1 June 1987, ACT UP–New York and groups from other cities demonstrated outside the White House during the International AIDS Conference. Michael Callen reported that the arrestees had filled out their bail forms before they were arrested. Apuzzo, Sweeney, and sixty other people were arrested. The police were wearing yellow rubber gloves, which made some demonstrators angry but many chanted, "Your gloves don't match your shoes. You'll see it on the news."[89]

The day after an October 1987 march, ACT UP groups from all over the nation formed ACT NOW, the AIDS Coalition to Network, Organize, and Win, to coordinate demonstrations. Major demonstrations targeted power centers that were blocking the development of a cure or charging exorbitant amounts for promising treatments; the demonstrations took place at: Wall Street; the FDA in Rockville, Maryland; the National Institutes of Health, where in 1990 twenty-one demonstrators occupied the office of the Director of AIDS Research; and at the manufacturer of AZT, Burroughs-Wellcome, where demonstrators infiltrated its North Carolina headquarters in 1989.[90] New York City and New York State governments were also targeted. Between twenty-five hundred and three thousand demonstrators surrounded City Hall and blocked traffic in lower Manhattan to demand more funding and services.[91]

Some of the demonstrations were zaps and others were campy. The tactics people used "often flaunted their 'gayness' as a shock tactic"[92] When the U.S. Commission on Civil Rights held a hearing on whether or not AIDS was a disability, ACT UP demonstrated outside while members inside "donned clown masks at various points during the hearing."[93] To draw attention to the impact of AIDS on women, a large group went to a baseball game at Shea Stadium in May 1988. As the huge screen flashed "Women and AIDS Day," members unfurled banners saying "Men Wear Condoms" and "AIDS Kills Women."[94] Protesting Burroughs-Wellcome's refusal to lower the price of AZT, five ACT UP members infiltrated the New York Stock exchange by using fake ID's from

brokerage firms and chained themselves onto a platform overlooking the trading floor. When the bell rang to start the day's trading, the protesters unfurled
a banner that read, "SELL WELLCOME."[95]

Not all actions and protests were dramatic or even campy, and some
included a mixture of insider and outsider strategies. When members of the
AIDS community protested the membership of the President's Commission on
the HIV Epidemic, ACT UP members met with members of the commission
along with several other groups and chartered two buses to give testimony.[96] In
May 1990, ACT UP mounted a boycott of Philip Morris to protest corporate
contributions to Senator Jesse Helms, who blocked funding for AIDS education. The boycott ended nine months later when the company announced that
it would double its contributions to AIDS research and education. Unwittingly,
ACT UP created an opportunity for the company to use corporate philanthropy
to gain good will and attract gay and lesbian customers.[97] During the Gulf War,
demonstrations over twenty-four hours during a "Day of Desperation" included disrupting three major news programs, marches in downtown Manhattan, Harlem, and the Bronx, and closing down Grand Central Station during
rush hour, carrying signs that proclaimed, "Money for AIDS, not for War."[98]

ACT UP carefully orchestrated media coverage and public attention, drawing on the expertise of Robert Rafsky, who left his job at a high-profile public
relations firm to volunteer for ACT UP on a full-time basis. David Barr, an ACT
UP member who worked in GMHC's policy department, pointed out that
"What distinguishes us from earlier protest movements is our ability to transform what we do into media events. Many of us are in graphic design, public
relations, and media, but instead of selling soap, we're selling ACT UP." Journalist Michaelangelo Signorile, stated, "We manipulate the media the same
way the government does."[99] Members chronicled the group's history with
video activism, forming a media collective called "Testing the Limits" in 1987
and, later, DIVA TV (Damned Interfering Video Activists).[100] In 1990, stickers
with ACT UP's symbol, the words SILENCE=DEATH on a black background
beneath a pink triangle, were "ubiquitous reminders on cash machines, news-
stands, tollbooth buckets, and pay phones."[101] This logo benefited ACT UP in
another way: the sale of stickers, t-shirts, and sweatshirts generated one-third
of ACT UP's 1990 income.[102]

Some demonstrations combined protest, mourning, and powerful death
imagery. Demonstrators wore cardboard tombstones. ACT UP mounted political funerals featuring actual corpses in caskets. At one political funeral, a dead
member's ashes were thrown over the White House fence.[103] Political funerals
enabled participants "to express grief and carry out the wishes of the dead and

those closest to them, . . . to enable them to recognize these deaths in the way they thought was morally necessary."[104] According to rhetorician Kevin DeLuca, the die-in combined with interrupting a Mass conveyed that group members were "using their gay and lesbian bodies to intervene in a public policy debate," which had the effect of increasing a sense of urgency, personalizing AIDS discourse, and giving a face to statistics.[105]

Powerful emotions—a fear of dying, mourning, anger, and the sense of being outsiders—led to increasingly outrageous tactics. Staley told a reporter in 1988 that "We're all very angry, and every year that goes by, we're going to up the ante." One leader explained: "If ACT UP doesn't keep screaming it, no one will hear."[106] Increasingly, the targets were not only power centers but individuals.

ACT UP members put stickers on vending machines all over the city that noted, "GINA KOLATA OF THE *NEW YORK TIMES* IS THE WORST AIDS REPORTER IN AMERICA." Protestors demonstrated outside the official residences of the mayor and the governor, and at the summer home of U.S. President Bush. After estimates of the numbers infected with HIV were cut in half, ACT UP targeted the city's health commissioner, Stephen Joseph, occupying his office and calling for his resignation. Members intruded on his personal life—picketing outside his house, calling him up in the middle of the night with threats, and throwing paint on his house—when he called for contact tracing for those who were infected.[107]

Targeting individuals included allusions that they had the power of life and death. Gina Kolata was criticized because she wrote an article noting that clinical trials were having difficulty recruiting volunteers because people could obtain the same drugs through a preliminary drug release called the parallel track. One member saw Kolata as having an almost magical quality, announcing "That woman is killing me." When Bill Clinton was running for president in 1992, Tom Duane, an HIV-positive city council member, pointed out, "I don't think I have a chance to live if he doesn't get elected." Larry Kramer told people attending an AIDS Institute–sponsored conference in 1993, most of whom were staff in community-based organizations, that they were "desk killers," likening them to office workers in Nazi concentration camps.[108]

A demonstration at St. Patrick's Cathedral in December 1989 marked a major turning point in the group's history. ACT UP's tactics began to alienate people inside and outside the AIDS community. This was not the first demonstration at the cathedral; Dignity, an organization of gay Catholics, protested there once a month during most of 1987.[109] The ACT UP demonstration was cosponsored with the Women's Health Action Mobilization (WHAM), a reproductive rights group. It took place during Advent, a reflective time when many Christians await the anniversary of Jesus's birth. There were protests outside the cathedral, and protestors disrupted a Mass, threw condoms in the air, and carried signs referring to Cardinal O'Conner as Cardinal O'Condom and declaring "Keep your rosaries off my ovaries." Perhaps the most shocking aspect was that one demonstrator allegedly desecrated a host.

Criticism of the demonstration came from many quarters, including ACT UP members. *Time* magazine described the event as a "sacreligious scene." An editorial in *The Economist* pointed out that the demonstration "harmed the cause it sought to promote." A bystander told a reporter that the action was "sickening" and "shows what bad judgment and weak character they have. Disrupting a religious service is simply not an acceptable way to disagree." Another observer described the demonstration as carnival-like, stating "They're making a party out of this, like they're having fun. How can anybody take them seriously?"[110] Larry Guttenberg, a board member of the PWA Coalition and an active member of the Atheist AIDS Ministry, pointed out that "We, the diagnosed, have a say on our movement's public image. . . . As a PWA, an atheist, and a civil libertarian, I share the rage of the protesters at St. Patrick's Cathedral. . . . The issue is bigger, however. . . . [T]he act did provide the mass media with a focal point away from the issues."[111]

The Saint Patrick's Cathedral demonstration underscored the group's inability and lack of desire to exercise discipline over the behavior of its members. Staley called the demonstration an "utter failure" and a "selfish, macho thing."[112] Democracy combined with unbridled anger meant that, even though some actions were carefully planned, "at many others, people simply show up and act naughtily. This lack of control is an aspect that makes some feel liberated, others frightened; any single member's actions can and will be attributed to the group. This is one reason many of the original founders, frustrated and burned out, are no longer active members."[113] Efforts to create some structure, like electing an administrative committee to make some decisions, were unsuccessful.[114]

Actions at several international AIDS conferences also illustrate the group's crossover from camp to irreverence, and from raising issues and fostering dialogue to creating what Stephen Joseph called "brownshirt tactics."[115] ACT UP members first demonstrated at the 1987 Conference, and they interrupted numerous sessions at the 1989 Conference, including Joseph's opening address, in which he announced support for contact tracing of the partners of people who tested HIV-positive. After the speech ended, the audience gave Joseph a standing ovation. Reporter Randy Shilts commented that ACT UP members were "so obnoxious. . . . The protesters' message was overshadowed by their tactics."[116] The following year, in San Francisco, members of the AIDS community attended the conference as protesters and as participants. Larry Kramer had called for riots at the conference, and some groups, like GMHC, boycotted the meeting to protest U.S. immigration policies requiring HIV testing.[117] Despite efforts to include the group in the program—Peter Staley gave a major address and there were a number of papers describing the organization and its goals—ACT UP members routinely disrupted the proceedings. They shouted down Secretary of Health and Human Services Louis Sullivan at the closing session and showered him with paper missiles. A *Los Angeles Times* headline asked, "Did AIDS Protest Go Too Far?" David Kirp, a professor at Berkeley, added, "[I]t was undoubtedly an act of personal integrity and authenticity, and I am sure that it made them feel better. But sometimes, personal authenticity and political effectiveness are incompatible." Kirp noted that had ACT UP members listened to Sullivan's speech, they would have hear him say, "We must learn to listen to each other, to learn from each other and to work together. Our frustration must never drive us to close our ears or our hearts."[118]

By the middle of 1990, there were fundamental divisions within ACT UP and the organization began a slow decline. As many as fifty-four cities in the United States and ten abroad had chapters at ACT UP's height, in 1991. In 1997, there were thirteen chapters.[119] ACT UP–New York met at Cooper Union for a year, then returned to its original space in the Lesbian and Gay Community Services Center; meetings attracted 500–600 people in 1990, but this figure decreased to an estimated 250 in 1993 and 50 in 1997.[120]

ACT UP's decline, both locally and nationally, can be traced to a number of factors. First was the combination of lack of a cure, continued deaths, and the inability to sustain the level of anger or to keep the organization focused on important issues. Key members were dying and others became too sick to participate. Many people had the same motives as Vito Russo, that "One of the reasons I helped start ACT UP is I didn't want to die," but the actions and even the progress did not stop the dying. Although it propelled action, anger had a corrosive impact. John Weir pointed this out after the death of writer and ACT UP member David Feinberg: "Anger is the orthodoxy of the self-proclaimed AIDS activist community. . . . Anger is seen as wholly reliable because it is so intensely felt. The fundamental sentimentality of it is the belief that emotions always tell the truth. . . . Like David, I thought that if I got angry enough, he would not have to die. I was wrong and so was he."[121]

The political opportunity structure had also changed. Some of the activists' demands—for faster drug release and expanded funding to care for people with AIDS—were met, and the government had become more responsive and more willing to work with members of the AIDS community. As some observers noted, the in-your-face politics of ACT UP had become less newsworthy. The extreme statements of AIDS activists became more hollow as the state responded. Larry Kramer noted in 1993 that "Just 20 people and an open coffin outside the White House is no longer a big enough show."[122] For writer Andrew Sullivan, the rhetoric itself was self-limiting since "Once you debate the currency of language, how do you have somebody take you seriously? Can everyone be evil all the time? Is everyone a Nazi?"[123]

Reporter Donna Minkowitz concluded that ACT UP was "struggling to contain its political divisions" in 1990. There were forty committees and working groups in 1990, and some discussions focused on broad social issues unrelated to AIDS. There were seven administrative committees and thirty committees, working groups, and caucuses in 1995.[124] ACT UP's agenda began to become too unfocused for some members, who left to form other groups. An informal survey of former ACT UP leaders in 1990 indicated that this was the most common reason most of them had left.[125] Many were interested in concentrating on treatment issues. For them, the urgency was enormous since they wanted to save their lives and get "drugs into bodies." Larry Guttenberg, the PWA Coalition president, stated "Beware! Some among the ranks of AIDS activists are invariably HIV negative." Although, he agreed, these were noble causes, "AIDS organizations must prioritize the pandemic. Our compromised immune system can't compromise our focal point."[126]

For others, the AIDS agenda was too narrow. They thought that ACT UP ought to be addressing structural issues like racism, sexism, and homophobia. They had a different perspective: "It's not about getting drugs into bodies, it's about the people whose bodies those drugs are going into."[127] The increasingly broad agenda combined with a lack of structure also reduced the group's ability to be task oriented, and made the meetings more difficult to attend. Minkowitz pointed out: "An ACT UP meeting is . . . daunting—both in the topics covered and the group dynamic. Audience members often illustrate points with an AA-style confessional or rephrase what's already been said. . . . As much cruising goes on as real work; meetings are rife with sexual puns and joking. . . . Frequently the meetings wallow in virulent disagreement over side issues. Is ACT UP co-opted by being granted a seat on a government panel? Must every piece of literature be translated into Spanish?"

———

ACT UP's lack of racial diversity reduced its legitimacy. Members were overwhelmingly gay white males, and the group had an overtly gay organizational culture. A survey done by Gilbert Elbaz in 1989 found that about 80 percent of ACT UP–New York's members were men, 91 percent were lesbian, gay, or bisexual, and 78 percent were white.[128] The criticism that ACT UP was not receptive to people of color surfaced early and, despite the large number of members concerned with broad social issues like racism, sexism, and homophobia, many African Americans and Latinos found the group hard to penetrate. Greg Broyles, a staff member at the Black Leadership Commission on AIDS, pointed out, "We wanted to be more involved and it is being met with some resistance."[129]

The tensions between blacks and gays, and between the insiders and the outsiders, surfaced around the appointment of Woodrow Myers as New York City's commissioner of health in 1990. Soon after Mayor Dinkins announced the appointment, ACT UP member Gabriel Rotello's magazine, *Outweek,* published an article documenting that Myers had supported mandatory name reporting and contact tracing, used quarantine when he was the health commissioner of Indiana, and supported the closure of gay bathhouses, bookstores, and bars. The AIDS community split along racial lines. Both Myers and Dinkins were African Americans, and several influential African Americans continued to support Myers. GMHC and Tim Sweeney were caught in the middle. ACT UP vilified Sweeney, who had been on the selection committee. The afternoon before GMHC's executive director, Jeffrey Braff, attended an ACT UP meeting to defend Sweeney, he received an anonymous phone call warning him that his safety could not be guaranteed if he showed up at the meeting.[130]

Another contentious incident between ACT UP and minorities working as insiders involved the accusation by ACT UP's Latino Caucus that the Hispanic AIDS Forum, especially its executive director Miguelina Maldanado, failed to provide leadership and make "an effective programmatic commitment to the struggle against AIDS in the Latino community." The Latino Caucus criticized HAF's location in a business area, not a Latino neighborhood, and the fact that none of HAF's board members were publicly identified as being HIV-positive. The group printed dollar bills with Maldonado's picture on one side and "In HAF We Trust" on the other, as well as "Wanted Posters" accusing her of "Criminal Negligence, False Representation, & the Misuse of Public Funds."[131] HAF's board responded in a long and thoughtful letter that indicated that their board was diverse and that "We believe that sexual orientation and HIV status are private, personal matters. . . . The Board does not and will not, in the foreseeable future, require that candidates for membership, or present members, make such personal facts about themselves known."[132] When Yolanda Serrano, ADAPT's executive director and a HAF board member, went to an ACT UP meeting to try to clarify the situation, she was booed, hissed, and called a liar.[133]

This situation created conflict between ACT UP and other organizations. The executive directors of several other AIDS organizations circulated a letter supporting Maldonado, which noted that "We all value the need for public dialogue. . . . We are, however, deeply upset by the vicious and dehumanizing nature of the personal attacks against one of our colleagues." Rod Sorge apologized to Yolanda Serrano, with whom he was working on the issue of syringe exchange (chapter 9), and said "I know that other members of ACT UP are equally upset about what happened. . . . Although I'm sure your relationship with ACT UP will now be very different from the way it was in the past, I hope you and I can continue working together."[134]

ACT UP's irreverence toward the Catholic church also overlooked the sensibilities of African American and Latino communities, who, despite differences and disagreements, had enormous respect for religious institutions. Journalist Chris Norwood, the founder of Healthforce, a Bronx organization serving women with HIV, observed that "By desecrating an institution important to multitudes of high-risk persons in New York, ACT UP violated the rule that AIDS prevention is supposed to be culturally sensitive. This largely white male group seems also to have no idea how appalling an attack on any church would appear to the black community—within which churches are deeply honored. No act could have made the whole difficult subject of AIDS seem more alien and threatening to those communities now at highest risk than the spectacle of phalanxes of white males invading a church."[135] Jim Eigo, an ACT UP member, also recognized the impact of this event, noting "If you force a twenty-year-old Hispanic woman to choose between the Church, which has been her only consolation in life, and ACT UP, she's going to choose the Church. We may have alienated a young Latino woman who needs us more than she knows."[136]

As more and more people living with AIDS came from communities of color, ACT UP lost its legitimacy as the voice of the AIDS community. When Staley interrupted Stephen Joseph at the 1989 International AIDS Conference, Joseph questioned Staley's ability to speak for people with AIDS, saying, "I don't know who 'we' is, my friend. Because the person who is infected in New York City today is quite different from you."[137]

The demonstrations and the rhetoric also diluted the group's legitimacy because they alienated some of the institutional activists who supported the

AIDS community. Continuing to call these insiders enemies and saying they had "blood on their hands" began to backfire. A striking contrast was ACT UP's relationship with staff in the New York State AIDS Institute, the sponsors of the conference where Kramer announced that AIDS organization staff members were "desk killers" and where several sessions on the agenda focused on AIDS activism including the current status of ACT UP. When ACT UP members visited AIDS Institute Director Nick Rango on his deathbed, they told him about their plans to "disrupt his annual state AIDS conference. . . . [A]s always when we let him in on our secret plans, he told us who we should target and exactly how he thought we should go about it."[138] Demonstrations and lobbying were not only orchestrated by activists, but sometimes guided by state officials. When funds were cut during one round of state budget negotiations, activists took over the State Bureau of the Budget and got assistance from AIDS Institute staff, who "were aware of who we were meeting with and when we were meeting with them. And as they became aware of obstacles, they informed us about the obstacles or really who the obstacles were . . . and if we didn't get anywhere with them lobbying, then we had a big demonstration."[139]

In 1990, ACT UP–San Francisco split into two chapters, one pursuing a broad agenda and another focusing on treatment issues.[140] New York's chapter splintered into many groups, rather than splitting in two. Members created new organizations that focused on specific issues. In that respect, ACT UP had an additional important role, since it mobilized, and served as a training ground for, people who started other organizations, including some hybrid groups that combined insider and outsider tactics.

One affinity group became Queer Nation in 1990, an organization that, like ACT UP, existed in other major cities, including Boston and Chicago. Its members believed that ACT UP had lost its strong ties to gay liberation.[141] The group had a relatively brief existence in the early 1990s, when its members "flaunted their sexual identity" at "kiss-ins" at heterosexual bars and demonstrations outside the homes of gay bashers, and "outed" homosexuals who were in the closet.[142] At about the same time, another group in New York, the Pink Panthers, began to patrol Greenwich Village to reduce antigay violence.[143]

The HIV Law Project, founded in 1989, evolved from the Women's Caucus, which started in 1988 as a result of a highly inaccurate article about women and AIDS in *Cosmopolitan* magazine. Its members picketed the magazine, sponsored teach-ins, published a book, and pressured the federal government to sponsor a national conference on women and HIV in December 1990.[144] Demonstrations combined with litigation led to a change in the CDC's surveillance definition of AIDS, so that women could be eligible for disability benefits.[145] The women's caucus also had an impact on a second issue, the routine exclusion of premenopausal women from clinical trials.

ACT UP members also founded Housing Works in 1990. Filling the need for housing for PWAs was one of ACT UP's early demands, mentioned in its first flyer and at a demonstration at the Trump Tower, a luxury apartment building, in 1988.[146] Housing Works was established when several ACT UP members realized that "no one was going to house them unless we did."[147] It also provided services and housing to an underserved group, homeless people—including active drug users. The agency grew rapidly, and by 1995, it was the second largest AIDS service provider in the city. It combined, and as of this writing still combines, insider and outsider strategies, and advocacy and services challenging the quality of services provided by the city.

Like GMHC, Housing Works combined advocacy and services, but it took far riskier political positions than GMHC. When New York Mayor Giuliani announced in 1994 that he would recommend the abolition of the city's Division of AIDS Services (DAS), Housing Works took the lead in a series of protests, including a march across the Brooklyn Bridge that shut down the bridge and stopped traffic. Housing Works engaged in personal attacks, plastering posters with photographs of city officials that called them murderers and criminals.[148] After the issue was resolved, with the New York City Council passing legislation to assure continuation of the agency, Housing Works filed a series of successful class action lawsuits that required the city to provide appropriate housing and services for PWAs and that led to a court-ordered monitoring of the city's Division of AIDS Services and Income Support.[149] Episodes of contention between the city and Housing Works continued under Mayors Giuliani and Bloomberg. The city canceled Housing Works' contracts because of alleged misuse of funds, but, in response to a lawsuit, a judge ordered the city to allow the agency to bid for contracts. It also successfully overturned Giuliani's decision to ban demonstrations from the steps of City Hall. Housing Works has continued to carry the torch of direct street activism in New York, mobilizing hundreds of its clients for its marches—achieving something ACT UP was never able to accomplish, the mobilization of large numbers of people of color.[150]

One secession, the 1992 departure of some members of ACT UP's Treatment and Data Committee (see chapter 8), was especially significant. The departure of these treatment activists challenged ACT UP's expertise on precisely the issue that accounted for the long-term commitment of its members and the focus of many of its demonstrations: finding a cure.[151]

Chapter 8

Finding a Cure

It takes nine years to get a new
drug approved by the FDA. We've
got two years to live.

—Thomas Hannan

We can't approve something that
isn't there.

—Dr. Frank E. Young

As the epidemic neared the end of its first decade, reporters and scientists were pointing out that the AIDS community had radically changed the rules for testing and approving new treatments.[1] A *Washington Post* reporter observed that "AIDS patients and their relentless advocates have in less than three years transformed the way experimental drugs are tested in the U.S."[2] Robert Wachter, who coordinated the 1990 International AIDS Conference, noted in the *New England Journal of Medicine* that "the entry of AIDS activists into the health care scene has added jarring new dimension to what was previously a genteel dialogue between patient advocates and clinicians, researchers, and policy makers."[3] These claims illustrate the conventional wisdom that the AIDS community mobilized and scientists and the government acceded to their wishes. Yet, the reality is far more complex. It took much longer than three or four years for these changes to occur, and, though the AIDS community was an important catalyst, it hastened a process already underway.

This chapter traces the culture and the evolution of AIDS treatment advocacy, describing the development of four interconnected and mutually reinforcing activities: buyers' clubs, community-based research, street-based activism, and treatment advocacy. The AIDS community accelerated interest in an issue already on the public agenda, the "drug lag," and directed attention to a second issue, the high cost of drugs, that has become even more prominent since the epidemic began. Although journalistic accounts stress the central role of ACT UP, a broad range of influences was at work, including insiders, outsiders, and two types of allies: government scientists and drug companies. In addition to street activism and political protest, the culture of the AIDS community led it to exercise another type of power: its ideas about "fighting" for one's own life promoted noncompliance and the prospect of destabilizing the system of testing and distributing new drugs. The organized advocacy and the informal collective action of the AIDS community, combined with the influence of drug companies and government officials, led to radical changes in the system of testing and releasing new drugs.

The AIDS epidemic started at a time when it seemed as if modern medicine had unlimited capabilities. According to historian Bert Hansen, enormous faith in the capacity of medicine to find cures for most diseases dates back to the first modern medical "miracle," Pasteur's discovery of a vaccine for rabies in 1885.[4] Infectious diseases could be cured by antibiotics. Medical procedures and drug therapies that were recently experimental had become routine: cortisone, coronary bypasses, and kidney dialysis. Surgeons were performing operations that would have recently defied the imagination: microsurgery, organ transplants, artificial joints, and procedures like bypass surgery were routine. Given the realities of the power of modern medicine, and a tendency to overlook its limits, people in the AIDS community found it hard to believe that doctors were baffled by AIDS, that people were dying, and that a cure did not exist. In a speech to the U.S. Conference of Local Health Officials in 1982, Assistant Secretary for Health Edwin Brandt pointed out: "The first factor alarming the public about AIDS is medicine's inability to understand it or to protect people against it. People have written and telephoned to ask if it is really true—that we do not know what this disease is. The public's confidence in American biomedical science is extremely high. It is so high that most people simply have a hard time understanding that we just do not know very much about some immediate things."[5] Early patients, their friends, family, and doctors found the rapid and unexplained deaths surprising and frightening. Participants in the AIDS community expected scientists and physicians to find a cure quickly. They were shocked and alarmed that this was not the case, and many began to believe that this was because not enough was being done.

Even without much funding, there were rapid and enormous advances in the basic understanding of the disease, and researchers forwarded some important findings.[6] Journalist and GMHC founder Nathan Fain noted in 1982 that, "If the gravity of this fear cannot be overstated by its victims, the outbreak is balanced by a gathering excitement in medicine. Dozens of researchers in several branches of health have begun to blaze new paths in the hope of answering not only the immediate questions but even more significant ones, such as what causes cancer? . . . [S]everal doctors are mindful of the glory that awaits the hero of the moment, the Jonas Salk of cancer."[7]

Doctors tried existing medications and treatments. Some were benign; others were toxic. In spring 1983, doctors were experimenting with bone marrow transplants, gamma globulin, and plasmapheresis, removing impurities from a person's blood.[8] With guarded optimism, articles in the *Native* in 1983 and 1984 reported that "Incipient AIDS May Be Reversible" and "Possible Cure Found for AIDS Patient."[9] There was remarkable progress despite limited funds. Research operated on a shoestring, and funds were allocated from other projects to study AIDS. The $5.5 million earmarked for 1982 was much less than for other health emergencies, Legionnaires Disease and a Swine Flu epidemic that never took place.[10]

AIDS advocates recognized that federal funding for AIDS research was critical. The federal government had been the major source of funds for scientific and medical research since the end of World War II. Even the polio vaccine, which collective memory attributes to the March of Dimes, relied heavily on support from the National Institutes of Health.[11] The AIDS community also expected that major scientific advances would occur in the United States, as the world's center for biomedical research, since, according to David Dickson, "Almost half of the Western world's research and development is carried out in the United States, which . . . spends more money on science than Japan and the industrialized nations of Europe combined."[12] Even before the AIDS community began to lobby for funds, federal support was increasing. By July 1983, when 1,600 cases had been diagnosed, AIDS funding was greater than the total spent for Legionnaire's Disease and toxic shock syndrome.[13] Many scientists began to study AIDS: the First International AIDS Conference in 1985 attracted 2,100 people.[14]

People in the AIDS community tried to prolong their lives by pursuing alternative treatments and improving their outlook (chapter 2). But they put most faith in mainstream treatments. There was reason for optimism. By the mid-1980s, some promising treatments were in the approval stages and it was possible to gain access by traveling abroad, to countries where the drug approval process was less stringent. News about these possibilities spread quickly, and people from a number of countries, including Rock Hudson and perhaps one hundred other Americans, traveled to Paris to try HPA-23 and three other experimental drugs.[15] French scientists were especially optimistic about

HPA-23; one patient treated for a year and a half seemed to have had the virus disappear, if only temporarily.[16]

Since the cost of traveling abroad was prohibitive for most people, members of the AIDS community developed an underground distribution system, importing drugs to the United States. The AIDS underground started in 1984, when several gay men in California started to purchase ribavarin and isoprinosine in Mexico for themselves and for friends and acquaintances. One, Martin Delaney, founded Project Inform in San Francisco in the fall of 1985, the first organization in the United States to provide treatment education and advocate for faster drug testing. The AIDS underground was centered in Los Angeles and New York. FDA officials and customs agents overlooked this smuggling as they had in the past when cancer patients imported laetrile, and only intervened when drugs were toxic.[17] By 1987, the AIDS underground was operating in forty cities.[18] With the enormous growth of the underground, the FDA announced that people could import a three-month supply of drugs for one's own use in person or through the mail, a policy that, it should be noted, already existed.[19]

The AIDS underground also included guerilla laboratories producing unapproved medications.[20] A handful of men in New York became interested in AL721, which was already in the pipeline for FDA approval. It seemed especially promising because Robert Gallo, the codiscoverer of HIV, wrote about it favorably in a letter to the *New England Journal of Medicine*.[21]

Interest piqued when one PWA, Michael May, experienced remarkable improvement after a trip to Israel, where the substance had been developed. May traveled to the airport in a wheelchair when he left, and said his final goodbyes to family and friends, but walked off the plane when he returned three months later. The following year, he reported, "I have no more physical symptoms. The infections have gone; the night sweats have stopped; I have no more fevers. I am able to eat again, and my weight is back to normal."[22]

Two PWAs, Stephen Roach and Tom Hannan, began to explore ways to increase access to AL721. They encouraged the U.S. patent holder to release it as a food, since FDA approval requirements were less stringent for foods than for drugs, but the potential profits would be lower. After an unpleasant and hazardous effort to produce their own AL721, they located a company able to manufacture it and, with Michael Callen, formed the PWA Health Group to distribute it. The first batch involved two hundred kilos distributed to one hundred buyers in May 1987.[23] Considering recent ACT UP demonstrations, they expected to make the distribution a media event involving arrests and closure. But there was no response from public officials.[24]

The PWA Health Group met an enormous need: it distributed unapproved substances and it increased access to approved medications by importing them from abroad and selling them at lower cost than did pharmacies. This was also true for underground clinics that sold pirated versions of AZT from Korea for one quarter of the cost in the United States.[25] Buyers' clubs were an alternate route to obtain new treatment for people who did not fit the criteria for clinical trials. In 1993, the Health Group was selling nineteen substances.[26]

Buyers' clubs empowered PWAs, giving them access to potentially lifesaving treatments on the premise that "PWAs and their physicians have the right to make their own treatment decisions. . . . [I]n its simplest terms: if a substance cannot hurt and may help, the PWA Health Group believes every PWA (or anyone else) should have the opportunity to acquire it."[27] At the same time, there was an important political dimension. PWA Health Group members were told that "every time you buy something here at the PWA Health Group, you're performing a political act. Throughout the history of the AIDS crisis in the United States, people with HIV/AIDS have refused to accept the limited wisdom of our government, the medical profession, and the drug companies. We question, we argue, we confront, and, through all of this, we make individual, empowered treatment decisions that are right for us."[28]

Buyers' clubs operated in a grey area. They were legal because they were agents for people who were purchasing drugs for their own use.[29] For the first several years, Federal and state agencies monitored the buyers' clubs to make sure that that they were not selling dangerous or fraudulent drugs.[30] Postal agents and customs inspectors allowed the groups to mail and to import drugs not on the FDA's list of toxic medications. The buyers' clubs were viewed as credible because they were not profiting from their sales and, according to one FDA official, "There are doctors involved in many of them."[31]

As the AIDS underground expanded, with buyers' clubs importing a larger number of drugs, the FDA reexamined its policies. One FDA official stated in 1991 that initially the clubs "distributed things like vitamins, minerals and nutritional supplements at little or no cost . . . [but] in the last few months, we have heard reports of them dealing in other types of products, clearly drugs. They seem to be getting into large-scale importation, and possibly commercialization. We need to evaluate whether these things are occurring and whether they are in violation of the law."[32]

The issue came to a head when buyers' clubs began selling pirated versions of ddC while the drug was undergoing clinical trials. There was enormous demand for the drug because many people were unable to tolerate AZT and access to ddC through clinical trials was limited to people diagnosed with

AIDS. In addition, a study released during the summer of 1991 indicated the positive benefits of combining AZT and ddC. People participating in clinical trials were not officially permitted to combine the drugs.[33] In the fall of 1991, as many as ten thousand people were buying ddC from the underground.[34] The FDA began to inspect buyers' clubs more closely to determine if they were profiteering from the sale of the drugs or were making "unrealistic promotional claims." Visits to three buyers' clubs in early 1992 led to the discovery that the drugs they were selling had significant potency problems. An FDA official announced that "underground ddC is produced under poor manufacturing conditions and that the overall safety and purity of underground ddC is suspect."[35] The FDA "strongly urged" the clubs to "cease the sale or distribution of underground ddC and to notify their clientele of FDA's findings." The buyers' clubs complied with this request, and the PWA Health Group informed its buyers that the ddC it had been selling varied from 64 percent to 188 percent of its "declared value."[36] A month later, ddC's manufacturer announced that it would distribute the drug free "in response to the needs of the AIDS community."[37]

FDA surveillance continued, and in 1993 the FDA sent a letter to a dozen buyers' clubs indicating that it would continue to closely monitor them because of a lack of involvement by physicians and the sale of "unproven and potentially dangerous products." They were also told that they were not to be involved in "excessive promotion or commercialization of their products that could constitute health fraud."[38] The PWA Health Group continued to provide medications and challenge the status quo by selling unapproved treatments like thalidomide and importing nitazoxanide (NTZ), which was seized by U.S. customs agents.[39] After a dozen years, the PWA Health Group closed its doors, in April 2000. A second New York–based buyers' club, the Direct Access Alternative Information Resources (DAAIR), which opened in 1991, closed down in 2003. In 2005, a handful of buyers' clubs remained. The underground and the buyers' clubs were critical when treatment options were limited. With the identification of the cause of AIDS in spring 1984, researchers began to actively pursue a magic bullet, and PWAs began to think more seriously about clinical trials as a treatment option.

Drug companies responded slowly to a disease not viewed as an emergency or a large source of profit. National Cancer Institute (NCI) researcher Samuel Broder contacted drug companies asking them to send him promising compounds because his laboratory was equipped to handle the virus.[40] By the mid-1980s, Broder's lab was testing products from fifty companies and laboratories, including Compound S, or AZT.[41] While some accounts suggest that AZT was randomly selected, simply taken off the shelf since the company had nothing to lose, other versions point out that a Burroughs-Wellcome researcher, Jane Rideout, began studying AZT in the early 1980s. After the cause of AIDS was identified in 1984, she realized AZT was a good candidate because its structure was similar to the kinds of chemicals that retroviruses needed to reproduce. Early tests with mouse and cat retroviruses supported her claim.[42]

After Broder discovered, in 1985, that AZT stopped the virus from multiplying in a test tube, tests on 19 patients with AIDS or ARC had startling results. During the first six weeks of the trial, immune function improved in fifteen; they gained weight and their cell cultures showed no evidence of the virus.[43] In February 1986, 282 people were enrolled in a classic clinical trial at twelve medical centers, in a double blind experiment where half received the medication and half were given a placebo. The early results were so remarkable that the experiment ended after six months and the control group too was offered AZT. Only one person receiving AZT had died, compared to 19 people in the placebo group. One year after beginning treatment, the mortality rate of those who originally received AZT was 10.3 percent. In contrast, the mortality rate of the original placebo group nine months after the study began was 39.3 percent.[44]

By the time the results of this study were announced, the demand for AZT was increasing. The federal government was under enormous pressure to find a cure. In the fall of 1986, Burroughs-Wellcome expanded access to AZT and the drug was already the standard treatment for AIDS. Patients could receive the drug at no cost if they had been diagnosed with PCP, a condition affecting two thirds of all people with AIDS.[45] Despite the fact that the drug had significant side effects and was not a cure, optimism was so great that future AZT trials would not involve placebos.[46] The urgency of finding effective treatments was so powerful that AZT was approved in record time; an advisory panel recommended approval in January and the FDA approved the drug in March 1987. The lone dissenter on the FDA advisory panel felt that the approval might later be regretted since the side effects were substantial. Approval did not preclude future testing, but this was not required.[47]

Federal funding for AIDS research increased dramatically while AZT was being tested. The fact that Americans like Rock Hudson needed to go abroad for treatment underscored the inadequacies of the American research effort and the slowness of FDA testing. In July 1986, one year after Rock Hudson's AIDS diagnosis became public, three thousand PWAs were enrolled in clinical trials, nearly one-third of the country's twelve thousand cases.[48] Thirty new drugs were under development and six new drugs were being tested.[49] Federal funding for AIDS research continued to increase and AIDS treatment units were established to test new medications.[50]

The expansion of clinical trials combined with the underground, increased treatment options enabling PWAs to gain a sense of control. Acording to medical ethicist George Annas, "human experimentation has been transformed from a suspect activity into a presumptively beneficial activity."[51] Unapproved medications were viewed as promising cures, not risky treatments. As a scientist, Mathilde Krim gave this viewpoint legitimacy. She asked, in 1986, "Do we have the right to refuse a dying person a small measure of hope or the dignity to fight to the end . . . even a few extra months of life are very meaningful for those with a short time to live."[52] She expressed a common view in the AIDS community, that "Placebo-controlled trials in patients with full-blown AIDS are . . . morally unacceptable" as well as "inhumane and unethical [because] many patients don't have the time to wait until all the answers are in."[53]

Patients also began to frame access to experimental treatment as a right. They were willing to take risks because, in the words of one PWA, "You're going to die from the disease one way or another so anything you can do to prolong your life is worth a try. It's my body. My choice. I can't wait for the FDA."[54] Doctors, too, needed to be cognizant of the fact that many of their patients were taking advantage of unapproved treatments. Readers of *Patient Care* were told, "Your AIDS patients probably know more about underground therapies than you do. You can strengthen the doctor-patient bond if you learn what they and many others with HIV disease are doing to empower themselves." The doctors were advised to continue to treat patients who were taking unlicensed drugs, possibly against their advice, and to "remember that monitoring doesn't imply agreement with this choice—only support for the patient's general well-being."[55]

With the rapid approval of AZT, a powerful idea began to circulate in the AIDS community: a cure for AIDS might already exist. After attending the 1989 International Conference on AIDS, Larry Kramer told the readers of the *Village Voice* that

> promising treatments that could keep us alive, that could end the AIDS epidemic, are so close we can almost touch them. The delays that are keeping these drugs from us are not scientific. They are bureaucratic. Drugs that could save us are sitting in laboratories when they should be in your local pharmacies. . . . [T]hey are out there waiting for us, these life-saving treatments. But we are not getting them. We are being held

prisoners by the Food and Drug Administration and the National Institutes of Health, by callous, greedy pharmaceutical companies, and by government regulations that leave us to die.[56]

This idea seemed plausible, since AZT was first developed in the 1960s and, in the minds of many in the AIDS community, was sitting on a shelf waiting to be discovered.[57] It also meant that a cure might be within reach if only a major obstacle could be removed—the slowness of gaining FDA approval for new drugs. AZT's rapid approval was an example of how this process could be streamlined.

One way to hasten a cure was to increase the number of drugs being tested. Synthesizing two ideas, the merits of research by community-based physicians (like Joseph Sonnabend) who had the trust and respect of their patients, and the self-empowerment ideas of the PWA Coalition, Sonnabend, Callen, Krim, and gay activist Ron Najman proposed a Community Treatment Initiative (CTI) in November 1986 as an alternative to the dominance of university-based drug testing. In some ways, this was an expanded version of the clinical research Sonnabend was already doing in his medical practice with small sums from the AIDS Medical Foundation (AMF), which he had founded with Mathilde Krim.[58] Combining the energy of PWAs with the expertise of physicians in private practice, the CTI could expand access to treatment and hasten a cure. The projected costs were modest: about twenty-five thousand dollars in salaries and operating expenses for the first six months, plus the cost of donated office space.[59] The idea quickly bore fruit and the group received the state's permission to develop an institutional review board. Renamed the Community Research Initiative (CRI), the project was established in May 1987 and was originally part of the PWA Coalition. The PWA Health Group and the CRI, formed at the same time, both empowered PWAs to save their lives.

The idea of expanding enrollment in clinical trials was not altogether new. Starting in 1976, the National Cancer Institute began to test promising medications at small community hospitals and, by the late 1980s, 40 percent of the data on new cancer treatments was coming from community-based oncologists.[60] A San Francisco group, the County Community Consortium (CCC), was also in the planning stages.[61] Yet CRI was unprecedented: for Thomas Hannan, a founder of the PWA Health Group and CRI's first administrator, "the most exciting aspect of this project is that it originates from the AIDS community, empowering ourselves to participate in the research that may save our lives and dramatically expand the number of patients who have access to experimental drugs."[62]

CRI wanted to test drugs that prevented the opportunistic infections that were major causes of death for PWAs—unlike AZT, which presumably kept the virus from replicating. The proposal for CRI noted that "Federal efforts at the present time are aimed almost exclusively at those who are already quite sick. We believe that finding interventions which will halt disease progression *prior* to the development of full-blown AIDS [are needed]."[63] For its founders, CRI represented "the first time in history that people with a disease have taken the initiative to organize research to find a solution to a disease."[64]

CRI experienced start-up problems because it attracted limited funding. Most of its support came not from individuals but from organizations, including GMHC, the Krim Foundation, Broadway Cares, and the Design Industries Foundation for AIDS. Its first major trial was Aerosol Pentamidine, which prevented pneumocystis carinii pneumonia, a major cause of death for people with HIV illness. The contract with the drug's manufacturer provided CRI with a major infusion of funds, totaling four hundred thousand dollars.[65] CRI, along with the CCC in San Francisco, achieved an early strategic success testing aerosalized pentamidine; because this success was the first of its type, and was a vivid reminder of how PWAs were fighting for their lives, it received a great deal of media attention, including a nationally televised documentary, "AIDS: Changing the Rules," and newspaper and magazine articles like "Doctors and Patients Take AIDS Drug into Their Own Hands."[66] CRI's approach also received a major boost when the President's Commission on the HIV Epidemic noted that CRI "offers the possibility to combine the technical expertise of the research community with the outreach potential of community health clinics and physicians in community practice."[67]

CRI was the prototype for a $1.4 million AmFar-sponsored program and a $9 million federal initiative. It received funds from AmFar but not from the federal government, because federal funds went to three groups in the city with stronger ties to communities of color.[68] By fall 1989, CRI lacked cash and, according to Callen, was in "grave danger of going under."[69] CRI rebounded and experienced a sharp rise in revenue, which peaked at $3.4 million in 1990.[70] It experienced leadership and staffing problems that led to its closure in 1991 and the establishment of a successor group, the Community Research Initiative on AIDS, one year later.[71] Now called the AIDS Community Research Initiative of America, the group continues to stress the importance of empowerment of PWAs to "take an active role in their own treatment," but is a smaller organization, with a $1.8 million income in 2003.[72]

Community-based research organizations would be successful recruiting subjects for trials because they could build on the trust between community-based physicians and subjects. This factor would increase enrollment and compliance.[73] There was a need to expand enrollment since, by the end of the 1980s, according to Mathilde Krim, university-based trials were a "bottleneck . . . in our ability to test all the drugs identified as having potential."[74] By the time CRI was established, university-based researchers were having difficulty enrolling people in clinical trials of AZT, because prospective patients were unwilling to chance getting a placebo but also because they were concerned about the drug's toxicity.[75] Community-based trials would also be a way to deal with a second set of problems which had not been explored empirically but were frequently discussed in news accounts: people were lying to get into trials; they were not adhering to the prescribed regimens; and they were obtaining drugs on the underground that they were not reporting to researchers.[76]

The efforts of the AIDS community to help people to gain access to unapproved and experimental treatments had the effect of destabilizing the existing system in which new medications were tested with experimental groups receiving treatment and control groups given a placebo. ACT UP's Jim Eigo pointed out that patients would be more likely to comply with clinical trials if they perceived them as operating under fair rules.[77] Research protocols began to eliminate another important barrier to participation, the use of placebos. Unlike past generations of patients, who accepted the expertise of physicians and willingly participated in clinical trials in an effort to help themselves and to advance science, PWAs and people with other diseases became selective about the clinical trials they joined, because they were understandably more concerned about fighting for their lives than simply advancing scientific knowledge.

The problems of low enrollment and noncompliance were not resolved. Journalistic accounts and AIDS activists themselves continued to point to the low levels of cooperation and cheating in clinical trials, in the mid-1990s. Particularly because members of the AIDS community viewed scientific research as political and guided by profits, it was not uncommon for people involved in clinical trials to place self-interest over the interests of science. Placebos were eliminated, since withholding experimental drugs was viewed as denying therapy, not risky treatment. Nevertheless, cheating to get into a trial and cheating while in a trial was not uncommon. No data support the claims about cheating and noncompliance, but anecdotal evidence provides ample evidence of what Dale Brashers calls "mindful nonadherence."[78] Some trials ended with less than half of their original participants.[79] In the very first AZT trials in New York, patients took capsules to laboratories and had them analyzed to see if they were placebos. An article in the PWA Coalition *Newsline* recounts the experience of a man who purposely lowered his T4 cell count the night before being screened for a clinical trial, by staying out all night and getting no sleep. Once in the study, he stockpiled the drug he was being given by taking it on his own schedule, rather than the schedule required in the treatment protocol. His overall assessment was that "one has to cheat, lie, and who knows what else to obtain what you need to live."[80] For Phil Zwickler, this was acceptable because "If a person feels that it's an issue of life or death, then all the rules go out the window. . . . When you talk about cheating, that implies that they're being fair also. . . . But when you think about how slow the drug approval process is and how little the Government has cared about the plight we face, should we be asked on top of everything to also play fair, by the rules? How much can you ask of us?"[81]

A combination of changed views about access to treatments and to clinical trials altered the traditional contract between patients and researchers. This change was not limited to the AIDS community.[82] Expanding access to experimental treatment through community-based research organizations, buyers' clubs and the underground created a range of pressure points that focused attention on the need for a cure. Noncompliance in clinical trials was a logical outgrowth of a central article of faith in the AIDS community: the virtue of doing what seemed necessary to save one's own life while awaiting a cure. An important turning point, which represented the dark side of the AIDS community, was the trial of Compound Q. This unauthorized trial, which began in the spring of 1989, was organized by Project Inform in San Francisco and involved thirty patients and nine doctors in New York, San Francisco, Los Angeles, and Miami. Testing a drug smuggled from China, the effort operated on the boundaries of a legal action—the importation of a drug for personal use—and an illegal one, conducting a clinical trial without the approval of an institutional review board. Three months after the trial began, news reports revealed that one patient had died and another had committed suicide. The underground trial ended but was later resumed as a standard clinical trial.[83]

The AIDS community was an important catalyst in a process of reexamining the drug approval system in the United States. Although expanding access to clinical trials was an important intermediate goal, advocates were primarily interested in FDA-approved treatments so that private insurers, Medicaid, and the federally subsidized but state-run prescription program for PWAs called ADAP (AIDS Drug Assistance Programs) would pay for them. The federal government's oversight of drugs dates back to the first decade of the twentieth century, but the Food, Drug, and Insecticide Administration was not established until 1927. Initially focused on preventing the sale of adulterated foods and, to a lesser extent, patent medicines, its major goal was to keep drug manufacturers from making false claims. Its role was expanded to include drug approval, which required demonstrating that the drugs were safe (beginning in 1938) and effective (starting in 1962).[84] After the thalidomide scandal of the early 1960s, when the FDA's intransigence prevented the kinds of severe birth defects that took place in countries where the drug had been approved, the FDA became extremely cautious. David Vogel offers a cogent explanation for this, noting that "the political costs to the FDA of approving a drug that turned out to be unsafe or ineffective were far higher than those incurred by delaying the approval of a drug that turned out to be safe."[85] The number of new drugs being tested began to decline; the time it took for approval expanded; and more drugs were tested outside the United States.[86]

In the decade before AIDS activists discovered the inadequacies of the FDA, the agency was already under scrutiny. Legislators requested a Government Accounting Office review of the FDA in 1977, a review that documented the agency's lengthy approval time and identified strategies for reducing it.[87] Walking a fine line between having stringent standards to protect people, promoting innovation, and allowing access to promising medications, the FDA had a difficult task, which its Commissioner, Frank Young, described as a conflict between "compassion and good science." Moreover, the agency was governing an industry with high development costs and very high profits that constituted a growing share of consumer spending.[88]

By the time the AIDS epidemic began, many observers charged that the FDA's caution resulted in a drug lag. As a result of the 1962 amendments, it took four times longer to approve a new drug in the United States than in any of five European countries and Canada.[89] This was especially problematic for drugs for life-threatening diseases. At the same time, the costs of developing and testing new drugs rose dramatically, from $1.3 million in 1960 to $50 million in 1979, according to the American Enterprise Institute (AEI), a conservative think tank. Longer approval time and increased costs would reduce innovation, decrease doctors' ability to treat patients, and lead to unnecessary deaths. According to the AEI, an average of fifty new drugs were approved annually between 1955 and 1960, compared to seventeen per year between 1965 and 1970. A study cited in the conservative *Cato Journal* estimated that the human cost of the FDA's slowness in approving beta blockers to prevent second heart attacks was as high as seventy thousand lives.[90]

Proposals to speed up the FDA's review of new drugs date back to the Nixon administration. A sustained effort began in 1975, with the appointment of the Review Panel on New Drug Regulation; its 1977 report concluded that the 1962 law was not responsible for the drug lag and that, in fact, many of the medications available outside the United States were not significant therapeutic advances. Responding to the charge that the FDA was dominated by the pharmaceutical industry, the final report concluded that the legal framework was neither pro- nor anti-industry; the FDA was "fundamentally sound" but nonetheless needed "substantial improvement."[91] A second report that same year, by the Secretary of Health, Education, and Welfare, reached different conclusions: that the FDA "has not kept up either with scientific advances or changing needs of society," and FDA procedures increased drug costs and did not provide consumers with adequate information.[92] Congressional hearings (1979), a GAO study (1980), a congressional study panel (1982), and a National Academy of Engineering study (1983) all documented that FDA approval was too slow. In 1981, the FDA commissioner made a commitment for the agency to begin to speed up drug approval. More drugs were approved that year (27) than the year before (12), and in 1985 thirty new drugs were approved. The average time from application to final approval also declined, from 37.5 months in 1979 to 31.2 months in 1981.[93] A series of rule changes between 1982 and 1985 were designed to speed up the review process by reducing record-keeping requirements and unnecessary paperwork, using electronic data submission procedures, and shortening the length of time for clinical trials.[94]

Another important reform affecting the development of new medications was the Orphan Drug Act, which took effect in 1984. Orphan drugs were those for diseases affecting fewer than 200,000 people or drugs unlikely to be profitable. In the early 1990s, 20 million people with five thousand diseases were potential users of orphan drugs.[95] Designed to provide incentives for companies to market drugs with a small demand, the Orphan Drug Act provided generous tax credits for clinical trials, a seven-year exclusive marketing license, extensive assistance by the FDA in developing studies to obtain approval, and federal grants and contracts that would support clinical trials.[96] The passage of the Orphan Drug Act provided significant incentives for testing AIDS drugs. By the mid-1990s, thirteen of the nineteen drugs licensed to treat AIDS were orphan drugs and seventy orphan drugs were under development. Two early AIDS treatments, intravenous pentamidine and AZT, were approved as orphan drugs, and Burroughs-Wellcome gained exclusive right to market AZT until the year 2005.[97]

Even while efforts were made to speed up drug approval and stimulate the development of new drugs, the AIDS community was skeptical of the federal government's commitment to finding a cure. Shortening the drug approval time did not respond to the reality of the lives of PWAs who expected to die quickly. The ethos of the AIDS community, the idea of the active health care consumer rather than the passive patient, created an alliance between the AIDS community and libertarians and conservatives who had been claiming that the drug industry was overregulated. A 1988 report by the conservative Heritage Foundation suggested that physicians should be able to prescribe drugs that had been certified as safe but had not completed clinical trials indicating that they were effective.[98]

Like conservatives and libertarians, people in the AIDS community believed that once a drug was proven safe, patients ought to be able to choose the level of risk they would undergo. The FDA became a target for the frustration that had welled up in the AIDS community. At the October 1988 demonstration at the FDA, one ACT UP demonstrator declared, "The experimental research they regulate is about to become the health care system."[99] In instances where people were suffering from life-threatening diseases, as Rothman and Edgar point out, there was a curious historical coincidence:

> Just when patients secured greater autonomy—the right to know a diagnosis, to accept or refuse treatment—the experts at the FDA and review boards controlled the right to regulate new drugs and research protocols. In a period when individual liberties were increasingly respected, this heavy paternalism flourished until the challenge of the eighties. . . . Patients with AIDS and their advocates reject the paternalism and risk-averse attitudes of the FDA-review board establishment. And they reject the view that the vulnerable and easily exploited in society need protection from the risks of participation in experimental protocols. From their perspective, experimentation is not a burden but a form of treatment.[100]

Over the course of nearly a decade, the FDA modified its policies, allowing patients to get medications more rapidly. By the time the epidemic began, drug companies were already giving patients unapproved treatments under a policy of "compassionate use," in which drug companies provided medications for free but were unable to use data on these patients for FDA approval. In July 1985, HHS Secretary Margaret Heckler announced the development of new rules to simplify and formalize compassionate use. As a result, twenty-five thousand patients were treated with two drugs later approved for heart disease and four thousand patients obtained AZT.[101] This procedure was further formalized and expanded in 1987 with the creation of a new category called Investigational New Drug for Treatment (Treatment IND), permitting drug companies to charge for drugs that had been approved for safety but not for efficacy when no alternative treatment existed.[102] All new drug applications would be reviewed in less than 180 days, and staff in drug companies could consult with the FDA "to facilitate more timely, effective, and efficient clinical studies and FDA reviews." The FDA also created a special designation for AIDS treatments ensuring them "first place in the review process" and giving them "prompt consideration for orphan drug status."[103]

Despite drug companies' initial interest in the idea of Treatment INDs, members of the AIDS community viewed this move as a failure, a "public relations exercise," since only eighty-nine patients were receiving trimetrexate, the only Treatment IND for AIDS. Ellen Cooper, the FDA official who oversaw AIDS drugs, suggested that members of the AIDS community had "mistaken expectations" that there was a "backlog of drugs."[104] ACT UP had a different view: "The drug companies hate Treatment IND because they have to make the drug available to patients they would rather have in their clinical trials."[105]

The first demand listed at ACT UP's first demonstration was "Immediate release by the Federal Food & Drug Administration of drugs that might help save our lives." Memorial Sloan Kettering Hospital in New York was selected for an early demonstration because it was an NIH-sponsored AIDS Treatment Evaluation Unit and the action would "exert pressure on NIH to immediately release lifesaving drugs caught up in the bureaucratic pipeline."[106] On 11 October 1988, between six hundred and fifteen hundred demonstrators from fifteen cities demonstrated at the "Federal Death Administration" because "Many Federal agencies, not to mention local and state ones, have been derelict in the fight on AIDS. . . . Yet only one agency, the FDA, is actively blocking the delivery of promising drugs to PWAs and people with HIV infection. Other agencies sin by omission, they aren't doing enough. Only the FDA sins by commission: it is doing the wrong things and they are deadly wrong. And only the FDA has the power *under existing laws* and regulations to change direction and provide many of our demands immediately."[107] Chanting, "We die, they do nothing" and "We're now the experts also," the demonstrators made demands that were cogent: "Release the drugs . . . open the trials. . . . Guarantee freedom of information." Closing down the building and stopping traffic on nearby roads, the demonstration led to 176 arrests. Vito Russo, a film critic and leader of ACT–UP New York, told a reporter, "I know there are drugs out there that can safe my life, and I want the FDA to do it quickly."[108]

A week later, the FDA affirmed its commitment to speed the approval process by permitting approval after two stages of testing (to prove safety and efficacy), and granting conditional approval before a third stage (requiring large clinical trials) if drug companies would do postmarketing studies. This was quite similar to the recommendation in the 1980 GAO report. In addition, trials could proceed more smoothly, since FDA staff would regularly consult with drug company representatives on how to design trials. The AIDS community saw the announcement as politically motivated, since it was made several weeks before a presidential election, and hollow, since, in the words of Mathilde Krim, "They come without significant dollars attached."[109] With the announcement in 1989 that HIV was mutating to "elude" AZT, the AIDS community was reminded that, eight years after the first AIDS cases, there was only one drug approved to fight AIDS and two more about to be approved.[110]

Demonstrations at the International AIDS Conference in Montreal and at the NIH, publicized AIDS activists' claim that the federal government was not interested in finding a cure. In Montreal, demonstrators "refused to leave the auditorium . . . giving notice that PWA's were 'inside' the conference to stay. . . . Activists had come to Montreal to influence more than just policy. We were there to hold science itself accountable to PWAs."[111] At a four-hour demonstration at the NIH, protestors carried cardboard tombstones and put "red tape" on nearby trees to symbolize the deaths being caused by bureaucratic delays.[112]

Two changes increased access to promising treatments. In June 1989, National Institute of Infections and Allergic Diseases Director Anthony Fauci announced his support for a "parallel track" in which individuals ineligible for clinical trials and unable to take approved medications could have unapproved medications prescribed. Data on the effect of drugs on individuals in a parallel track could be used to support drug approval.[113] The first drug released under this procedure, DDI, was approved only three-and-a-half months after its application was submitted.[114] In 1992, the FDA developed a new category of drug approval, called accelerated approval. This was in reality a conditional approval, but was given a different name since "conditional" implied that the drug was still in an experimental phase. Accelerated approval would also move drugs from being experimental to being eligible for coverage by private drug insurance plans and for Medicaid or Medicare coverage.[115]

All these changes moved toward an intermediate goal of "drugs into bodies." But a major source of optimism and a driving force behind AIDS activism—the belief that a cure was out there and simply needed to be tested and approved—no longer seemed so realistic. Even though AIDS had become a more manageable disease and life expectancy between diagnosis and death was longer, the sense of disaster and urgency continued. Leaders of the AIDS community felt they were still in the midst of a plague, and a cure seemed more distant. Scientific data on the fact that the virus had the ability to mutate meant that the very nature of HIV was still not completely understood.

Within ACT UP–New York, a great deal of the work on access to treatments was carried out by a small group in the Treatment and Data Committee (T & D), an affinity group founded in 1987.[116] Drawing on the expertise of Iris Long, a pharmaceutical chemist who had volunteered for CRI and the PWA Health Group, several members became "treatment activists," lay experts on current and promising AIDS treatments who developed cogent critiques of the FDA. The group produced one-page handouts and, in early 1988, Jim Eigo began researching clinical trials in the New York area, research that led to the establishment of the AIDS Treatment Registry, a listing of clinical trials. Long testified in Congress and to the President's Commission on the HIV Epidemic, recommending a national registry of clinical trials.[117] Members of the T & D Committee continued to participate in ACT UP demonstrations, but were increasingly becoming insiders as they took their place at the table with scientists and politicians and as members of the Treatment Action Group (TAG).

TAG member Mark Harrington described how his work drew on important ideas from Michel Foucault: to "master and appropriate the jargon of science," to "be flexible tactically but stubborn strategically," and to "'listen to the data' and change course when new findings make it necessary."[118] Harrington and other TAG members taught themselves basic science to understand AIDS and some political and policy issues related to drug testing and approval and to scientific research. As lay experts who mastered scientific language and knowledge, they were able to join clinicians and researchers "inside." Steven Epstein identifies several other aspects of their influence: they "presented themselves as the legitimate, organized voice of people with AIDS or HIV infection"; they "yoked together methodological (or epistemological) arguments and moral (or political) arguments, so as to multiply their 'currencies' of credibility"; they also "took advantage of pre-existing lines of cleavage within the scientific establishment to form strategic alliances."[119]

The TAG members' expertise, along with their legitimacy as representatives of the AIDS community and as people living with AIDS, formed a powerful combination. Scientists and politicians respected them because they had done their homework. Louis Lasagna, who headed the National Committee to Review Current Procedures for Approval of New Drugs for Cancer and AIDS, told sociologist Steven Epstein, "I'd swear that the ACT UP group from New York must have read everything I ever wrote."[120] Increasingly, the operating methods of T & D were at variance with the highly decentralized and democratic approach of ACT UP. One T & D member described its meetings: "there were stacks of Xeroxes covering almost every imaginable technical aspect of the HIV virus—bizarre abstracts of mind-numbing complexity. It was all either jargon or junk, and I had no idea how to discriminate between what was worthwhile and what was gibberish. In the center of the room, a group of eight or so people—the core—feverishly tossed acronyms at each other. . . . In their more accessible moments, they would complain that they were overloaded, burned out, and in need of help. I sat in the back of the room with the mostly silent majority of 20 or 30, waiting for a revelation."[121]

Treatment activists developed alliances with several disparate groups including former enemies. An AmFar-funded conference at Columbia University in July 1989 represents a turning point. The conference was sponsored by CRI and the CCC in San Francisco. Treatment activists and government scientists met to discuss common goals. Larry Kramer, for example, developed a good working relationship with Anthony Fauci, whom he once had called a "murderer."[122]

In addition to using, critiquing, and synthesizing scientific information and developing policy analyses and reform strategies, treatment activists represented patients who had a distinctive source of power, which, according to Arno and Feiden, was that "patients held a crucial bargaining chip—their bodies. The researchers could not run trials without their participation. Knowing they held that singular advantage, patients educated themselves in the arcane details of scientific studies until they were prepared to negotiate with investigators on equal footing."[123]

Treatment activists found themselves agreeing with conservatives who felt that government regulation ought to be reduced: groups like the Heritage Foundation whose 1988 report on the FDA was, according to John James, the editor of the widely circulated *AIDS Treatment News*, "the best call ever written for major reform of the FDA drug-approval process. The AIDS community might consider using this proposal as a rallying point."[124] But treatment activists were careful about these alliances. ACT UP's *FDA Handbook* noted that "AIDS advocates must be careful to keep their agenda, supporting earlier access to promising life-saving drugs for life-threatening disorders, from becoming confused with the Bush deregulation/*Wall St. Journal*/Heritage Foundation agenda of sweeping drug industry deregulation."[125]

Anthony Fauci's announcement of his support for the parallel track was another milestone in the history of treatment activism. Fauci's 1987 meetings with representatives of the AIDS community, including GMHC's Richard

Dunne and Michael Callen, had been adversarial.[126] Fauci's support for the idea of a parallel track, an idea developed by ACT UP–New York member Jim Eigo and San Francisco's Martin Delaney, was indicative of the growing alliance between the AIDS community and certain institutional advocates. Congressional hearings on the idea, in July 1989, included positive testimony from Assistant Secretary for Health James O. Mason and FDA Commissioner Young, as well as Fauci and Broder.[127]

Eigo had developed the idea of a parallel track in spring 1988 and presented it to a federal committee investigating cancer and AIDS drugs, headed by Louis Lasagna, the following year. By spring 1989, Fauci was discussing the concept with ACT UP–New York members.[128] He realized that scientists could learn from treatment activists. He recalled, "In the beginning, those people had a blanket disgust with us. And it was mutual. . . . When the smoke cleared we realized that much of their criticism was absolutely valid." In 1990, he stated "We will have as much dialogue as we possibly can with activists. . . . Some are better informed than many scientists can imagine," offering a "special insight" which can "be helpful in the way we design" research protocols.[129] Michael Callen agreed: "After a lot of shouting, we have all decided we have more to gain from listening to one another. It is a marriage between the brain trust and the people in the trenches."[130]

After a small group of ACT UP members took over the offices of AZT's manufacturer, Burroughs-Wellcome, in April 1989, the members of T & D and the drug manufacturers became more cooperative. Peter Staley, one of the demonstrators, was "the driving force" behind a $1 million donation from Burroughs-Wellcome to AmFar for community-based drug trials. Staley pointed out that "the industry will help build an invaluable network of research sites. . . . The federal research effort is not working. We'll take help wherever we can get it. This is a desperate situation." A Burroughs-Wellcome representative pointed out that "We as an organization have come to realize that the goals of ACT UP—most notably, the discovery of treatments for HIV disease—are not all that different than ours."[131] David Barr, an ACT UP and TAG member doing policy research for GMHC, wrote about the benefits of this kind of collaboration, indicating that "Working directly with pharmaceutical companies also is a way advocates can ensure that the most promising drugs are researched first."[132]

The Burroughs-Wellcome donation contributed to a split within ACT UP. After 1989, when T & D began to be consulted by government officials on a regular basis, a growing schism had been developing between T & D and other groups within ACT UP. For Mark Harrington, the dozen treatment activists were "determined to focus their efforts on research and treatment advocacy.

Infighting was getting in the way of that focus."[133] In the early part of 1991, the "Renegade Caucus" offered a critique of T & D in the *Newsline,* stating: the group hid information; members were "riddled with conflicts of interest"; the group was "dominated by a small group of people" and did not focus on treatment issues affecting women; and it "pays only lip service to many types of treatments which might be viable."[134]

Early in 1992, several key members of T & D formed the Treatment Action Group (TAG), a group that resembled a think tank. The differences between TAG and ACT UP were strategic, philosophical, personal, and organizational, and represented fundamentally different views of how lesbian and gay organizations ought to promote social change. ACT UP focused on outsider tactics, and its agenda expanded. TAG members believed that the combination of activism and treatment advocacy was no longer effective. Mark Harrington observed that "We'd won more power within research than other groups within ACT UP. . . . So where was the cure? The inside/outside strategy (demonstrations followed by meetings) began to be questioned. Demonstrations and zaps against drug companies stopped working; both the media and the industry were bored by them." The differences were also strategic. TAG had already begun to move in a different direction: it was becoming a think tank. TAG members thought ACT UP was more interested in sound bites and vague proposals than in detailed policy analyses.[135] Peter Staley pointed out, "Our policy initiatives are rarely as simplistic or as popular as Ross-Perot-like sound-bites," such as demands for an "AIDS czar" or a "Manhattan Project" for AIDS.[136] ACT UP continued to maintain an outsider position, fiercely criticizing its enemies and especially vilifying the government. TAG experienced a transition, and its members felt more comfortable operating as autonomous insiders. Harrington reflected back on this evolution, noting that "We started . . . with civil disobedience and demonstrations, but we ended up forming partnerships between activists and researchers which turned out to be both enduring and very useful."[137]

The idea of becoming collaborators, not remaining outsiders, was problematic to many ACT UP members. Members of the Women's Action Committee proposed a "six-month moratorium on face-to-face meetings with government officials" in 1991.[138] By then, treatment activists were not willing to give up their place at the table. Mark Harrington had been a member of the Community Constituency Group of the AIDS Clinical Trials Group since the fall of 1989. In 1990, representatives of the AIDS community were attending meetings once closed to them, had gained voting rights comparable to principal investigators, and had seats on all AIDS Clinical Trial group committees, including the executive committee. When President Clinton appointed panels to hasten the search for new drugs and to assess federal AID research, the membership included TAG founder Staley. In 1999, the NIH adopted a policy that encouraged peer review panels to include lay members.[139]

Some ACT UP members were skeptical about the ability of treatment activists to maintain their autonomy once they were having dinner and drinks with "the enemy." Hence, ACT UP New York prominently noted on its website for several years that "Our job is not to be invited to coffee or to schmooze at a cocktail party. . . . Our job is to make change happen as fast as possible and direct action works for that." Returning to the Holocaust imagery, Kiki Mason wrote in *POZ* magazine in 1995 that "I am being sold down the river by people within this community who claim to be helping people with AIDS. . . . 'Activists' now negotiate with drug companies just as the Jewish [Council] in the Warsaw ghetto of World War II negotiated with the Nazis."[140]

Differences of opinion over the idea of a Manhattan Project illustrate the growing divergence between ACT UP and TAG. The vision of a Manhattan Project—a government-sponsored centralized research project like the one that created the atom bomb—began circulating in the AIDS community in the 1980s. A Washington-based gay and lesbian organization, the Fairness Fund, began operating a hotline, in the summer of 1987, on which callers could use a prerecorded announcement that would be transmitted to public officials as mailgrams, including a message supporting a "New Manhattan Project on AIDS" since "Such a no-holds barred approach is needed now to combat the AIDS crisis."[141] In 1987, *U.S. News and World Report* noted that the idea was "gaining momentum among scientists, politicians, and public health officials," but was dismissed as unwise by Admiral Watkins of the President's Commission on HIV, who thought that more funding was needed for investigator-initiated research.[142] Nobel Prize winner David Baltimore pointed out that creating a small, elite research unit—the method used by industry to create specific results—was superior to the highly decentralized and loosely coordinated method currently being used.[143] Supporting an elite group of scientists who would not need to attend to organizational and funding constraints could hasten the discovery of a cure. Larry Kramer believed that "Only the Federal government can manage the project to find, as quickly as possible, the cure that top scientists believe is there."[144] The concept seemed to be gaining momentum when Bill Clinton endorsed it during the 1992 presidential primaries.[145]

The members of ACT UP–New York thought that a Manhattan Project would speed up the discovery of a cure because the NIH's AIDS research programs were "self-perpetuating research machines which contribute only marginally at best to uncovering effective treatments." Such a project would reduce the impact of conflicts of interest when scientific researchers received generous support from drug companies, and would reduce the power of drug companies to determine projects. It would bypass the "system of secret, competing proposals," the main goal of which was to "get money to pay the electric bill of the researcher's university," and in which researchers tended to submit "safe" proposals. It might also enhance collegiality. In this way, it would stimulate creativity and innovation. They renamed the idea after Barbara McClintock, the Nobel laureate who had received limited financial support and recognition for her early work.[146]

TAG's Mark Harrington, who met with NIH officials about the concept in 1992, became critical of the idea. He believed that a cure was not so close and that there was a need for basic science research before mounting a specific and goal-oriented project. He pointed out that that the mathematical model that was the blueprint for the Manhattan project existed before the project began.[147]

TAG's shift to an emphasis on basic research represented a recognition that seeking a cure by putting drugs into bodies did not stop the dying. Keeping people alive while awaiting a cure seemed a good strategy in the late 1980s, but the magic bullet no longer seemed so close. Two studies released in 1991 cast serious doubt on the long-term impact of AZT on slowing down the progression of HIV.[148] Although people were living longer, the idea of AIDS being chronic if manageable was premature. TAG members began to question the "drugs into bodies" approach. Until this point, the strongest critic of this approach in the AIDS community had been Michael Callen, a strident critic of AZT who retired from AIDS activism in 1991.[149] Within the next several years, TAG members began to be critical of widely held views in the AIDS community. Harrington, for example, recalls that he realized that "the AIDS community, in its understandable desperation, was being manipulated by industry to demand the expeditious approval of inadequately tested drugs."[150]

In the autumn of 1993, TAG member Gregg Gonsalves told an FDA advisory committee, "We have arrived in hell. . . . AIDS activists and government regulators have worked together, with the best intentions, over the years to speed access to drugs. What we have done, however, is to unleash drugs with well-documented toxicities into the market, without obtaining rigorous data on their clinical efficacy." Several months later, another TAG Member, Spencer Cox, testified that there was far too little data on another drug nearing approval, d4T. Cox later told reporters that "Simply making drugs available is not enough." He realized that "We were naïve. There are standards for a reason," and came to believe that "We need to go back to the way we did studies, or move forward to new study designs that answer concerns about control studies."[151]

TAG began to look more closely at basic scientific research and modified its understanding of the barriers to finding a cure. Rather than seeing the issue as a matter of the FDA blocking the approval of existing drugs, TAG came to realize that there was a need to develop a better understanding of the disease. TAG recommended better coordination of AIDS research, a recommendation made by an Institute of Medicine report the previous year.[152] In response, the federal government did provide greater coordination of AIDS research. The 1993 NIH Revitalization Act stipulated that all AIDS research funds, then totaling $1.3 billion, would be coordinated by an Office of AIDS Research. William E. Paul, a well-respected immunologist but a newcomer to AIDS research, was appointed the director. At the beginning of his tenure, he pointed out that "Thoughtful scientists analyzing the current status of our progress against the disease and the state of research have concluded that the limited progress made thus far is due to an inadequate knowledge base. . . . As we now enter a phase requiring the development of new basic knowledge and in which research budgets are no longer rapidly increasing, I am committed to increasing that fraction of the AIDS budget that supports unsolicited investigator-initiated research grants."[153]

As saquinivir, the first of an entirely new class of AIDS drugs called protease inhibitors, began to near approval, a letter to the FDA coauthored by TAG, GMHC, and AIDS Action Baltimore objected to the drug's premature release, questioning the "inappropriately low standards" of drug approval being used.[154] TAG members recommended to an FDA panel the need for large simple trials, in this case a trial of eighteen thousand people with liberal entry requirements, and a diverse group of participants to provide detailed data on the safety and efficacy of the drug. This would be an improvement over a system in which there was no incentive for drug companies to complete follow-up studies after FDA approval. TAG also recommended a feature that had once been anathema to the AIDS community: that one third of participants receive placebos. Harrington reflected back on this decision:

> Most people with HIV are not the polypharmacy maniacs who tended to show up at drug company meetings and FDA hearings. Many treatment activists represent a vocal segment of the community which is intoxicated with access, and has abundant access to health care and the latest information and experimental treatments. Most people with HIV, however, lack such access, and many do not want to take drugs which are

toxic, expensive, inconvenient, and for which no clear evidence of benefit exists. From a public health standpoint, we felt we had a responsibility to confront the drug industry, the FDA, and the community activists with whom we disagreed, to force them to design studies which would provide whether a given new drug was worth taking or not.[155]

David Barr amplified this idea: "It's not just me who has to take the drugs, not just a group of informed people, but doctors and patients all over the world need to know what works. . . . And this is not just for today. In five years there'll be a whole lot more people looking for treatment options. . . . Part of what we're doing is not just for ourselves, but is, unfortunately, planning for them also."[156]

With the approval of the first protease inhibitor in 1995—and a new form of treatment, HAART, in 1996, consisting of combinations of the two major types of AIDS treatments, protease inhibitors and nucleoside analogues—it seemed as if a cure had been found.[157] The number of AIDS deaths declined rapidly. AIDS seemed more manageable, but the drugs had other side effects, costs were high, and the treatment regimen was complicated. There were a possible 120 combinations of drugs, and studies demonstrated that many physicians made serious errors prescribing the drugs. A very substantial proportion of patients, between 20 percent and 40 percent, developed resistance to existing treatments, and the virus continued to mutate. And it was no longer clear when treatment ought to begin or whether or not people would benefit from planned interruptions or "holidays." A conventional wisdom about HIV treatments was no longer true: it was not clear that early intervention was highly effective in maintaining a person's viral load.[158]

TAG's increasingly cautious stance was enormously criticized by other members of the AIDS community. By the end of the century, however, other influential members of the AIDS community shared their position. When Martin Delaney was asked his opinion about an FDA advisory panel's decision to reject a new HIV treatment because of its limited efficacy and extensive side effects in 1999, Delaney responded, "Nobody has worked harder than we have to get new treatments approved. But with fourteen other drugs out there, we now tend to look a little more harshly at the new ones."[159] As of this writing, the AIDS community remains optimistic about the discovery of more effective treatments and a vaccine. According to the Pharmaceutical Research and Manufacturers of America, 102 new medicines were being developed for HIV in 1999 and 79 in 2004. Twenty new medications were approved in 2004.[160]

The AIDS community's early years were marked by a sense that the capabilities of medicine and of science were unlimited. In the rush to obtain experimental treatments, defined as promising rather than risky, patients in general and AIDS patients in particular created a crisis in the testing and the development of new medications.

The impact of the AIDS community on finding a cure has been complex. The FDA has become "modernized," a process that was already underway but was dramatized by the demands of the AIDS community. For several years, a larger number of drugs was approved and approval was faster than in the past—121 new drugs in 14.4 months in 1997—but most were modifications of existing compounds.[161] The number of drugs withdrawn from the market has increased and there is serious concern that the approval process may be too rapid and that too few drugs continue to be studied once approved.[162] The FDA is now becoming much more cautious and is issuing more warnings for drugs that have been approved.[163] A major FDA official testified to an Institute of Medicine Committee that the drug safety system in the United States had "pretty much broken down," and the FDA created a scientific advisory panel in 2005 to warn patients about unsafe drugs.[164] More and more, drug testing has become the province of practicing physicians, not just those in university settings, but this raises the concern that patients may be pressured by their doctors to take new drugs, and there is a conflict of interest when doctors are paid to recruit their patients for drug trials.[165] It is also not altogether clear that participating in clinical trials has a positive impact on people's longevity.[166]

The AIDS community created a host of organizations that collaborated and used a range of tactics to challenge the system of testing new drugs, and that questioned the high cost of prescription drugs. A broad coalition including the AIDS Action Council, local AIDS service organizations like GMHC, and activist groups like TAG and ACT UP have been central to this effort. Summing up the forces that led to the passage of the NIH Reorganization Act, TAG member Gregg Gonsalves pointed to the central role of the National Academy of Sciences, the science journal *Nature*, and a broad coalition including "The Treatment Action Group, the AIDS Action Council, the American Foundation for AIDS Research, the Pediatric AIDS Foundation, and Gay Men's Health Crisis, along with over two hundred AIDS researchers."[167]

With the development of new medications and increased life expectancy, the pool of people living with HIV has risen exponentially. This has created serious concerns about preventing transmission by the fastest growing group of people living with HIV: individuals infected by sharing equipment used to inject drugs.

Chapter 9

Clean Needles Save Lives

I can tell you from experience, the man on the street may not be able to quit, but he doesn't want to die."

—Michael Sehested, ADAPT

The black community saw an empty needle. The advocates saw a full needle. There was the whole crux of the issue. The needle is empty. That means the person is going to go out and get some drugs. Hook it up. Put it in this needle. Shoot it in his veins. Wreak havoc on the community. . . . They're saying that the needle is clean. That he'll continue to do all this. . . . That's why there's so much controversy.

Preventing HIV transmission to injecting drug users was complex and contested.[1] In August of 1985, New York City Health Commissioner David Sencer recommended a simple but controversial way to save lives: to allow drug addicts to obtain clean needles and syringes to inject drugs.[2] He urged Mayor Koch to lobby for a change in the state law banning the over-the-counter sale of syringes without a doctor's prescription. He also recommended that substance abuse treatment programs become "arrest-free zones" where addicts could exchange used needles for new ones. The proposal unleashed a firestorm of protest, and it was quickly dismissed.[3] All of the district attorneys in the city opposed it and the president of the City Council described it as "ill advised and misguided." The director of the Addicts Rehabilitation Center in Harlem said that it was "almost like an endorsement to go out and help yourself to drugs."[4] Public officials believed that distributing syringes meant that the state would be encouraging drug use. It was also contrary to the received wisdom of drug treatment professionals and substance abuse researchers who, like State Commissioner of Health, David Axelrod, assumed that sharing needles was "a pattern of social behavior that is hard to break."[5] There was some support, however. The director of the New York State Division of Substance Abuse Services thought the proposal was worth considering since addicts were getting needles from the black market." A *New York Times* editorial, "Choosing between Two Killers," pointed out that it was worth a try because "Drug addiction is a scourge, but AIDS is a scourge that multiplies."[6]

Fifteen years later, the New York State legislature enacted a policy that was quite similar to Sencer's proposal. Under an Expanded Syringe Access Program (ESAP), a "temporary" policy adopted for two years beginning in 2001 and later extended until 2007, adults could purchase up to ten syringes without a prescription. ESAP and an earlier approach, legal syringe exchanges (established in 1992), give drug injectors access to sterile syringes. In contrast to the early strident public discussion of needle exchanges, ESAP was enacted with no public debate.[7] Few news stories discussed the legislation, its implementation, or its extension. The same was true for needle exchanges, once they became legalized in New York in 1992. The passion surrounding the issue had dissipated.

Syringe access is an interesting case study precisely because public discourse was originally passionate and public opinion remains divided.[8] The AIDS community and institutional advocates used a range of strategies, in a process of policy learning and a shift in the drug policy paradigm from abstinence to harm reduction. Initially a vanguard if not unthinkable social policy, the policy of New York and other states allows drug addicts access to sterile syringes to reduce the transmission of HIV and other diseases, combining a social service approach with a market-based solution.

Early in the epidemic, drug addicts began to take steps to reduce their chances of being infected by inhaling rather than injecting drugs, by reducing needle sharing, by changing the kinds of drugs they used, and by purchasing what they thought were new syringes. Early outreach efforts by ADAPT included teaching addicts to clean their equipment with bleach, and encouraging them to enter treatment. Expanding treatment was the first policy seriously considered as a way to fight AIDS among drug users. It was also consistent with the country's "war on drugs." Funding for substance abuse treatment increased by $160 million for 1987 and 1988, and this amount plus $40 million was allocated for 1989.[9] With an ever-growing number of people being diagnosed with HIV as a result of drug use—and serious concern that men would infect their female sexual partners and their newborn children—it became apparent that other strategies were needed. Expanding drug treatment would take several years and, despite serious concerns about the impact of drug use on society, would cost more than the American public might be willing to spend.[10] There was also community resistance to expansion of drug treatment.

A first step might be to modify treatment to quickly expand enrollment and to lower costs. This strategy was used in a pilot Interim Methadone Maintenance program in Harlem that was sponsored by Beth Israel Medical Center.[11] The pilot program was not "treatment," because it lacked the psychological and social services mandated for methadone programs.[12] It faced fierce opposition from local politicians and Harlem residents, who believed that it created a "methadone black market outside its doors." A member of the local community board thought it was "one of the worst things that I've seen on 125th Street in the past twenty years—it's out of control. The people are drinking and selling the methadone. It's all over the streets." Harlem Congressman Charles Rangel, chair of the Select Committee on Narcotics Abuse and Control, pointed out that "Methadone is no panacea for heroin addiction."[13]

Federal officials were seriously considering the idea of expanding Interim Methadone Maintenance, however, since the approach was working in Hong Kong, and the evaluation of the pilot program in Harlem documented that participants reduced their use of heroin. But the idea of developing methadone-only programs lost favor after a negative report from a GAO study of twenty-four methadone programs showed that they had serious problems.[14] A high proportion of those in the programs for more than six months used heroin, between 1 percent and 47 percent, and "many of the patients used other drugs, primarily cocaine."[15]

Despite the negative reaction to Sencer's proposal, the idea of expanding access to syringes was not completely off the public agenda. Drug addicts in New York had the highest HIV rates in the country.[16] When a reporter asked Sencer's successor, Stephen Joseph, about expanding access to syringes, at his first press conference, in early 1986, Joseph replied that the idea was worth considering.[17] The concept gained momentum and legitimacy during 1986. ADAPT issued a position paper supporting a trial needle exchange, and the New York Bar Association's Committee on Medicine and Law recommended that the state should "legalize the purchase of hypodermic needles and syringes without a prescription."[18] James Curran, the director of the CDC's AIDS program, endorsed a test program of needle distribution and noted that "The problem we face is bigger than politics." A report issued by the World Health Organization indicated that needle exchange could play an important role in stopping the spread of HIV.[19] Perhaps the strongest influence on state and city officials was a National Academy of Sciences report, issued in November 1986, that argued "It is time to begin experimenting with public policies to encourage the use of sterile needles and syringes by removing legal and administrative barriers to their possession and use."[20] This report influenced Mayor

Koch and the state health commissioner. Koch explained that he had changed his mind because giving addicts access to clean needles was like putting a patch on a tire and that "Reality forces us to come to grips with the fact that an addict not in custody or a successful treatment program is going to use drugs."[21]

Joseph reasoned that a successful pilot needle exchange would decrease political resistance by demonstrating the feasibility of giving needles to drug injectors. However, the state rejected the city's request in May 1987.[22] Advocates became impatient. ADAPT's executive director, Yolanda Serrano, decided to force the issue. The group had been teaching drug addicts to clean their injection equipment with bleach, a method the group saw as feasible but ineffective. One board member recalled that "it was criminal not to be able to give people access to sterile syringes."[23] Without the backing or approval of ADAPT's board, Serrano told a *New York Times* reporter that the agency was willing to break the law and distribute clean needles and collect used ones. The front-page story indicated that they were willing to risk their funding and tax exemption "to protect the public and save lives."[24] ADAPT's board met that evening and the following day's *Times* included a statement from Serrano that "preferably, we would like to do it within the law." The board clarified its position and sent telegrams to public officials indicating that the agency intended to ask the state commissioner of health "to designate and authorize ADAPT to implement a carefully monitored sterile needle and syringe exchange and controlled distribution program in shooting gallerys [sic] and other areas of New York City where there is an extremely high incidence of intravenous drug abuse."[25]

Serrano's announcement had its intended effect: it reopened the public conversation. Commissioner Joseph pointed out that, even though he didn't condone Serrano's original statement, it "underscores the urgency and importance of what we have been asking to do for over a year." New York Governor Cuomo sent out a trial balloon, noting that the issue was "tormenting me" and, at the end of the month, approved the plan.[26] By then, new data documented the incidence of HIV among newborns.[27] Scientific evidence from Holland, Australia and the U.K. was also giving the idea of needle exchange greater legitimacy, although some were skeptical about whether these data shed any light on the situation in the United States, where drug use was associated with an underclass.[28]

It took most of 1988 to iron out the details, and the pilot needle exchange opened its doors on November 7. This was the second legal needle exchange in the country, but the first operated by a city government. The idea of syringe exchanges was enormously unpopular, and Los Angeles, Chicago, and Boston considered and rejected the idea.[29] In 1988 Congress passed legislation banning the use of federal funds for programs that provided needles or syringes to inject illegal drugs.[30] New York's project involved a compromise, because of community resistance. It was located in a Department of Health building in the city hall area, far from the four neighborhoods with high levels of drug use where it was originally supposed to operate. The location was a handicap, and so was the requirement that needles would only be given to people who were waiting to enter drug treatment. Participants were required to be tested for tuberculosis, sexually transmitted diseases, and HIV.[31] The early response was modest: 2 addicts came on the first day and only 160 in the first seven months.[32] But, by its very existence, the program could achieve one important objective: to answer critics who claimed that addicts would not be willing to make the effort to obtain clean needles.

A strong countermovement emerged in the city, which contributed to the pilot needle exchange's rapid demise. Supporters of the war on drugs believed that needle exchange would encourage drug use or was a poor substitute for drug treatment. Drug treatment professionals, like Mitchell Rosenthal, the president of Phoenix House, which provided drug-free treatment, thought that the plan was unworkable since "These are the most disordered people in society. To think this person is going to get on a bus or a train and travel across Manhattan to register and appear regularly flies in the face of what we know."[33] Cardinal O'Connor viewed the program as a "quick fix because we are not spending the dollars on fighting narcotics."[34] One month after the pilot began, the City Council voted, 31 to 0 with one abstention, to stop the program.[35]

The strongest criticism came from African American community leaders and politicians who labeled the program racist and "genocide." Three weeks before it opened, an Ad Hoc Committee to Stop the Distribution of Needles and Syringes to Addicts pointed out in the *Amsterdam News* that the program was "completely lacking in merit as a scientific experiment, or as a medical or public health measure. . . . It is a recklessly dangerous experiment on human beings, which will have consequences directly counter to those proposed."[36] This elite group had considerable legitimacy since its members included several public officials, including Congresspersons Charles Rangel and Floyd Flake. The City Council's Black and Hispanic Caucus thought the pilot program illustrated the mayor's insensitivity to their community, because they had not been adequately consulted. Beny Primm, who headed a large methadone maintenance program and had been a member of the President's Commission on the HIV Epidemic, believed that needle exchange was a poor substitute for expanding drug treatment and gave people "license to engage in aberrant behavior."[37] Rangel saw it as a "band aid" that would "accomplish little but to prolong drug addiction," inconsistent with the goal of becoming a "drug-free society," and as promoting "death on the installment plan."[38] City Council member Hilton B. Clark argued that "If the i.v. drug population was anywhere close to being integrated . . . you can be sure we would not have this program; we'd find money for drug treatment." Another elite group, the Black Leadership Commission on AIDS, took a similar position, claiming that the city ought to expand drug treatment and stating that needle exchanges sent the wrong message to IV drug users and to young people.[39] Special drug prosecutor Sterling Johnson believed that users would sell the needles and that the plan might be the first step in creating "city-supervised shooting galleries" in "an attempt to make zombies out of people."[40]

Roy Innes, the head of the Congress of Racial Equality, was the only African American leader who endorsed needle exchanges. He told a Congressional committee in the spring of 1989 that the government should not be in the business of distributing needles but that injection equipment should be available. He proposed that needle possession and distribution ought to be decriminalized and that nonprofit organizations should distribute needles.[41]

A report of the pilot needle exchange's activities over ten months showed that, even though the pilot study had some shortcomings, the idea could work. Despite a smaller than anticipated enrollment, about three hundred people, it was clear that the addicts who came to the exchange were making an effort to protect their health and that the program was reaching a high-risk population, since half were HIV-positive, one third were homeless, eight in ten had shared injection equipment, and 62 percent had shared equipment within the past month. The pilot program was described as a bridge to drug treatment and, in fact, most of those who responded were interested in drug treatment and some never got needles.[42] The project was more than a way to distribute needles, then; it was a model for a new approach to working with drug addicts, called "harm reduction," which was gaining support and would become an ideological anchor for providing increased access to syringes.

The needle exchange closed soon after the 1990 inauguration of Mayor David Dinkins, who had promised to end it during his campaign because he believed that providing needles was "to surrender" to drug use.[43] He and his new commissioner of health, Woodrow Myers, agreed with other African American leaders that bleach and needles promoted drug use and were a poor substitute for getting people into treatment. Myers, whose appointment was highly contested (chapter 7), supported the principle of drug treatment on demand and strongly opposed over-the-counter sale of syringes because he did not think it was the city's responsibility to help people to safely inject drugs.[44] Dinkins announced the end of the pilot needle exchange soon after he took office.

Dinkins and Myers were less successful in their effort to bar the use of city funds to teach drug addicts how to clean their syringes with bleach. The commissioner of health asked ADAPT to modify its $861,000 contract to reflect this change; city officials assumed that the agency would be able to continue to do this work with funds from New York State. ADAPT's board voted to sign the contract with the altered language, but Serrano, believing that ADAPT ought to be more committed to advocacy, marshalled support from other AIDS organizations, the city's comptroller, and the president of the City Council, and successfully challenged the Health Department's proposed changes.[45] At the same time, and perhaps unbeknown to its supporters, the Department of Health was also concerned about ADAPT's management, especially its fiscal procedures, but wanted to renew the contract because of the agency's ability to carry out needed programs.[46]

Thirteen AIDS organizations sponsored a demonstration and press conference that included Dr. Mathilde Krim, Serrano, and the executive directors of HAF and the MTFA.[47] MTFA (the Minority Task Force on AIDS) took a different position from other African American organizations, such as the Black Leadership Commission on AIDS, which meant that, as one leader put it, "we caught hell."[48] At the press conference accompanying the demonstration, MTFA's executive director, Ronald Johnson, requested that the Department of Health "continue to support the work of the Association for Drug Abuse Prevention and Treatment, including ADAPT's efforts to reduce the risk of HIV transmission through the distribution of bleach kits."[49] The MTFA distinguished between teaching addicts about bleach, which they endorsed, and giving them needles, which they continued to oppose. Dinkins and Myers retreated from their position, and ADAPT's contract was renewed without any changes.[50]

The AIDS community also challenged Dinkins' decision to end the needle exchange. ACT UP members mounted a test case to force the city and the state to legalize the exchanges. The idea was to establish an illegal exchange, get arrested, and be acquitted. This was part of a larger effort of civil disobedience carried out by the National AIDS Brigade. Starting in 1987, volunteers in the National AIDS Brigade began to purchase needles where they were legal and transport them to other states in the Northeast that, like New York, banned over-the-counter purchase of syringes without prescriptions, to court arrest and mount test cases.[51] A month before ACT UP started New York's exchange, its leader, a Yale graduate student in public health and former addict named Jon Parker, had been acquitted in Boston.[52]

Just after Dinkins ended New York City's pilot exchange, ACT UP and the AIDS Brigade began exchanging needles on the Lower East Side, in East Harlem, and in Williamsburg. One month later, ten ACT UP members were arrested in a carefully orchestrated event preceded by two newspaper articles announcing that needles would be distributed at a major intersection of the Lower East Side and inviting the press and the police.[53] Officials offered to drop the charges if the defendants did one day of community service and promised not to violate the law for six months. The exchangers refused this offer: they preferred to bring the case to trial.[54]

Between the arrest and an acquittal in June 1991, ACT UP operated illegal exchanges in the Bronx, Harlem, Brooklyn, and the Lower East Side of Manhattan, with limited police interference. One exchanger recalled that "In the beginning we had a lot of hassles" but over time "we reached a tacit truce. If we kept the works under the table, they would leave us alone."[55] There were obstacles and problems: one exchange sometimes ran out of money to buy needles and did not have enough help assembling the kits.[56] Beginning with one hundred needles each week, ACT UP was distributing two thousand per week by the end of 1990 and estimated they had contact with forty thousand people in 1991.[57] The needles were tagged to track how many were returned, and people coming to three of the exchanges assembled their own bleach kits, since "making their own bleach kit directly engages drug users, and again encourages them to think about their behaviors as they assemble the kits." Even when the organizers did not have needles, exchanges remained open because "Our main goal was to remain consistent, even if we didn't have any supplies we would go out. If we only had a hundred works we would hand them out and then sit there the rest of the day giving out bleach kits and answering questions."[58] People could exchange as many as fifteen syringes, or, if they had no needles to exchange, they could get three. Used needles were turned over to the Department of Health.[59]

As the ten exchangers awaited trial, the idea of making syringes accessible was becoming more acceptable. ACT UP members produced, and GMHC distributed, a video called *Clean Needles Save Lives,* which provided a sensitive look at addicts, including one person who noted that "lots of people think addicts are not concerned about their health but they [are]," and pointing out that needle exchanges do not condone drug use but simply provide clean needles. The American Civil Liberties Union supported the ten exchangers, noting that the penal law under which they were arrested "was adopted long before the emergence of the AIDS epidemic and was not intended to apply to those who, like the ten defendants, possess and distribute needles . . . in the best traditions of Good Samaritanism."[60] Several researchers and public health officials were expert witnesses, including Don Des Jarlais from Beth Israel and Ernest Drucker from Montefiore, and Joseph, who noted that the group was performing a "needed public service."[61] The city had one witness, Dr. Laurence Brown, who was affiliated with Harlem Hospital and the Addiction Research and Treatment Corporation. He pointed out that there was a need for more research on the safety and efficacy of needle exchange and that this was a "band-aid approach to the drug problem."[62]

The New York needle exchangers based their case on a necessity defense, that "Conduct which would otherwise constitute an offense is justifiable and not criminal when such conduct is necessary as an emergency measure to avoid an imminent public or private injury."[63] It is also important to recognize that the exchanges were not simply distributing clean needles; they were taking contaminated needles out of circulation.[64] The judge's decision noted that "AIDS has created an imminent crisis in New York City. There is no dispute that use of clean needles by addicts prevents the spread of HIV infection. . . . When coupled with AIDS education and counseling, a needle exchange program serves as a means for convincing addicts to avoid other risk-related behavior, to get medical care and ultimately to discontinue use of drugs. . . . It is equally apparent that there were no meaningful available options . . . insufficient drug programs exist for the number of addicts in New York and there is no reason to believe more treatment slots will come into existence in the near future.[65]

Behind the scenes, members of the AIDS community began to pressure the city to legalize needle exchanges. Two weeks after the court decision, ACT UP members brought used syringes to a Board of Health meeting to demonstrate their support for legalized exchanges. ADAPT sponsored a forum at Lincoln Hospital in the Bronx in late August, and the Minority Task Force on AIDS changed its position and urged Dinkins to legalize needle distribution.[66] The American Foundation for AIDS Research announced that it was planning to donate three hundred thousand dollars for four needle exchange programs in the United States.[67]

Less than five months after the court decision, Mayor Dinkins reversed his position and announced that he would approve legal needle exchanges in the city. He realized that he could no longer ignore AIDS' devastating impact, and described the needle exchanges as "only one component of a more comprehensive effort to fight the overlapping epidemics of AIDS and drug abuse." He pointed out that 2,573 new drug treatment slots had been added during his administration and more were planned.[68] His announcement was accompanied by a report from a needle exchange working group that pointed to positive findings of a study done in New Haven (released just after the court decision) that documented that syringes distributed through a needle exchange "were less likely to be contaminated with HIV than those obtained on the street or in shooting galleries," and that the exchange reduced the rate of HIV infections by 35 percent.[69]

Dinkins' decision was also based on another reality: although the city's leadership was still divided, there was growing support from civic leaders, black and white, including the City Council president, the Manhattan borough president, and James Dumpson, the chair of the city's Health and Hospitals Corporation, who was also the chair of the Black Leadership Commission on AIDS.[70] Several African American elected officials endorsed needle exchange, including State Senator Velmanette Montgomery from the Bedford Stuyvesant neighborhood of Brooklyn, who introduced a bill in the state legislature to decriminalize needle possession.[71] Dinkins was also influenced by the decision of another African American mayor, John Daniels from New Haven, who reversed his position because "I had to deal with the grim reality that AIDS was decimating my community."[72] Even the idea's fiercest foe was no longer so strident; Charles Rangel admitted that it was hard to oppose an effort designed to reduce the incidence of a terminal disease.[73] As a group, African American leaders supported increased access to syringes for purely pragmatic reasons; they viewed it as the lesser of two evils.[74]

Several of the city's illegal needle exchanges began operating above ground in June 1992, with funding from the American Foundation for AIDS Research and from New York State. They were able to serve more people and no longer faced the shortage of supplies that had plagued the illegal exchanges. Public and foundation funding allowed them to expand but ended their ad hoc and informal quality, and the organizations became more bureaucratic. One staff member told program evaluators, "It's like you're coming up to a welfare counter or to a doctor's office. . . . It's a physical barrier, as opposed to when we just had bags and there was a person, and there was a provider, and there was nothing between them."[75] Funders required a higher level of professionalism, and collecting data was not just done for accountability but had a significant advocacy dimension, since favorable evaluations gave this highly contested policy greater legitimacy.

New York's experience was duplicated in other cities. In May 1992, there were illegal needle exchanges in San Francisco, Santa Cruz, Oakland, Boston, and Philadelphia, as well as legal exchanges in Seattle, Spokane, and Boulder.[76] Between 1988 and 1995, there were fourteen test cases in eleven cities. In nearly all of them, defendants were acquitted on the basis of a necessity defense or the cases were dropped. After that, the strategy was less effective as a way of pressuring officials to change policies. Defendants were convicted in several cases in New Hampshire and New Jersey.[77] The number of legal and illegal exchanges expanded rapidly. From a single exchange in the United States in 1987, the number rose to 33 in 1993 and to 148 in 2002.[78]

The establishment of legal syringe exchange programs (SEPs) in New York City was part of a paradigm shift taking place to deal with HIV and substance abuse. In its first report on the operation of needle exchanges in New York State, the AIDS Institute described needle exchanges as part of a broader effort of harm reduction, a conceptual framework that emphasized helping clients "where they are" rather than only providing assistance to those who were clean and sober.[79] Although the major purposes were to help people to inject safely and to teach them about HIV risk reduction, needle exchanges also functioned as low-threshold entry points into the health care and social service system, helping addicts to obtain identification to access public benefits, obtain housing, and enter substance abuse treatment.

Two harm reduction advocates, Richard Elovich and Michael Cowing, point out that substance abuse treatment programs traditionally assumed that people hit bottom before they began treatment.[80] Programs were also unforgiving of relapse. In extreme cases, such as Synanon, the response was to impose shame and stigma by shaving a person's head.[81] The relapse rate of drug treatment programs was quite high; in fact, eight in ten of the participants in Beth Israel's Interim Methadone Program had been in treatment at an earlier time.[82]

Harm reduction was developed in Holland and in the United Kingdom to assist people who were not ready to "cure" their addiction. It was designed to help addicts "through a difficult phase in their lives, while it is hoped that one day they may overcome their addiction either through treatment or natural recovery."[83] The first objective was to help people to reduce the harm they experienced in using drugs. A second major premise was that recovery from addiction would be a long term process, with relapse a common if not normal part of the process. One theorist observed that the approach involved "an acceptance of the reality that some injecting will continue and that any initiatives should be accompanied by efforts to reduce the damaging nature of this continued injecting."[84] Just as needle exchanges began to expand, a number of scientific studies began to cast doubt on the effectiveness of cleaning syringes with bleach. Cleaning equipment with bleach had its greatest impact when HIV seroprevalence was low.[85] It was not clear that injectors were cleaning their equipment properly, even though many of them thought they were. A joint statement by the CDC, the Center for Substance Abuse Treatment, and the National Institute of Drug Abuse (NIDA) in 1993 recommended a complex procedure for cleaning equipment, an approach probably not practical since compliance was reduced when the complexity of the process increased.[86] A subsequent study supported earlier work concluding that "bleach use as employed by IDUs in everyday life in New York City has not been protective against HIV seroconversion."[87] In 1995, a National Academy of Sciences panel recommended that "Bleach use is clearly an intervention to be used when injection drug users have no safer alternative."[88]

Recognition of the limits of cleaning syringes with bleach made other options more important. The most visible advocacy—by activists, and by institutional advocates like the social scientists doing research on the subject—focused on increasing syringe exchanges. Advocates anticipated that favorable evaluations of syringe exchange programs would pave the way for federal funding and rapid expansion to meet the demand. This did not occur, however, despite growing evidence and additional endorsements by a varied set of individuals and professional associations.

Most research on SEPs had positive findings. Even if it was not really possible to untangle the causes and the effects, it appeared that SEPs had numerous benefits and relatively few drawbacks. Drug injectors made use of the exchanges, participants used new syringes, and participants returned the syringes they received; also, people who used the exchanges were less likely to become HIV positive.[89] And potential hazards—increases in drug use or violence—did not occur.[90] The policy was endorsed by the American Public Health Association, the American Bar Association, the American Medical Association, the Academy of Pediatrics, the American Nurses Association, the National Institutes of Health, the Association of State and Territorial Health Officers, and thirty-two drug researchers who had been studying the issue.[91] Eight major reports, including several released by the National Academy of Sciences, one created for the CDC in 1993, one GAO report, and a study done by the surgeon general in 2000 all supported the policy.[92]

Despite the evidence and elite support, President Clinton decided not to overturn a congressional ban on federal funding for SEPs. There was growing pressure to overturn the ban, and AIDS advocates became more optimistic. The National Coalition to Save Lives, a group that included ACT UP–Philadelphia, the North American Syringe Exchange Network, the Harm Reduction Coalition, and New York City–based organizations like the Latino Commission on AIDS,

Housing Works, and Exponents/ARRIVE put pressure on the administration.[93] A 1997 report issued by the U.S. Department of Health and Human Services observed that syringe exchange programs "can be an effective component of a comprehensive strategy to prevent HIV and other blood-borne infectious diseases in communities that choose to include them."[94] A demonstration at the Department of Health and Human Services in 1997 led to twelve arrests. The press estimated the crowd at two hundred, but the organizers claimed that more than six times as many people were present.[95]

The Clinton administration moved cautiously. The idea of providing federal funds for syringe exchanges moved onto the federal agenda in 1994, but, three years later, it was not included in the administration's six AIDS policy goals.[96] In addition to the political objections, the scientific evidence was not airtight. Of the forty-two studies published before 1999, "28 found positive effects associated with use of syringe exchange, two found negative associations, and 14 found either no association or a mix of positive and negative effects."[97] Few studies established causality, since a number of confounding factors, like the availability of syringes through pharmacies, could have influenced the results. Even if people did not share syringes, other practices increased HIV risk, like sharing equipment used to prepare and to split drugs.

The issue came to a head in April 1998. According to *Washington Post* reporters, the administration was about to announce an end to the ban, citing "airtight" evidence, but changed its mind at the last minute, opting to follow the lead of drug czar General Barry McCaffrey, who claimed that syringe exchange "sends the wrong message." Clinton was concerned that Congress might overturn his decision, and decided to change course. Shalala finessed the issue, announcing that the administration endorsed the concept of syringe exchanges but that the federal ban on funding would continue.[98] The following July, ten ACT UP members chained themselves to the furniture in the AIDS czar's office.[99] Clinton had another opportunity to end the ban on federal funding when a *Surgeon General's Report* in 2000 noted, "there is conclusive scientific evidence that needle exchange programs, as part of a comprehensive HIV prevention strategy, are an effective public health intervention."[100] Curiously, the strongest criticism of Clinton's decision came from the Congressional Black Caucus, which called SEPs "life-saving . . . a new tunnel to draw into treatment hard-core addicts who are often responsible for the relentless spread of AIDS in our community."[101]

Given the limited likelihood of expanded funding for SEPs under the current administration, it seems quite likely that they face limits on their growth. The actual number of SEPs has increased, and they rely on local funding and support from a number of private sources, including AmFar and a $1 million commitment from philanthropist George Soros. Public funding actually declined by 18 percent between 2000 and 2002.[102] The actual number of SEPs needed so that IDUs use a new syringe for each injection, as recommended by the CDC, would require the distribution of 1.2 and 1.6 billion syringes each year by between five thousand and ten thousand syringe exchanges.

A combination of lack of federal funding and divided public opinion meant that SEPs were unlikely to expand to meet demand. Although syringe exchanges have many benefits, since they provide a range of services and attract a self-selected group of addicts who inject more frequently, the exchanges could not meet the demand for sterile syringes without a major infusion of funds. The CDC's 1997 announcement that IDUs ought to use a new syringe for each injection would mean that a total of 1.2 and 1.6 billion syringes were required each year, and that between five and ten thousand syringe exchanges were needed.[103]

On a local level, there is also considerable community resistance to SEPs. Two boroughs in New York City, Queens and Staten Island, had no exchanges for a number of years, and, after a great deal of controversy, one was established in Queens in spring 2005; however, Staten Island continues to have no exchange. Even in neighborhoods where exchanges have been operating for a number of years, like the Lower East Side of Manhattan, community residents were critical of the policy, because they thought that the syringe exchange was a magnet for drug sales.[104] In addition, some people are concerned that the exchanges represented the beginning of a slippery slope since some of the supporters also advocate legalizing drugs.

Despite the growth of SEPs, only 2.5 percent of drug injectors had obtained their most recent needle from an exchange in 1995. This was far smaller than the 22 percent of injectors who had received it from someone else.[105] The overall impact of syringe exchanges in New York City was even lower. They provided less than 2 percent of the syringes that were needed for the city's addicts to have a new needle for each injection.[106] Large numbers of addicts still did not have access to sterile needles and were obtaining their needles from friends and from "the street." In fact, the most common source of syringes, for 38 percent (or one million) of the IDUs in the United States, was a pharmacy.[107]

The political history of the New York State bill that allowed over-the-counter sales of syringes and the distribution of syringes by health care providers has a great deal to do with the culture of New York's legislative politics, not only with the realization that the policy was needed. The state's legislature is tightly controlled; relatively few bills have hearings, and not one of the 11,474 bills that reached the floor between 1997 and 2001 was voted down. A recent study concluded that the legislature "systematically limits the roles played by rank-and-file legislators and members of the public in the legislative process."[108]

Convinced that there was a need to change state law, Richard Gottfried, chair of the State Assembly Health Committee began to introduce a bill allowing pharmacy sales every year, starting in 1991. Because of the institutional advocacy of staff in the AIDS Institute and support from an influential Republican state senator, the Republican governor, George Pataki, became highly committed to the bill. Widely circulated rumors attributed his support to financial contributions he allegedly received from a syringe manufacturer. One key informant rejected this interpretation and claimed that Pataki's support stemmed from his recognition of two pragmatic potential benefits of the policy: saving lives and reducing the ever-spiraling costs of HIV. The link between lack of access to syringes and HIV rates was extensively documented, and increasing access to syringes had a high cost-to-benefit ratio: rates were significantly lower in states and localities where syringes could be purchased in a pharmacy.[109]

By the time the New York State legislature voted on it, the policy was not as risky as in 1985. Since the beginning of the epidemic, eleven states deregulated the sale of syringes or decriminalized syringe possession.[110] Marshalling support from the Republican leadership, Pataki waited until a nonelection year and buried the legislation in the state budget. The potential for controversy was so great that the bill was printed without its Assembly sponsor, Richard Gottfried, knowing about it. In a late-night session with no debate in the Senate and heated debate in the Assembly, over-the-counter syringe sales—called the Expanded Syringe Access Program (ESAP)—became a temporary law in New York State. The bill decriminalized syringe possession and allowed adults to purchase up to ten syringes at once without a prescription, either from a pharmacy or from a health care provider. The bill also required that vendors accept used syringes. The policy was much more popular than syringe exchange programs: in 2000, six in ten Americans thought it would be a good idea if an IDU could purchase a syringe from a pharmacy or get a prescription for a syringe from a doctor.[111]

There were important barriers to the policy's implementation, especially significant resistance by pharmacists, who were critical to its success. Less than half of pharmacists in neighborhoods with high rates of drug use in New York City were willing to sell syringes to any IDU, but many more (72 percent) were willing to sell syringes to an IDU "with a referral card from an agency or clinic."[112] As a result of extensive outreach and collaboration with schools of pharmacy, professional societies, and local health departments by the state's health department, many pharmacies enrolled as providers, and barriers decreased. Pharmacists became more positive about the program and were more willing to sell syringes. Access was limited in some neighborhoods, and in some cases pharmacists required identification (which was not required in the law). Overall, the ESAP program was deemed successful and has been extended until 2007.[113]

Expanding over-the-counter sales is a viable policy because it reduces the incidence of HIV without expanding public costs, as it places the economic burden on the drug user. Syringes are relatively inexpensive, between two dollars and eight dollars for a package of ten.[114] By employing a public health approach allowing people to purchase syringes wherever they wish at whatever time of day they want, the ESAP approach expands access to syringes and destigmatizes the process of obtaining them.[115] Pharmacies are far more dispersed and accessible than needle exchanges; entering a pharmacy or even purchasing syringes in one is less stigmatizing than going to a needle exchange.

A broad range of factors led to the expansion of syringe availability, including a process of policy learning, the influence of activists and institutional advocates who carefully marshalled empirical data that responded to the objections of the policy's opponents. The decision to increase access to syringes was clearly influenced by activists and advocates, but was also based on another important calculus in the politics of AIDS: a desire to save lives. As the epidemic neared the beginning of its third decade, it was becoming increasingly clear that, despite the enormous gains in containing the epidemic, new prevention strategies were needed.

Chapter 10

HIV Stops with Me

We must eliminate the false dichotomy between civil liberties and public health.

—Stephen Joseph

We've analyzed this thing to death. We must move from mass analysis to mass action.

—Rev. Jesse Jackson

June 2001, the twentieth anniversary of the AIDS epidemic, was an occasion for journalists and public health officials to take stock of the epidemic's past and consider its future under a newly elected Republican president.[1] Over 775,000 people had been diagnosed with AIDS in the U.S.; 58 percent of them had died and between 800,000 and 900,000 people were living with HIV.[2] The number of new HIV infections each year had stabilized at 40,000, a significant reduction from an estimate of 150,000 in the late 1980s, but double what the CDC's 2001 strategic plan projected for 2005.[3] An article in the *MMWR* pointed out that "The twentieth year of AIDS is a milestone. . . . It is a time to remember persons who have become ill and died and to reflect on the progress made in both HIV prevention and treatment. A way to commemorate those persons who have died from AIDS is to accelerate efforts to stop HIV transmission. . . . New strategies are needed to maintain and accelerate progress in HIV prevention."[4]

That month, the CDC introduced a blueprint for reducing HIV transmission that focused on expanding HIV testing to reduce the number of people who were HIV-positive but were unaware of their serostatus, linking them to treatment, and reducing HIV transmission to their partners. This was a significant change in how people were approaching HIV prevention. As this policy evolved over the next several years, the AIDS community objected to the policy, to the process involved in its development, and to what it revealed about the changing political context.

The uncertainty of the epidemic's early years and the sense of panic during the late 1980s were replaced by a perception that the epidemic was changing in

177

many ways. Gay men and IDUs radically altered their behavior, the number of new AIDS cases declined, fewer people were dying, transmission rates declined, and people were living longer.[5] Newspapers were reporting fewer AIDS deaths, and media coverage declined.[6] People were no longer attending so many funerals and memorial services. The epidemic moved from center stage in the public mind to being one of a host of endemic, if not insoluble, social problems.

A posthumous article by reporter Jeffrey Schmaltz published in the *New York Times Magazine* in 1993 asked "Whatever Happened to AIDS?" The article pointed out that AIDS had been normalized, "part of the landscape. It is at once everywhere and nowhere. . . . The world is moving on."[7] Three years later, journalist Andrew Sullivan pointed out that, even though the plague was not over, "something profound has happened in these last months . . . H.I.V. infection is not just different in degree today than, say, five years ago. It is different in kind. It no longer signifies death. It merely signifies illness."[8] In a front-page article in the *Wall Street Journal*, David Sanford described his Lazarus-like experience as an early user of newly approved protease inhibitors—an image similar to the earlier description of AL721, but in this case not an illusion. Sanford "stopped the presses" on his obituary and gained back twenty-five pounds over ten months. In his view, "I am probably more likely to be hit by a truck than to die of AIDS."[9] In 1997, AIDS was no longer one of the ten major causes of death in the United States. The number of AIDS deaths declined 46 percent between 1996 and 1997.[10]

The decreased sense of urgency was accompanied by a decline in private funding. It was becoming harder for AIDS organizations to raise money from individual donors. GMHC's income plummeted from $29.5 million in 1996 to $19.4 million in 1999.[11] The impact of downsizing and restructuring was profound; one key staff member noted that not only was the organization's capacity decreased but "our soul was very injured."[12]

At the same time that some were envisioning its end if not its normalization, the epidemic was clearly not over. Longer life expectancy created a growing pool of people living with HIV, which meant that there were more people alive who could infect other people. In the last several years of the 1990s, news articles and research projects were reporting the continuation of, and a possible decrease in, condom use among men who had sex with other men including sex in public venues like bathhouses.[13] The safer-sex messages once so evident in gay communities were also less apparent. Fewer posters, brochures, and condoms were being distributed.[14] Being HIV-positive meant having a manageable illness that could be controlled with medications. Numerous observers noted that magazine ads for protease inhibitors, ads that were plastered all over subway stations and on bus shelters during the second half of the 1990s, provided an overly positive view of living with HIV: people skiing, climbing mountains, and declaring that they were feeling great. This created what playwright Harvey Fierstein called a "culture of disease," a situation in which efforts to reduce the negative connotations of HIV may have created a "generation embracing AIDS as its gay birthright." In contrast to these positive images, Fierstein pointed out, "AIDS is not fun. It's not sexy or manageable. . . . H.I.V. drugs can bring on heart, kidney, and liver disease. . . . Unlike the photos in the ads we see, most of my friends who are on the drug cocktails are not having the time of their lives. They spend mornings in the bathroom throwing up or suffering from diarrhea. They spend afternoons at doctor's appointments, clinics, and pharmacies."[15]

The declining death rate and the prospect of living with AIDS for a longer period of time changed the calculus of risk for many Americans, and led to a concern about HIV/AIDS complacency.[16] A small number of gay men reported that they were more willing to engage in risky sex without a condom since the introduction of new medications, because they believed that the treatments made them less infectious.[17] A growing body of research was also documenting that a large number of people who were HIV-positive did not know they were infected. Not only might they miss the chance to obtain adequate healthcare for themselves, they could infect other people.

After a rapid decline in the early years of the epidemic, the incidence of sexually transmitted diseases (STDs) began to rise in the mid-1990s.[18] There were new opportunities for risky sex, since some HIV-positive gay men were able to meet prospective partners over the internet and others were "barebacking," having sex without using a condom, and there was the thought that some men might be "bug chasers," taking risks in perhaps an unconscious or even conscious attempt to become HIV-positive.[19] Among IDUs, risky behavior continued even when syringes were readily available: an evaluation of ESAP indicated that only 47 percent of African American IDUs in Brooklyn and Queens reported having purchased at least one syringe from a pharmacy in the previous six months.[20]

It was also becoming clear that HIV prevention efforts were not having sufficient impact in communities of color. The prevalence of HIV among black and Latino men and women was alarmingly high. Between 1985 and 2001, blacks moved from being one quarter of all AIDS cases to half of new HIV cases. One in 50 black men and one in 160 black women were HIV-positive. In contrast, the rate for white women was one in 3,000. The differential in prevalence rates was striking: it was five times higher among blacks than whites in 1991, and thirteen times higher in 2001.[21] In the 1980s, a majority of HIV-positive women had been infected through their own drug use; by the end of the century, most had been infected by a sexual partner.[22] The prospect of new infections, re-infection, or "superinfections" led many to conclude that, even though the strategies used to fight HIV had been effective—providing information, encouraging men to use condoms, holding safer sex workshops—new approaches were needed, especially among young men of color who had sex with other men. The executive director of Bronx AIDS Services pointed out, in 1997, that "AIDS education as we have done it traditionally is basically a failure. . . . We have a huge problem getting people to take it seriously. For many young people in the Bronx, the threat of AIDS is part of a whole constellation of problems that they just have to deal with . . . AIDS is just another one of the things that is likely to get you."[23] New methods of fighting AIDS were needed. A series of parallel developments became part of this rethinking.

A case in upstate New York created enormous alarm about the potential spread of HIV, and served as a focusing event crystallizing the need for changes in public health policy in New York State.[24] In 1997, Nushawn Williams, an African American man from Brooklyn, was alleged to have infected between ten and thirteen women in the small upstate city where he was living.[25] Following the lead of public health officials in twenty-nine other states, and facing the opposition of many organizations in the AIDS community, the New York State legislature passed the HIV Reporting and Partner Notification Act in July 1998, which took effect two years later.[26] The law required mandatory reporting of the names of people with HIV infection, HIV-related illnesses, and AIDS by physicians and other medical providers. Individuals with HIV or AIDS would be asked to identify the names of their sexual and needle-sharing partners, and either the Health Department or the individual would contact them.[27] GMHC supported the HIV reporting portion of the act because of the need to have more accurate information about HIV, not only about AIDS, to plan prevention and services, but only if unique identifiers, not names, were used.[28] Other groups, like Housing Works, called the legislation intrusive and coercive, claiming that "HIV name reporting will deter people from testing [and] will not produce the accurate data that are needed."[29] After the law was passed, Housing Works called upon "everyone to take the pledge to participate in civil noncompliance."[30]

The AIDS community had long resisted such laws because of fears that name reporting would lead to breaches of confidentiality and to discrimination, and would drive people away from the health care system. In fact, New

York State began using names in tracking AIDS cases in 1985 "with no known breaches of confidentiality."[31] Lawrence Gostin, a researcher and member of the CDC's advisory committee, pointed out that "Partner notification is the one thing that the AIDS community deeply fears, that intimate sexual partners will be talked to and that their names will be given to the government."[32] But he thought the time right for HIV name reporting because the epidemic had changed. In a 1998 article, he and a coauthor stated:

> We have long opposed named HIV reporting for many of the same reasons offered by the community of persons living with HIV/AIDS. HIV infection, however, was at one time quite distinct from other infectious diseases. There were strong and justifiable reasons for rejecting named reporting: HIV infection was not transmissible through the air like tuberculosis; it was not treatable like hepatitis; and persons could not be rendered non-infectious as they could with syphilis or gonorrhea. HIV/AIDS was also unique because it engendered the kinds of fear and associated discrimination that demanded privacy and respect for human rights. We have changed our mind about named HIV reporting, not because we have changed, but because the epidemic has changed. We value civil liberties but, perhaps more important, we value the health and lives of persons living with HIV/AIDS.[33]

New York's changed position on HIV reporting and partner notification was consistent with a nationwide trend in which more states were instituting traditional public health measures for HIV. This marked a shift away from a strategy that Ronald Bayer labeled AIDS exceptionalism. During the first several years of the epidemic, the gay community's fear that AIDS might serve as a pretext for discrimination had led to its opposition to standard public health procedures for sexually transmitted diseases—procedures like mass screening, HIV testing, and partner notification. When, in that period, President Reagan and Vice President Bush suggested that large numbers of people should be tested for HIV, they were "booed and hissed" at the Third International Conference on AIDS (Bush) and a dinner for AmFar (Reagan).[34] Some CDC officials recommended contact tracing and mass HIV testing, but these positions were not seriously considered because they seemed anachronistic and ineffective.[35] For the first several years after the procedure was licensed, gay men were urged not to take the HIV test—a position that changed once there were legal protections against discrimination, and once research documented that early intervention in HIV illness could slow down the progression of the disease.[36]

The AIDS community's claim that standard public health methods would drive people underground made contact tracing seem infeasible.[37] The association of some traditional public health measures with the extreme Right and a lack of consensus among public health officials also trumped serious consideration of these methods. At the end of 1988, only eleven states had instituted contact tracing.[38]

The strongest voices in favor of standard public health measures conflated these recommendations with moralistic views of the epidemic, or extreme suggestions like William Buckley's idea of tattooing people who were HIV-positive. An article coauthored by Congressman William Dannemeyer concluded that the "education-only" public health approach to the epidemic "has failed miserably with respect to the urban underclass, the second wave of the AIDS epidemic."[39] Dannemeyer's political capital was greatly affected by his other extreme positions, including support for quarantine, massive HIV testing, banning children with AIDS from school, and criminalizing blood donations by gay men. He routinely criticized the morality and the lifestyles of gay men, proposing that they abstain from sex, recommended the expulsion of a gay congressman, and stated that "A whole political movement has been created and sustained on a single notion: sodomy." He had also suggested, in 1988 when the evidence for HIV transmission was quite clear, that it was possible that "deep kissing might transmit AIDS."[40] The association of traditional public health measures with figures like Dannemeyer and Senator Jesse Helms reinforced the AIDS community's contention that there was a need for exceptional measures to protect the civil liberties of people with HIV.

Organizations representing public health officials, including the Association of State and Territorial Health Officials and the National Association of County Health Officials, did not support mandatory partner notification.[41] Even a proposal to notify people whose partners had died was described as "treacherous terrain" potentially violating "rights of privacy of the deceased and family members," by Thomas Stoddard of the Lambda Legal Defense Fund.[42] New York Health Commissioner Steven Joseph was vilified by ACT UP for his support of partner notification; he noted, in a memoir of these years, that "AIDS is the first major public health issue in this century for which political values rather than health requirements set the agenda. The political definition of the epidemic—defined first by gay men and later modified by a stream of civil libertarians and political spokesmen—drove and determined the medical and public health response until well after the epidemic was in full flower."[43] When the New York City Board of Health requested that the state allow it to do name reporting for contact tracing, Tim Sweeney, from GMHC, argued that "it's not going to bring people into the health system, but will in fact drive them away."[44]

In 1991, Ronald Bayer offered a prophetic analysis of the politics of AIDS, noting that the "potency" of the "alliance" that originally supported AIDS exceptionalism had "begun to wane," and that the initiation of classical public health measures—testing and screening, name reporting, partner notification, and even quarantine—were being recommended by public health and medical professionals because of the changing face of AIDS and "notable advances in therapeutic prospects."[45] Over the course of the 1990s, it became apparent that there were at least two other reasons for questioning AIDS exceptionalism: a significant proportion of HIV-positive people were not being tested, and more women were being infected by partners who either did not say or did not know that they were HIV-positive.[46]

State legislatures were becoming more concerned about protecting the public from infection while maintaining the civil liberties of people with HIV. Some viewed the new laws as the result of a backlash, though others, including the Queens congressman who sponsored a federal HIV partner notification law, pointed out that "advocates had put aside public health concerns for too long."[47] With the recognition that giving pregnant mothers AZT would reduce perinatal transmission, the CDC recommended in 1995 that HIV testing be a routine part of all prenatal care. The 1996 reauthorization of the Ryan White CARE Act required states to engage in "good faith efforts" to notify the spouses of HIV-positive people of possible exposure, to demonstrate reductions in perinatal AIDS cases, to provide HIV testing of 95 percent of women receiving prenatal care, and to have mandatory testing of newborns whose mothers who had not been tested.[48] In 1997, New York State began reporting the test results for all newborns, another policy that was implemented after several years of discussion and against the judgment of some organizations in the AIDS community, including the HIV Law Project.[49] A larger proportion of women opted for voluntary prenatal HIV testing after the law was passed (83 percent) than before (74 percent), and there was no evidence that HIV testing was a deterrent to receiving medical care.[50]

Some members of the AIDS community continued to oppose standard public health strategies. Ravinia Hayes-Cozier of the Harlem Directors Group called New York's passage of a partner notification law a "quick fix solution, the offspring of a dangerous combination: election year politics and editorial-board-driven policy proposals."[51] Critics of partner notification claimed that it would subject women to physical violence.[52] Chris Norwood supported contact tracing; she pointed out, "It is unprecedented in modern health history to know so absolutely that literally thousands of people are at risk of a fatal disease and not take ordinary public health measures which can significantly slow its spread."[53] Norwood noted that 18,000 people learned that they were HIV-positive but only 359 partners were notified in 1993. This was troubling because "in the bleak disparity between these two numbers are literally thousands of lives that should haunt us all." Norwood also observed that many of the people involved in the "changing face of AIDS" had different needs, "a real hunger" for the kinds of services associated with standard partner notification and wanted "the state to supply the processes, counseling, and public health personnel for notification to proceed as a *universal service.*"[54]

There was little published empirical data on people's attitudes toward public health practices. Dannemeyer made reference to studies of methadone clients at Greenwich House and Harlem Hospital who "strongly supported traditional public-health measures to control contagious diseases," measures such as routine voluntary testing and even mandatory testing and partner notification, but he was not specific about the source of these data.[55] Another study, based on focus groups and personal interviews with fifty-seven people, including drug users, counselors, and clients in methadone programs, counselors in a sexually transmitted disease clinic, and nine experts in HIV partner notification and substance abuse prevention and treatment, noted, "although drug users are critical of existing partner notification programmes, most acknowledge the need for this type of intervention and are willing to participate as long as it is completely voluntary.[56]

In the wake of the Nushawn Williams case and reports of a resurgence of risky sex, there was increasing interest in rethinking HIV prevention. A number of government agencies began moving in the direction of prevention for positives, including an NIH Consensus Conference Panel that recommended more funding for research on effective prevention strategies for HIV-positive people.[57] A CDC-initiated Institute of Medicine (IOM) panel, charged to develop "a visionary framework for effective HIV prevention," also supported prevention for positives, noting that "Every new HIV infection begins with someone who is already infected—yet current prevention programs do not emphasize directing prevention to individuals who are HIV-infected and who may still engage in risky behavior."[58] The CDC started an internal review of its programs toward the end of 1998, brought together "external collaborative partners, expert academicians, and organizational representatives" in early 2000, and issued a strategic plan in January 2001 that pointed out that the forty thousand new infections each year was *"unacceptably high"* and that "A new strategic plan for HIV prevention and control is timely and essential," setting a goal of reducing the number of new infections by half and eliminating racial and ethnic disparities.[59]

Three articles by CDC staff in June 2001 issues of the *American Journal of Public Health* and the *MMWR* described the rationale and features of another policy initiative. An article called "Are We Headed for a Resurgence of the HIV Epidemic among Men Who Have Sex with Men?" noted that there was "the potential for a resurgence in HIV infections among MSM" because of a rise in STDs and in unprotected anal sex.[60] Additional confirmation of this disturbing trend appeared in a brief analysis of a study of young men (ages 15 and 22) in seven cities, which documented a "high prevalence of HIV and associated risks" and suggested a "resurgent MSM epidemic among young MSM."[61]

The third article outlined a policy model to respond to these trends, a Serostatus Approach to Fighting the Epidemic ("SAFE") model involving five steps: increasing the number of positives who knew their HIV status; increasing their "use of health care and preventive services;" "high quality care and treatment;" improving "adherence to therapy by individuals with HIV;" and expanding "the number of individuals with HIV who adopt and sustain HIV-STD risk reduction behavior."[62] The program would also include referrals to prevention programs for "High-risk individuals who test negative, particularly those whose partners are living with HIV."[63]

This was a new approach, since HIV prevention programs had "historically been based on behavioral risk factors and demographic characteristics." One third of states and cities applying for CDC funding in the late 1990s specifically mentioned that they included HIV-positive people as a priority. The SAFE strategy was already being tested in a Primary HIV Prevention for HIV-Positive Persons project that had begun in 1999 in San Francisco, Los Angeles County, Wisconsin, and Maryland.[64]

Pilot efforts to rethink prevention strategies included funding for "HIV Stops with Me," a social-marketing initiative by an advertising agency working closely with a community advisory board and with community-based organizations in San Francisco and Los Angeles.[65] A key element of the campaign was to identify and reach unknowing positives and to "support positive people in reducing their risk of infecting others while leading full, healthy, and (if desired!) lusty lives." It used television commercials, distributed postcards in doctors offices, and developed print advertising, public relations, and outreach measures. Working with a number of organizations, like the Stop AIDS Project, B.A.Y. Positives, and the AIDS Health Project in San Francisco, as well as Being Alive–Los Angeles, the Gay and Lesbian Center and Being Alive–Long Beach, and the Minority AIDS Project in Los Angeles, the project was intended to "help build a culture in which it is the norm for HIV+ people to take responsibility for preventing new HIV infections in sexual and needle sharing partners."[66]

The plan also built on the work of a number of other programs and ideas generated in 2000 at a conference, "Designing Primary Prevention for People Living with HIV," at the University of California, San Francisco. The conference presenters and attendees included representatives of several AIDS organizations (the National Association of Persons with AIDS, ACT UP–Golden Gate, and STOP AIDS–San Francisco), along with public health officials and researchers. There were presentations and discussions of ongoing research projects and prevention for positives programs at AID Atlanta, AIDS Action in Boston, and CDC-funded prevention case management programs. The conference proceedings noted that "There is an urgent need—and sufficient expertise—to move forward with prevention campaigns focused on helping people living with HIV and AIDS avoid passing their infection along to others."[67]

The idea of expanding prevention for positives was gaining momentum, but funding was limited; the CDC spent $3.8 million in 2002.[68] Refocusing of HIV prevention moved to a new stage in April 2003 when the CDC announced Advancing HIV Prevention (AHP). Several developments in the previous two years led to this new proposal.

First was a transition to a presidential administration with a more conservative political agenda. The CDC's new director, Julie Gerberding, was about to embark on a major restructuring of the CDC, reducing administrative costs by $83 million, directing these savings to "frontline projects," and eliminating redundancy by "consolidating our 40 separate information hotlines into a single hotline."[69]

Two important trends in the epidemic were also related to AHP. The number of newly reported AIDS cases increased in 2001, the first time this had occurred since 1993.[70] HIV incidence was declining among injecting drug users and, even though they and their sexual partners comprised one third of all new HIV cases, this decline, in combination with a continuing increase in STD that was "almost exclusive among" MSM (a bellwether of continued risky sexual behavior), meant that rethinking HIV prevention was more urgent than in 2001.[71] And CDC officials were realizing that their target of reducing new HIV infections by half was not realistic.[72]

There was also an important change in medical technology. The AHP announcement noted that the existence of a "simple rapid HIV test . . . creates an opportunity to overcome some of the traditional barriers to early diagnosis and treatment of infected persons." Since nearly one third of HIV positive people did not return to learn the results when conventional tests were used, the rapid test, which provided results in twenty minutes, would increase the efficiency of HIV testing.[73] In addition, research demonstrated that condom use with partners who knew they were HIV-negative ranged between 78 percent and 96 percent, higher than with partners who did not know their serostatus.[74]

Four key strategies were outlined in the plan: "Make HIV testing a routine part of medical care"; "implement new models for diagnosing HIV infections outside medical settings"; "Prevent new infections by working with persons diagnosed with HIV and their partners"; and "Further decrease perinatal HIV transmission."[75] AHP was similar to SAFE in placing an emphasis on decreasing the number of unknowing positives, but it was much more specifically focused on people who were HIV-positive, making the proposal highly contentious.

The AIDS community's reaction to AHP was generally negative. When CDC and other public health officials and representatives of AIDS organizations met at the CDC's National HIV Prevention Conference in July, about 250 people caucused to discuss their criticisms and concerns.[76] CDC officials organized a series of meetings with members of the community afterward as "outreach to better explain what we're doing."[77]

One major concern was that the plan implied that funding for primary prevention for HIV-negative people was about to be reduced, and, according to a New York AIDS Coalition report, "Many hold that the failure to reach out to this population will cause a spike in infections."[78] Although the CDC claimed that the elements of the approach had been discussed, funded, and written about for several years, the AIDS community felt that the overall plan was a surprise and that the new guidelines were developed without the participation of "the community." The National Association of Persons with AIDS charged that "the CDC has NEVER convened any formal consultation with representatives of the diverse community of people living with HIV/AIDS. . . . Such a failure to involve positive people in shaping this important initiative can only add to the fears of many that rather than 'working with' us this will turn out to be something done to us."[79] They believed that the plan was developed by public health professionals and overlooked the important role of another group of experts, the consumers. One person at the 2003 CDC conference noted, "The community feels that we have rolled back to the era of Ronald Reagan when the government ignored this epidemic and did not talk to the people most affected by this disease."[80]

The response to two speakers at the closing session of a CDC prevention conference in July 2003 suggests additional reasons for the AIDS community's negative reaction to AHP. Attendees applauded former CDC researcher David Holtgrave, who called for $300 million more each year in prevention funding and charged that the government's unwillingness to fund science-based prevention programs was "public health malpractice."[81] The very presence of the other speaker, Deputy Secretary of Health and Human Services Claude Allen, a last-minute substitute for the CDC's director, was found objectionable. A former press secretary to Senator Jesse Helms, Allen was "a widely known opponent of comprehensive AIDS prevention" and a supporter of abstinence-only sex education. During his speech, thousands of participants stood up and held signs that said "Stop the War on HIV Prevention."[82] The contrast was striking: Holtgrave stressed the need for more resources while Allen symbolized an approach to public policy focused on "the strategic use of resources" and a moral agenda associated with the political right.

Holtgrave's call for more funds was consistent with central principles of the AIDS community: that more money was needed, and that, despite previous funding increases, resources were inadequate. The administration's commitment to targeting resources more effectively was contrary to this view. The AIDS community also viewed AHP as a political, not a scientific, decision, part of a shift to the right in the political climate, and a sign that the administration was not applying its standard of "compassionate conservatism" to domestic AIDS policy. AHP and Claude Allen's presence at the July 2003 CDC Prevention Conference were symptomatic of the growing dominance of political conservatives, who, the AIDS community claimed, were more concerned about traditional notions of morality than about public health. AIDS advocates strenuously objected to federal support for abstinence-only education, the George W. Bush administration's commitment to expanding funding for faith-based organizations, and the fact that the CDC's website pointed to the importance of abstinence and monogamy, rather than condom use, as "the most reliable ways to avoid becoming infected with or transmitting HIV."[83] ACT UP detailed a series of examples of the Bush administration's poor record, including flat funding for HIV programs, the AHP initiative, a proposal to block-grant Medicaid funding, efforts to "undermine confidence in the effectiveness of condoms," and audits of HIV prevention programs that, the group believed, were politically motivated.[84]

In addition to reflecting a rightward turn, AHP and other CDC policies challenged the AIDS community's autonomy in designing and implementing programs. GMHC's Ron Johnson pointed out "When 70 percent of new HIV infections in the country are among people of color, it's more important than ever to empower those most at risk to decide what will work and how it will be implemented."[85] Efforts at government accountability and oversight were framed as political acts by a conservative administration. Soon after the announcement of AHP, federal officials told San Francisco's STOP AIDS Project not to use federal funds for programs that promoted sexual activity contrary to federal policy. This determination was the result of a nearly two-year investigation involving a review of the organization's activities. The executive director of the National Association of People with AIDS labeled this move the work of "right-wing jihadists." Critics claimed that the CDC was bowing to the pressure of Representative Mark Souder, who initiated the review. Souder's spokesperson replied that Souder was not interested in obscenity but, rather, "We'd like to know why we should continue to fund the same programs if there is no proof they're actually working."[86] Several days later, the CDC proposed that all educational materials on the internet would require approval to determine if statements were "medically accurate" about "the effectiveness of condoms in preventing sexually transmitted diseases."[87]

The AIDS community was alarmed that AHP, designed as part of a move to create a more cost-effective approach to HIV prevention, might offer the promise of reducing if not dismantling the labor-intensive work of AIDS prevention, work that stressed the need for pre- and post-test counseling, often on a one-on-one basis, for everyone who chose to be tested. Public health officials, like New York City Health Commissioner Thomas Frieden, thought that HIV prevention could be handled like other diseases, since "an hour of counseling is not needed for a cholesterol check."[88] Rethinking HIV prevention might mean that funding could be redirected, and organizations would have to downsize. A letter from NORA to the CDC's director of HIV/AIDS prevention pointed out, "Organizations must not be forced to scale-back or cut other programs that they know to be effective in order to meet the CDC's new goals."[89]

In fact, there was a gap in scientific information on the dynamics of HIV disclosure and risk taking. Although it was clear that a large proportion of HIV-positive people took steps to protect their partners, more needed to be known since simply learning one's HIV status did not necessarily lead to radical changes in behavior.[90] The first empirical study of whether or not HIV-positive men disclosed their status to their sexual partners was published in 2003. Its authors, Robert Klitzman and Ronald Bayer, revealed that even among people actively engaged in the AIDS community who were employees of HIV organizations, nondisclosure was common and, at minimum, one third of the gay men in the small sample studied actually lied about their serostatus. People almost always told their long-term partners, but this was not the case for more casual or fleeting encounters.[91]

The AIDS community was also critical of the AHP's focus on HIV-positive people because it ran contrary to a central tenet that everyone was at risk and that prevention efforts needed to be broadly directed. Prevention education had primarily taught people to protect themselves, perhaps because it was thought that they had a greater stake than those already positive. The principles of voluntarism, individual freedom, and civil liberties were articles of faith in the AIDS community, which, from the earliest days of the epidemic, had been reluctant to preach about sexual restraint or abstinence (see chapter 3).

A small but vocal minority in the AIDS community had pointed to the need for HIV-positive people to exercise restraint and alter their behavior. Larry Kramer took this position, and so did Michael Callen and Richard Berkowitz, the inventors of safe sex, who pointed out emphatically in "How to Have Sex in an Epidemic" that "WE BELIEVE THAT AIDS PATIENTS HAVE AN ETHICAL OBLIGATION TO ADVISE POTENTIAL PARTNERS OF THEIR HEALTH STATUS."[92] In early 1993, the AIDS Action Council's Jeffrey Levi noted that changing the norms of the community was a "piece" that had been "woefully missing since the beginning of the epidemic."[93] In the late 1990s, a group called Sex Panic attracted about fifty people to its regular meetings in New York. The group challenged the "reactionary" position of a "new gay right" that included well-known authors like Kramer and Andrew Sullivan who "make the fundamentalist argument that AIDS is nature's revenge on gay men."[94] Emphasizing sexual restraint was associated with the kind of extreme positions taken by political conservatives like William Dannemeyer who stressed that the epidemic was the result of sexual mores that had strayed from the ideals of monogamy and sexual fidelity.[95]

AHP was also problematic in that it would target resources. A 1993 National Academy of Sciences report on the social impact of the AIDS epidemic took issue with the conventional wisdom that everyone was at risk, since

The convergence of evidence shows that the HIV/AIDS epidemic is settling into spatially and socially isolated groups and possibly becoming endemic within them. Many observers have recently commented that, instead of spreading out to the broad American population, as was once feared, HIV is concentrating in pools of persons who are also caught in the "synergism of plagues": poverty, poor health and lack of health care, inadequate education, joblessness, hopelessness, and social disintegration converge to ravage personal and social life; . . . many geographical areas and strata of the population are virtually untouched by the epidemic and probably never will be; certain confined areas and populations have been devastated and are likely to continue to be.[96]

The report's recommendation that resources ought to be targeted toward high-risk communities challenged a paradoxical aspect of AIDS policy. On the one hand, the assertion that everyone was at risk meant that prevention was directed widely rather than targeted toward those with the greatest chances of contracting HIV, especially since targeting resources might marginalize and stigmatize people and communities that were at high risk. On the other hand, numerous resources had been specifically directed toward people with HIV, who were in effect being targeted for special funds. Although the move was not called targeting, framing Ryan White Funding as disaster relief meant that funds *were* based on objective measures of which communities were hardest hit. In addition, people with HIV had access to health benefits, like prescription coverage through the ADAP program, that people with other diseases did not.

Two institutional advocates, June Osborne and David Rogers, the co-chairs of the National AIDS Commission, criticized the National Research Council's report, noting that targeting would lead "the vast majority of people outside those specific neighborhoods to deny the epidemic's threat, ignore the need for their own preventive actions, and thus accelerate the virus' spread through all segments of the society."[97] When asked about the idea of directing efforts to particular racial groups, Stephen Joseph replied that "I have no sensitivity about raising the issue of race but I don't agree that it's the place to focus attention. You need to understand the demographics of an epidemic in order to target resources. But it would be counterproductive from a public health point of view to see AIDS as a disease of one racial or ethnic group. It's a color blind message we want to get across. Anybody who engages in risky behavior is at risk."[98] Charles Caulfield took a more extreme position. He labeled the idea of directing resources as "zip code genocide" and asked "Are we to assume that these groups, potentially identified by their zip codes, whether infected or not, will not suffer decreases in the values of their houses, rejection of insurance coverage, difficulty finding employment, and other ostracization?" and that infected people living in such areas might be "allowed, perhaps assisted, to die out[?]"[99]

Minority organizations were less critical of AHP than were other voices in the AIDS community. Among the minority organizations, the idea of directing resources where they were most needed was no longer contentious or viewed

as "zip code genocide." In fact, minority AIDS organizations had long complained that they were not getting their fair share of AIDS funding in comparison to organizations founded by gay men, who were the first at the "table."
At a 1985 conference, "The Economics of AIDS: Blacks and Gays Competing
for a Shrinking Pie," one speaker stated, "The word in the black community
is that white gay men are getting the funding, while the number of black AIDS
patients skyrockets."[100] Leaders of African American and Latino AIDS organizations and some political leaders were critical of the distribution of funding,
noting that the gay community was more articulate, had more access to politicians, and was better organized. Enoch Williams, chair of the Health Committee of the New York City Council, had pointed out in 1992 that "it is clear that
the resources available to battle this epidemic must be shifted to where the
problem is worst. And here in New York City that means that black and Latino
community agencies must begin to get more of the limited resources that are
being distributed."[101] A 2001 study done by Housing Works found that 80 percent of people living with HIV were black or Hispanic but only 30 percent of
state funding went to organizations these minorities controlled.[102] There were
also geographic inequities. Services and funding continued to be concentrated
in Manhattan while the epidemic expanded in the city's outer boroughs. A
coalition representing organizations in the 718 area code—which comprised
all boroughs outside Manhattan—noted that, even though two thirds of adults
and nearly nine in ten children were outside Manhattan, they were not receiving an adequate portion of public funds, and noted, for example, that the state
spent 250 percent more on Manhattan programs than for programs in other
boroughs. This was also true for private funding, since only 30 percent of
funds from the New York City AIDS Fund went to organizations outside of
Manhattan.[103]

The Minority AIDS Initiative, spearheaded by the Congressional Black
Caucus, was a national effort to direct funds to the communities where they
were most needed. The idea of allocating funds to hard-hit communities without committing zip code genocide became even more urgent with the recognition that class, racial, and neighborhood effects created health disparities and
affected communities' well-being and ability to be economically productive.[104]

The National Minority AIDS Council (NMAC) was critical but also supportive of AHP. It questioned whether AHP would achieve its goals by
expanding testing without counseling, and without considering the stigma
associated with the disease. NMAC recognized, however, that AHP's goals
were consistent with the CDC's 2001 strategic plan, which NMAC had "played
an active role in developing." African American organizations became com-

mitted to AHP's goals and were active participants in expanding HIV testing. NMAC was a cosponsor of the CDC's annual National HIV Testing Day. Balm in Gilead, a faith-based group headquartered in New York, also coordinated its 2005 "Our Church Lights the Way" effort with this event, stating "we need all of our churches to light the way on HIV testing. . . . Help us save the lives of our people . . . HIV/AIDS is seeking to destroy all of us. However, we can stop this virus. . . . And we must support and embrace all of our family members who are affected." [105] Community-based organizations like Harlem United began to include prevention for positives into their programming.[106] African American leaders like Jesse Jackson promoted HIV testing, and Beny Primm observed, "The key to stemming the tide of this epidemic is to know your status as to whether you are HIV-positive. And if you are, to get into treatment and to practice safe sex. . . . And be monogamous."[107]

The objections to Advancing HIV Prevention were not sustained, and the idea of doing prevention with positives became central to HIV prevention. The CDC responded to criticisms by framing the plan as "a component of CDC's overall prevention portfolio."[108] In the first round of prevention funding after AHP was introduced, $23 million went to prevention for positives, $14 million was for counseling and testing, and $12 million was earmarked for outreach and education. An overwhelming portion—82 percent—targeted minorities. The earlier concern that some organizations would have their funding eliminated or reduced was correct. Two thirds of the organizations that received CDC funding did not receive support under the first round of AHP grants— among these, the STOP AIDS Project of San Francisco.[109]

Local and national public health officials had successfully shifted the paradigm for HIV prevention. New York State successfully implemented partner notification with little resistance from individuals or organizations.[110] The New York State AIDS Institute assessed its programs and reexamined its priorities in line with the "prevention with positives" approach.[111] The New York City Commission on AIDS 2005 report included several recommendations that indicate a commitment to mainstreaming HIV, including an expansion of prevention with positives, partner notification, and counseling programs, and supported "making HIV testing an integrated part of normal medical care." The report recommended "citiwide availability of HIV testing, especially rapid tests, in venues where high-risk populations can be found."[112] The city's department of health took steps to promote HIV testing in jails and in STD clinics, where more than half of the patients were not tested for HIV, but where, when they were, two thirds were discovered to be HIV-positive.[113] Public health officials thought that HIV testing ought to be a routine part of health care encounters, including emergency room visits and public hospital admissions. The health department also made a renewed commitment to broad distribution of condoms.[114]

HIV testing began to be introduced in places for people at high risk, but also in more pedestrian locations like the Six Flags amusement park in Dallas and the annual conventions of the Southern Christian Leadership Conference and the NAACP[115] For public health officials, AIDS prevention and treatment were a critical part of improving the health of citizens and were becoming mainstreamed into public health and health care. Local health departments and community organizations faced new challenges in counseling people who tested positive, since doctors who often had a high volume of patients were not able to take much time to counsel people who tested positive.[116]

In contrast to the initial development of safe sex, where the AIDS community took the lead, the AHP policy was designed by professionals. The AIDS community had moved from actively participating in creating new health policy paradigms to being consulted. Its place at the table had changed, as the nation moved from a concern with fighting the epidemic to reducing health disparities and directing public resources to where government officials determined they were needed.

Chapter 11

The Politics of Disease

We changed the course of the disease.

—Jeff Getty, AIDS Activist

This history of New York's AIDS community has traced its beginnings from the living rooms of its creators to various "tables" of decision making. It has considered several factors that had an impact on AIDS policy.

The first was the work of the AIDS community, which mapped out a response to the epidemic creating ideas, programs, and new organizations. A central feature of this community was that people were fighting for their lives and the lives of their friends and family, in the hope that more money, better access to medical care, and faster drug approval would prolong lives and lead to a cure. The community effectively deployed outsider and insider strategies and leveraged support from elected and appointed officials and elite allies.[1]

As the epidemic expanded, the second factor—the limitations of the voluntary sector and the need for a major infusion of public funding—became apparent, with the realization that AIDS was enmeshed with other urban problems threatening the viability of numerous cities as centers of commerce.

A third and equally important factor was the AIDS community's collective action frame. This community employed a powerful rhetoric that resonated with a central element in American culture, the tendency to allocate public resources to save lives.[2] At a time when most people lived well into their seventies, the shock of large numbers of people dying at young ages, and the surprise that diseases are still sometimes uncontrollable, made the politics of AIDS distinctive.

Numerous observers, dating back to de Tocqueville, have described the critical role of organizations and associations in building civil society and promoting democracy in the United States. Social and religious organizations have an important political role: they build social capital that, in turn, promotes civic engagement.[3] Citizen groups engage in a complex bargaining process with government and the corporate sector. The AIDS community's work is part of this longer political tradition. Self-help, social, service, and political organizations in the AIDS community relied on varied strategies (what Tarrow has called repertoires of contention), like civil disobedience, demonstrating and marching, writing letters, lobbying, and participating in advisory groups, to make issues vivid, urgent, and requiring a response.

The work of the AIDS community reflects an important trend in American life: an increase in the number of political organizations, particularly a rise in health advocacy groups, a growth that has been described as an advocacy explosion.[4] It is not clear, however, that the expansion in the number of nonprofit associations and advocacy organizations has promoted a higher level of citizen participation in the policy process. Advocacy work has been professionalized, and citizen participation is sometimes passive, limited to writing a check, rather than active involvement such as attending meetings, writing letters, or lobbying.[5] Some advocacy groups rely on patrons, like foundations and corporations, rather than on members.[6] Professional lobbyists have become an important force in American political life, especially in health policy, and much political advocacy is dominated by business interests rather than by the concerns of citizens. Between 1995 and 2005, the number of registered lobbyists more than doubled, and the greatest amount of money spent on lobbying was for health care.[7] The sharp rise in the number of paid lobbyists may mean that the growth of civil society organizations has some built-in inequities, privileging some groups and forwarding the interests of some citizens, but not of others. As E. E. Schneitschneider observed in *The Semisoverign People,* "the flaw in the pluralist heaven is that the heavenly chorus sings with an upper class accent."[8]

Just as the number of nonprofit organizations has increased, so too has the number of health- and disease-related organizations. Many of these organizations are what Deborah Minkoff calls "hybrid" organizations, since they provide information, advice, and services but also engage in advocacy and lobbying. Organizations serve and represent the interests of health consumers with the same disease, patients with common concerns (like those of the terminally ill), and caregivers. The actual or even estimated number of such groups has yet to be quantified.

Journalists and scholars claim that AIDS activism is distinctive and represents the beginning of a higher level of citizen involvement in health advocacy. They also point out that organizations for people with other diseases, most notably breast cancer, have modeled themselves after the AIDS community.[9]

The AIDS community is, in fact, distinctive in one very important way: it has addressed a much broader range of policy issues than other health and social movement organizations. But, the idea that the AIDS community's efforts are completely new overlooks several important past precedents.

In the 1970s, cancer patients, like AIDS patients later, traveled abroad for treatment, and pressured twenty-three state legislatures to legalize laetrile, a drug once viewed as promising but never approved. The Committee for Freedom of Choice in Cancer Therapy, which was involved in trying to legalize the drug, claimed thirty-five thousand members.[10] After a decade-long debate involving a small but influential group of advocates, Congress extended Medicare coverage to people with End-Stage Renal Disease in 1972. Advocates had successfully collaborated with journalists to tell their stories and one patient had himself dialyzed in front of a congressional committee, "a demonstration which apparently contributed to the willingness of Representative Wilbur Mills to support a kidney disease amendment to Medicare."[11] Another example of disease-related advocacy that predated AIDS was the passage of the Orphan Drug Act which was influenced by a coalition called the National Organization for Rare Disorders.[12] Finally, an alliance of "scientists, representatives of government agencies, patrons, the media, and members of the general public" joined with other advocates to lobby for research on Alzheimer's disease, and the Alzheimer's Disease and Related Disorders Foundation "kept the issue of Alzheimer's disease in the public consciousness and helped to recruit new allies to the cause."[13] Even though AIDS advocacy and activism is, therefore, not altogether new, it is an important example of certain major trends in policymaking—growing professionalization, and the fact that more association and advocacy groups are mounting public protests, a strategy associated with social movements and the disadvantaged.[14]

The nature of the AIDS community has shifted. In the first several years of the epidemic, it was actively involved in generating new ideas and knowledge; volunteers and professionals collaborated to create prevention and service models fashioning the safe-sex approach to reducing sexual transmission, and devising ways of reducing HIV transmission among IDUs (outreach, bleach kits, syringe exchanges). The community developed a philosophy about how to live with the disease, and recommendations about the system of testing and approving new drugs. As the epidemic continued, less of the AIDS community's work involved the creation of new ideas and strategies. Its early positions combined its own interests and social reforms with a potentially larger impact; in the course of representing members' own interests, the AIDS community offered critiques of public policies affecting a broader range of the population—critiques of, for instance, the inadequacies of the entitlements system, the lack of housing for the homeless, the slow process of drug approval, the high cost of prescription drugs.

The balance has now shifted, and the AIDS community is operating more as an interest group than a social movement, focusing its work on increasing funding and continuing AIDS exceptionalism. This shift has occurred for several reasons. Private and foundation funding for innovative programs decreased as major foundations moved to provide support for other policy issues, individual donors lost interest in an issue that no longer seemed as urgent, and AIDS organizations became more dependent on state funding. Many of the early leaders in the AIDS community—both activists and advocates—died, others moved on to other causes or issues, and some were focused on their personal and professional lives. Without a new generation of activists, the movement lost momentum.[15] Treatment activist Gregg Gonsolves pointed out that there had been a "brain drain," with a resultant need to recruit "new, smart, and practical policy 'wonks,'" while trying to reengage the alumni who were responsible for many of the advances during the first two decades of the epidemic."[16] Fewer leaders were volunteers; many more of the active participants in the AIDS community were paid staff members working for AIDS organizations. Even though some outsider tactics continued to be used, the volume had been turned down and the rhetoric had taken on a predictable quality. At a Housing Works rally in front of City Hall in 2003, for instance, participants chanted, "Bloomberg, billionaire! People with AIDS, HE DON'T CARE" and a familiar refrain, "He's killing us."[17]

A great deal of the energy of the AIDS community was expended on the yearly budget cycles of city, state, and federal governments. This was a necessary response to a funding structure that involved yearly allocations and CARE Act reauthorizations every five years. Political leaders relied on institutionalized activism to justify funding. A yearly cycle of lobbying events, local and national, were an important part of the AIDS community's calendar, including an annual lobbying day in Albany sponsored by NYAC and an annual AIDS Watch in Washington DC (which attracted seven hundred participants in 2005).[18] A shared interest in maintaining funding was the strongest unifying force in an otherwise diverse community.

One reason for the negative response to AHP was that it mainstreamed AIDS into the health care system and strongly linked AIDS prevention and services to the government's commitment to reducing health disparities. Maintaining the position that AIDS was distinctive and unique was also necessary to justify services funded by the CARE and Housing Opportunities for Persons with AIDS Acts.

The development of distinct funding streams for specific categories of people is a common feature of American social policy. As Smith and Lipsky point out, the identification of "emergency" policy areas is a way of justifying programs for specific problems rather than universalistic programs. The creation of services earmarked for people with HIV privileged them. They had access to medical and dental care, to housing, to prescription coverage and services that people who were HIV-negative did not.

As the epidemic neared the quarter-century mark, as survival time increased and the "face" of the epidemic changed, the AIDS community could no longer assume that it had its place at the table. The epidemic itself was changing and so was the policy context. Facing a rise in the number of new cases, and growing costs as more and more people living with HIV required increasingly expensive medications, the AIDS community was being called upon to defend AIDS exceptionalism. AIDS organizations serving the inner-city poor had become remarkably like other social service agencies. They provided legal services to help people fight evictions, deal with domestic violence, challenge decisions by welfare agencies, and help people with family problems. The executive director of one large AIDS organization in New York City observed in late 2003 that "we are basically an anti-poverty agency for people with HIV. . . . People come into us for service and they talk about their problems with housing, with food. . . . HIV is not the first thing in their constellation of problems."[19] For people affected by a host of problems not just HIV, the lines between the positive and the negative were not so clearly drawn. In fact, audits of seven agencies in New York City receiving Ryan White Funding for "Outreach and Risk Reduction" found that "these services were provided predominantly to individuals whose HIV status was unknown at the time the services were provided."[20]

The Bush administration's proposals for the 2005 reauthorization of the Ryan White CARE Act were criticized by AIDS advocacy groups. The reallocation of resources to areas where the epidemic was growing was described by the National Association of Persons with AIDS as "robbing Peter to pay Paul," and the executive director of NYAC claimed that the Bush administration's recommendations were "creating a breeding ground for declining health and widening health disparities among at-risk populations, especially communities of color."[21]

At the same time, there was growing fragmentation and much more redundancy among AIDS organizations. The major lobbying group supporting the passage of the Ryan White CARE Act was NORA, which was coordinated by the AIDS Action Council. In 2005, when a new Ryan White reauthorization was proposed, eighteen national organizations and two organizations in New York City offered "stakeholder recommendations" about the Act.

Disease-related advocacy has at least two important consequences for American political life. First, serious questions arise as to whether funds are distributed rationally and equitably. Critics of AIDS policy noted that AIDS was receiving more than its fair share of funding compared to the actual impact of the disease, and that a disproportionate amount of research funds were directed to studies of children, a small proportion but a highly sympathetic target population.[22] AIDS is not alone in this respect. A study of the allocation of NIH research funds indicated that AIDS, breast cancer, diabetes, and dementia "all received relatively generous funding" in comparison to several measures of the impact of these diseases.[23]

The existence of numerous organizations related to specific diseases and conditions may have deflected attention from the need to enact significant health care reforms, and contributed to a lack of grassroots mobilization for national health insurance.[24] Generally, organizations are much more concerned about expanding benefits for their constituents than with pressing for significant and profound changes. The AIDS community, for example, is, as of 2005, lobbying for the passage of the Early Treatment for HIV Act (ETHA). This would allow states the option of expanding Medicaid coverage for people who are HIV-positive. It would create an entitlement for health insurance that currently only exists for breast cancer and cervical cancer, two diseases given similar treatment in 2002 legislation.[25] Although it is understandable that AIDS advocates want to expand benefits for their stakeholders, the singling out of people with one disease at a time when 45.8 million Americans lack health insurance creates enormous inequities.[26]

The potential for greater collaboration among health advocacy organizations exists. Several organizations in the AIDS community have been involved in issue-specific coalitions. In 1990, AIDS organizations worked closely with disability rights groups in the passage of the Americans with Disabilities Act.[27] The AIDS Healthcare Foundation, a California-based organization providing primary care and prescription drugs, challenged the high cost of AIDS medications and placed an ad against one drug manufacturer in the *New York*

Times, along with the Coalition for Access to Affordable Prescription Drugs, Senior Action Network, the National Association of the Terminally Ill, and several other organizations.[28] Medicaid Matters, "a consumer-oriented coalition that advocates on behalf of New York's Medicaid program and the people it serves," includes the AIDS Treatment and Data Network, the New York AIDS Coalition, and GMHC. The AIDS Action Council belongs to the Coalition for Health Funding, a membership organization of fifty groups whose goal is "to ensure that funding for the programs and agencies that comprise the U.S. Public Health Service is adequate to meet public need."[29]

As this book goes to press, one thing is clear: certain aspects of the epidemic, the lives of the one million people living with HIV, and the AIDS community will continue to change.[30] A number of recent and impending developments promise to alter the nature of the disease and its transmission: a possible approval of a home HIV test; the approval of buprenorphone, and federal legislation to increase access to this method of treating heroin addiction; the proliferation of more strains of drug-resistant HIV; the use of "crystal," a drug associated with engaging in risky sex; a morning-after treatment for HIV infection that has been approved for health care workers; and the prospect of microbicides that block HIV transmission to women.[31] Members of the AIDS community are trying to promote a resurgence of direct action and a broader agenda. The first demonstration of the Campaign to End AIDS, for example, involved placing eighty-five hundred pairs of shoes on Pennsylvania Avenue to symbolize the number of people dying of AIDS throughout the world every day.[32] Although the work is today less often covered by the media, people in the AIDS community continue to fight for their lives, both individually and collectively, and remain hopeful that they will witness the end of the epidemic.

Notes

Introduction

1. Rodger McFarlane interview, 23 December 1988.
2. Lawrence Mass, "It Happened in Fragments," Lawrence Mass Papers, Box 14, New York Public Library.
3. Lawrence Mass, "Disease Rumors Largely Unfounded," *New York Native* (hereafter, *Native*), 18–31 May 1981, 7.
4. Albert R. Hunt, "Defining Events: World War II, Vietnam, AIDS," *Wall Street Journal*, 12 December 1997, R6.
5. M. S. Gottleib, H. M. Schanker, et al., "Pneumocystis Pneumonia—Los Angeles," *Morbidity and Mortality Weekly Report* (hereafter, *MMWR*) (5 June 1981): 250–252; A. Friedman-Kien, L. Laubenstein, M. Marmor, et al., "Kaposi's Sarcoma and Pneumocystis Pneumonia among Homosexual Men—New York City and California," *MMWR* (3 July 1981): 305–307; "Follow-Up on Kaposi's Sarcoma and Pneumocystis Pneumonia," *MMWR* (28 August 1981): 409–410.
6. Matt Clark with Mariana Gosnell, "Diseases That Plague Gays," *Newsweek*, 21 December 1981, 51–52; Kenneth Hymes, Jeffrey B. Greene, Aaron Marcus, et al., "Kaposi's Sarcoma in Homosexual Men: A Report of Eight Cases," *The Lancet*, no. 8247 (19 September 1981): 598–600.
7. Gina Kolata, "10 Years of AIDS Battle: Hopes for Success Dim," *NYT*, 3 June 1991, A14.
8. Herman Joseph interview, 12 May 1997; Randy Shilts, "Horror Stories and Excuses: How New York City Is Dealing with AIDS," *Native*, 25 March–7 April 1985, 22.
9. Lawrence K. Altman, "Rare Cancer Seen in 41 Homosexuals," *NYT*, 3 July 1981, A20.
10. Author interview, May 1990.
11. Lewis Thomas, "AIDS and the Immune Surveillance Problem," in *AIDS: The Epidemic of Kaposi's Sarcoma and Opportunistic Infections*, ed. Alvin Friedman-Kien and Linda Laubenstein (New York: Masson, 1984), 1.
12. "Doctors Tell of International Resurgence in a Variety of Infectious Diseases," *NYT*, 17 January 1996, A16.
13. Peter S. Arno and Karyn Feiden, "Ignoring the Epidemic: How the Reagan Administration Failed on AIDS," *Health/PAC Bulletin* 17, no. 2 (1986): 7–11; Sandra Panem, *The AIDS Bureaucracy* (Cambridge, MA: Harvard University Press, 1988); Charles Perrow and Mauro F. Guillén, *The AIDS Disaster: The Failure of Organizations in New York and the Nation* (New Haven, CT: Yale University Press, 1990).
14. Daniel Fox, "AIDS and the American Health Polity," in *AIDS: The Burdens of History*, ed. Elizabeth Fee and Daniel Fox (Berkeley and Los Angeles: University of California Press, 1988), 316–343; Lewis H. Kuller and Lawrence A. Kingsley, "The Epidemic of AIDS: A Failure of Public Health Policy," *Milbank Quarterly* 64, supp. 1 (1986): 56–78.
15. James Kinsella, *Covering the Plague: AIDS and the American Media* (New Brunswick, NJ: Rutgers University Press, 1989).

16. David Sencer," Tracking a Local Outbreak," in *The AIDS Epidemic*, ed. Kevin Cahill (New York: St. Martin's, 1983), 18; E. James Fordyce et al., "Causes of Death Contributing to Changes in Life Expectancy in New York City between 1983 and 1992," *Population Research and Policy Review* 16 (1997): 197, 199.

17. New York City Department of Health HIV Epidemiology Group, "25 Years of HIV in New York City: Lessons from Surveillance," *Journal of Urban Health* 78 (2001): 669–678; Centers for Disease Control and Prevention (hereafter, CDC), *HIV/AIDS Surveillance Report, 2001*, http://www.cdc.gov/hiv/stats/hasr1302.pdf, *accessed on 20 June 2005*.

18. *AIDS/HIV Semiannual Report* (New York: New York City Department of Health, June 2002): 7; CDC, *HIV/AIDS Surveillance, 2001*.

19. See Susan M. Chambré, "Redundancy, Innovation, and Fragmentation: HIV/AIDS Nonprofit Organizations in New York City, 1981–1992," *Policy Studies Journal* 27 (1999): 841, and "The HIV/AIDS Grants Economy in New York City, 1983–1992," *Health Affairs* 15 (1996): 250–260.

20. Ulrich Beck, *Risk Society: Towards a New Modernity* (London: Sage Publications, 1992). See also Christopher H. Foreman Jr., "Grassroots Victim Organizations: Mobilizing for Personal and Public Health," in Alan J. Cigler and Burdett A. Loomis, eds., *Interest Group Politics* (Washington, DC: CQ Press, 1995), 34–53.

21. See Bruce Wood, *Patient Power? The Politics of Patients' Associations in Britain and America* (Philadelphia: Open University Press, 2000); Phil Brown and Stephen Zavestoski, eds., *Social Movements in Health* (Malden, MA: Blackwell, 2005); Rob Baggott, Judith Allsop, and Kathryn Jones, *Speaking for Patients and Carers: Health Consumer Groups and the Policy Process* (New York: Palgrave, 2005).

22. Sidney Tarrow, *Power in Movement: Social Movements and Contentious Politics* (New York: Cambridge University Press, 1998).

23. "ACT UP Marks Tenth Anniversary Founding at Center," *Center Voice*, April/May 1997, 4.

24. For a review of the literature on the role of "frames" in social movements, see David Croteau and Lyndsi Hicks, "Coalition Framing and the Challenge of a Consonant Frame Pyramid: The Case of a Collaborative Response to Homelessness," *Social Problems* 50 (2003): 251–272.

25. Zachary Gussow, "The Role of Self-Help Clubs in Adaptation to Chronic Illness and Disability," *Social Science and Medicine* 10 (1976): 407–414.

26. "AIDS: Coping with the Unknown," *Emergency Medicine* (30 October 1983): 165–168, 177, 181.

27. Deborah B. Gould, "Life during Wartime: Emotions and the Development of ACT UP," *Mobilization* 7, no. 2 (2002): 177–200.

Chapter 1: Managing the Madness

1. "The History of Gay Men's Health Crisis, Inc.," *Circus* program,16, author's files.

2. Larry Kramer recalled that invitations were sent to "hundreds," but Mass had a lower estimate. Larry Kramer, GMHC (Gay Men's Health Crisis) oral history interview; Lawrence Mass, "Chronicles of the Violaceous Death: A Personal Journal of the Deadliest and Most Mysterious Epidemic in Recorded Medical History," 1982, 26, Mass Papers, Box 14.

3. GMHC, *Annual Report, July 2000–December 2001*.

4. Maureen Dowd, "For Victims of AIDS, Support in a Lonely Siege," *NYT*, 5 December 1983, B1; Jane Howard, "The Warrior," *Esquire* 102, December 1984, 272;

GMHC, *Annual Report, 1986/1987*; "Vital Statistics," *The Volunteer* (hereafter, *Volunteer*), December 1991, 9; "Vital Statistics," *Volunteer*, March/April 1992, 16.

5. Randy Shilts, *And the Band Played On* (New York: St. Martin's Press, 1987), 25–29, 91; author interview, 8 May 1990.

6. Nathan Fain, "Dream, Tragedy, and the Birth of Courage," speech on 15 June 1985 at Hunter College, New York, Mass Papers, Box 1.

7. Presentation by Martin Levine at a National Academy of Sciences panel on "Social Impact of the AIDS Epidemic," New York, 2 April 1990.

8. "History of Gay Men's Health Crisis," 16.

9. Michael VerMeulen, "The Gay Plague," *New York Magazine*, 31 May 1982, 62.

10. "Diseases of Immunodeficiency in the Gay Community" *New York Native*, 10–23 May 1982, 7.

11. James D'Eramo, "A Night at the AIDS Forum," *Native*, 20 December 1982–22 January 1983, 1.

12. Larry Kramer, GMHC oral history interview, 25 July 1990.

13. "Where Are We Now?" *GMHC Newsletter*, no. 2 (January 1983), 10 and 13.

14. Lawrence Mass, "The Epidemic Continues," *Native*, 29 March–11 April 1982, 1.

15. "Who We Are and What This Is," *GMHC Newsletter*, no. 1, July 1982, 1.

16. Ibid.

17. Marty Levine, "Fearing Fear Itself," *GMHC Newsletter*, no. 1, 14.

18. Mel Rosen, GMHC oral history interview, November 1989.

19. "A Letter from Your Gay Men's Health Crisis," *Native*, 24 May–6 June 1982, 5; "A Letter from Your Gay Men's Health Crisis" *Native*, 2 August–15 August 1982, 12; "A Letter from Your Gay Men's Health Crisis," *Native*, 13 September–26 September 1982, 22.

20. Elizabeth Midlarsky, "Helping as Coping," in *Review of Personality and Social Psychology*, ed. M. S. Clark (Newbury Park, CA: Sage, 1990), 238–264.

21. David Black, *The Plague Years* (New York: Simon and Schuster, 1986), 153; Rosen interview.

22. Hon. Richard C. Failla, "Board Members Speak: Words from Departing Board Members," *Volunteer* 7, July/August 1990, 10.

23. Lewis Katoff, "GMHC Launches New Fellowship Program," *Volunteer* 7, September/October 1990, 11.

24. Presentation by Arthur Myer, GMHC volunteer orientation, 9 January 1989; Mitch Cutler, GMHC oral history interview.

25. Sal Licata, "When AIDS Strikes the AIDS Professional," *PWA Coalition Newsline* (hereafter, *Newsline*), October 1987, 33.

26. "A Letter from Your Gay Men's Health Crisis," *Native*, 11–24 October, 1982, 14

27. "A Letter from Your Gay Men's Health Crisis," *Native*, 8–21 November 1982, 28.

28. "A Letter from Your Gay Men's Health Crisis," *Native*, 17–30 January 1983, 24; "Together This Is What We're Doing." *Native*, 24 October–6 November, 1983, 24 ; Dowd, "For Victims"; "Medicine, False and True: Aides for AIDS," *NYT*, 11 December 1983, A4, 20.

29. Richard Dunne, GMHC oral history interview, 16 March 1990.

30. Rosen interview.

31. Richard De Thuin, "Gay Men's Health Crisis," *Lesbian/Gay Pride Guide* (New York, 1983).

32. AIDS Committee of Toronto, "Report on Visit to Gay Men's Health Crisis in New York," 29 September 1983, Hansen Papers.

33. Sandi Feinblum, GMHC oral history interview.
34. Ken Wein and Diego Lopez, *G.M.H.C. Crisis Intervention Training Handbook* (New York: Gay Men's Health Crisis, June 1983); Lewis Katoff and Richard Dunne, "Supporting People with AIDS: The Gay Men's Health Crisis Model," *Journal of Palliative Care* 4 (December 1988): 88–95.
35. McFarlane interview.
36. GMHC, *Annual Report, 1987/1988.*
37. Barry Davidson, GMHC oral history interview.
38. Ken Wein, GMHC oral history interview, 11 May 1988.
39. Robert Cecci, "When the System Fails," *American Journal of Nursing* (January 1986): 47.
40. Feinblum interview.
41. James D'Eramo, "Dentists Refuse to Treat AIDS Patients and Gay Men; State Issues New Dental Guidelines," *Native*, 30 January–12 February 1984, 14.
42. "The City: Undertakers Unit Warns of AIDS," *NYT*, 18 June 1983, A27; David France, "Salvation Army Nixes AIDS Clothes," *Native*, 18 June–1 July 1984, 13.
43. "Coop Board Sued for Evicting AIDS Doc," *Native*, 10–24 October 1983, 6; "AIDS Doc Gets Preliminary Injunction," *Native*, 7–20 November 1983, 10–11 .
44. 10 November 1988 interview.
45. McFarlane interview.
46. GMHC, *Annual Report, 1987/1988.*
47. Levine presentation.
48. Davidson interview.
49. McFarlane interview.
50. Michael Quadland, GMHC oral history interview, 23 March 1990; Mark Senak, GMHC oral history interview, 21 April 1988.
51. Susan Kucklin, *Fighting Back: What Some People Are Doing about AIDS* (New York: Putnam, 1989), 29.
52. Mitchell Cutler, GMHC oral history interview.
53. Jed Mattes, GMHC oral history interview.
54. Wein interview.
55. Perrow and Guillén, *AIDS Disaster.*
56. 9 November 1988 interview.
57. "Fighting AIDS," *NYT*, 11 July 1983, II-3.
58. "Circus Benefit for AIDS," *NYT*, 14 March 1983, B4.
59. *Circus for Life* program, 27 March 1992.
60. "A Letter from Your Gay Men's Health Crisis," *Native*, 9–22 May 1983, 14; Michael Fischer, "The Last Crisis," *Native*, 14–27 July 1983, 5–6; GMHC Fundraising Letter, December 1982, Hansen Collection.
61. Michael Fischer, "Last Crisis," *Native*, 5–6; John Wallace, "State Grants $200,000 for Gay Health," *Native*, 11–24 April 1983, 9.
62. GMHC Fundraising Letter, December 1982, Hansen Collection.
63. *Circus* program, 10–11.
64. In 1983, GMHC raised $926,651 and spent $473,184. A total of $93,000 went for research, but more of the budget went for education ($165,276) and services ($110,021). GMHC tax returns, copies in the author's files.
65. Dowd, "For Victims," B1.
66. Jane Howard, "The Warrior," *Esquire*, December 1984, 272.
67. "Richard Dunne to Resign as Executive Director of World's First AIDS Organiza-

tion," GMHC press release, 20 March 1989, author's files; "An Interview with the New E. D," *Volunteer* 2, March/April 1985, 2.

68. The 1986 fiscal year only contained six months. These figures are derived from tax returns filed with the New York State Attorney General's Office.

69. William Booth, "Another Muzzle for AIDS Education," *Science* (20 November 1987): 1036.

70. "Interview with the New E. D."

71. Unpublished data from a survey by Philip Kayal, copy in the author's files; Suzanne C. Ouelette et al., "GMHC: The Volunteers and the Challenges and Hopes for the Second Decade of AIDS," *AIDS Education and Prevention* 7 (1995, supp.): 64–79.

72. Ellen Steinbaum, "Moving On," *Volunteer* 6, July/August 1989, 1.

73. Barry Adkins, "Building an AIDS Service Empire," *Native*, 28 July 1986, 10.

74. David Firestone, "A Monument to AIDS," *Newsday*, 29 December 1988, 54.

75. Joy [A.] Tomchin, "Challenge and Commitment," *Volunteer* 5, March/April 1988, 2.

76. Joy A. Tomchin, "A Board Member Speaks: Seeking Balance," *Volunteer* 6, March/April 1989, 2.

77. James G. Pepper, "Words From Departing Senior Board Members," *Volunteer* 7, July/August 1990, 10.

78. Jeff Soref, "Increasing Caseload, Adding Space," *Volunteer*, March/April 1992, 2.

Chapter 2: Fighting the Victim Label

1. Buddy Noro and Josef Scharf-Wilner, "AIDS: 1987," *Native*, 3–16 December 1984, 22–23.

2. Ronald Bayer, *Private Acts, Social Consequences: AIDS and the Politics of Public Health* (New Brunswick, NJ: Rutgers University Press, 1991).

3. Ulrich Beck, *World Risk Society* (Malden, MA: Blackwell, 1999).

4. Debbie Indyk and David A. Rier, "Grassroots AIDS Knowledge: Implications for the Boundaries of Science and Collective Action," *Knowledge* 15 (1993): 3–42.

5. Robert D. Benford and David A. Snow, "Framing Processes and Social Movements: An Overview and Assessment," *Annual Review of Sociology* 26 (2000): 611–639; Francesca Polletta and James M. Jasper, "Collective Identity and Social Movements," *Annual Review of Sociology* 27 (2001): 283–305.

6. Paul Lichterman, *The Search for Political Community: American Activists Reinventing Commitment* (New York: Cambridge University Press, 1996).

7. "6-Month Surge in AIDS Reported." *NYT*, 5 August 1983, A6; Morgan and Curran, "Acquired Immunodeficiency"; "New AIDS Forecast: A Long, Long Siege," *U.S. News and World Report*, 14 October 1985, 14.

8. Josh Barbanel, "City Expects Rise in AIDS Care Costs," *NYT*, 18 October 1985, A19; Jesus Rangel, "City Expanding Its Plan to Help Victims of AIDS," *NYT*, 30 March 1985, A27; Jack Sirica, "Regan: AIDS Underestimated," *Newsday*, 12 December 1985, 7.

9. "Around the Nation: Federal AIDS Hotline Is Swamped by Callers," *NYT*, 22 August 1983, A14.

10. Bayer, *Private Acts*, ch. 3; "Disease Stirs Fear on Blood Supply," *NYT*, 6 January 1983, B17; J. Oleske et al., "Immune Deficiency Syndrome in Children," *JAMA* 249 (1983): 2345–2349; Erik Eckholm, "Chief of Study on Victims' Families Doubts AIDS Is Transmitted Casually," *NYT*, 6 February 1986, B7.

11. Eleanor Singer et al., "The Polls—A Report: AIDS," *Public Opinion Quarterly* 51 (1987): 580–595; Erik Eckholm, "Poll Finds Many AIDS Fears That the Experts Say Are Groundless," *NYT*, 12 September 1985, B11.

12. James W. McNally and William Mosher, "AIDS-Related Knowledge and Behavior among Women 15–44 Years of Age: United States, 1988," *Advance Data* (14 May 1991): 3.

13. "Northwest Airlines Eases Policy on AIDS Travelers," *Wall Street Journal*, 15 September 1987, accessed from Factiva.

14. "Dr. Koop's AIDS Dissent," *NYT*, 25 October 1986, A26.

15. Thomas Morgan, "Amid AIDS, Gay Movement Grows but Shifts," *NYT*, 10 October 1987, A1.

16. This is an estimate combining information from testimony and reports from New York City and New York State: testimony of Katy Taylor, New York State Task Force on Gay Issues, 17 January 1985, Nimmons Papers; "Report on Discrimination against People with AIDS and People Perceived to Have AIDS, January 1986–June 1987," AIDS Discrimination Unit, New York City Commission on Human Rights, PWA Coalition Collection; letter from Mitchell Netburn, director, New York State Division of Human Rights, author's files.

17. "Buckley Retracts 'AIDS Tatoo' Proposal," *Native*, December 1986, 6

18. Larry Rohter, "11,000 Boycott Start of Classes in AIDS Protest," *NYT*, 10 September 1985, B1.

19. Dirk Johnson, "Ryan White Dies of AIDS at 18; His Struggle Helped Pierce Myths," *NYT*, 9 April 1990, D10.

20. Rubin Rosario, "Dying Patient Set Afire," *New York Daily News*, 14 March 1984, 5.

21. Sue Hyde, "Falwell Speaks, Cincinnati Responds," *Gay Community News*, 23 July 1983, 3.

22. "Most Americans Say They Are Religious, but Oppose Moral Crusades," Associated Press, 20 July 1986.

23. Gregory M. Herek, "AIDS and Stigma," *American Behavioral Scientist* 42: 1107; "Poll Indicates Majority Favor Quarantine for AIDS Victims," *NYT*, 20 December 1985, A24.

24. "ACT UP Marks Tenth Anniversary Founding at Center," *Center Voice*, April/May 1997, 4.

25. Philip M. Kayal, "'Morals,' Medicine, and the AIDS Epidemic," *Journal of Religion and Health* 24 (1985): 218–238.

26. Lawrence Mass, "Cancer as Metaphor," *Native*, 24 August–6 September 1981, 13.

27. George S. Tracy and Zachary Gussow, "Self-Help Groups: A Grass-Roots Response to a Need for Services," *Journal of Applied Behavioral Sciences* 12 (1976): 381–396.

28. Frank Riessman and Timothy Bay, "The Politics of Self-Help," *Social Policy* (fall–winter 1992): 28–38.

29. Peggy Thoits, "Stress, Coping, and Social Support Processes: Where Are We? What Next?" *Journal of Health and Social Behavior* ("Extra Issue") (1995): 53–79.

30. Kathryn P. Davison, "Who Talks? The Social Psychology of Illness Support Groups," *American Psychologist* 55, no. 2: 206–217; Alf Trojan, "Benefits of Self-Help Groups: A Survey of 232 Members from 65 Disease-Related Groups," *Social Science and Medicine* 29 (1989): 225–232; Dale E. Brashers et al., "Social Activism, Self-Advocacy, and Coping with HIV Illness," *Journal of Social and Personal Relationships* 19 (2002): 113–133.

31. Robert Cecci, GMHC oral history interview.

32. Peter M. Marzuk et al., "Increased Risk of Suicide in Persons with AIDS," *JAMA* 259 (1988): 1333–1337; Gregg Bordowitz and Jean Carlomusto, "PWA Power: Life after Diagnosis," GMHC Living with AIDS Show, 1988.

33. Luis Palacios, GMHC oral history interview, 2 September 1988.

34. Michael Callen, "People with AIDS–New York: A History," 19 March 1984, Callen Papers, Box 6, Folder 184.

35. Ibid.

36. "A Warning to Gay Men with AIDS," *Native*, 22 November–5 December 1982, 16.

37. Alan Burns, "H.E.A.L.," *Newsline*, November 1986, 21; Michael Callen, "Jim Fouratt: Unsung Hero," *Newsline*, December 1986, 35.

38. Remarks of Michael Callen to the New York Congressional delegation, 10 May 1983, repr. in Frederick P. Siegal and Marta Siegal, *AIDS: The Medical Mystery* (New York: Grove Press, 1983), 181–182.

39. Michael Callen, "AIDS as an Identity," in Michael Callen, ed., *Surviving and Thriving with AIDS* (New York: People with AIDS Coalition, 1987), 31; Ivan Illich, *Medical Nemesis: The Expropriation of Health* (New York: Pantheon Books, 1982).

40. "A Warning to Gay Men with AIDS," *Native*, 22 November–5 December 1982, 16; "A Warning to Gay Men with AIDS," *Native*, 6 December–19 December 1982, 29.

41. Phil Lanzaratta, "Why Me?" *Christopher Street*, April 1982, 15–16; Glenn Collins, "Facing the Emotional Anguish of AIDS," *NYT*, 30 May 1983, A-14; Craig Rowland, "Philip Lanzaratta (In Memorium)," *Newsline*, September 1986, 11.

42. Esther B. Fein, "AIDS and Its Victims: Support Networks Grow," *NYT*, 21 February 1985, B1; Frank J. Prial, "TV Crew Leaves Set of AIDS Victims' Interview," *NYT*, 28 March 1985, B6.

43. David Nimmons interview, 31 January 2001.

44. Callen, "People with AIDS."

45. "Founding Statement of People with AIDS/ARC: 'The Denver Principles,'" in Michael Callen, ed., *Surviving*, 128–129.

46. Arthur Felson and Michael Shernoff, "AIDS Groups Find Solidarity in Denver," *Native,* 14–21 July 1983, 28; Michael Callen and Dan Turner, "A History of the PWA Self-Empowerment Movement," in *Surviving and Thriving with AIDS: Collected Wisdom*, vol. 2 (New York: PWA Coalition, 1988), 291.

47. Callen, *Surviving AIDS*, 177.

48. New York City Department of Health, HIV/AIDS Surveillance Statistics, 2001, http://www.nyc.gov/html/doh/downloads/pdf/ah/surveillance2001_table1_and_2.pdf, accessed on 23 June 2005.

49. Letter from Centers for Disease Control to Gay Men with AIDS, 7 December 1983; Letter from Federico Gonzales to Michael Callen, Callen Papers, Box 7, Folder 208.

50. Michael Callen and Dan Turner, "A History of the PWA Self-Empowerment Movement," in *Surviving and Thriving: Collected*, 294–295 and 291–292.

51. "Brief History of PWAC," 2 August 1989, People with AIDS Coalition Papers (hereafter PWAC Papers), Box 13; fundraising letter for the PWA Coalition, November 1986, PWAC Papers, Box 28.

52. PWAC Coalition Bylaws, 24 November 1986, PWAC Papers, Box 5.

53. "At Long Last, a Newsletter!" *Newsline*, June 1985, 1; "Brief History of PWAC."

54. PWA Coalition Bylaws.

55. Max Navarre, "A Queen Screams," *Newsline*, November 1985, 11.

56. Wolf Agress, "GMHC's PWA Advisory Council Update," *Newsline*, March 1986, 2.

57. Kenneth William Meeks, "So What Are PWAs/PWARCs, Anyway? Chopped Liver?" *Newsline*, January 1986, 18.

58. Ken Meeks, "Panel Watch: Chopped Liver Ain't Found Only in the Deli," *Newsline*, February 1986, 7.

59. "History of the PWA Coalition," PWAC Papers, Box 13.

60. Notices in *Newsline*, June 1985, 12–13; Ken Meeks, "Oysters: A Raw Deal," *PWA Coalition Newsline*, July 1985, 9.

61. "*Newsline* Now on Computer!!" *Newsline*, February 1986, 1; "AIDS Information by Computer," *AIDS Treatment News* (8 May 1987), reprinted in John S. James, ed., *AIDS Treatment News, Issues 1 through 75* (Berkeley, CA: Celestial Arts, 1989), 133–138.

62. Letter from Christopher Babick to Michael Schimmel, n.d., PWAC Papers, Box 8.

63. "What to Look for in a Doctor: A Conversation between Michael Callen and Robert Herman," in Callen, *Surviving and Thriving*, 70–72; PWA Coalition, Final Community Service Report to the New York State AIDS Institute, 30 June 1988, PWAC Papers, Box 22.

64. Ken Meeks, "Speaker's Bureau Organized by PWAC," *Newsline*, December 1987, 1–2.

65. *Newsline*, February 1986, 2.

66. Randy Wicker, "Open Letter to Max Navarre," *Newsline*, February 1987, 10.

67. "Managing Editor's Note," *Newsline*, April 1986, 5.

68. Michael Callen, "Farewell," *Newsline*, September 1989, 2.

69. Michelle Cochran, *When AIDS Began: San Francisco and the Making of an Epidemic.* (Routledge: New York, 2004), ch. 7; Neenyah Ostrom, "Plague Island," *Christopher Street*, 4 January 1993, 16–18, 31.

70. J. A. Sonnabend, "Promiscuity Is Bad for Your Health," *Native*, 13–26 September 1982, 21, 49; Joseph Sonnabend, Steven S. Witkin, and David T. Purtilo, "Acquired Immunodeficiency Syndrome, Opportunistic Infections, and Malignancies in Male Homosexuals: A Hypothesis of Etiologic Factors in Pathogenesis," *JAMA* 249, no. 17 (6 May 1983): 2370.

71. "PWA Potluck Dinner!" *Newsline*, February 1986, 1; PWA Coalition List of Living Room Support Groups, 26 April 1988, PWAC Papers, Box 71; Ann-Marie Schiro, "A Haven for AIDS Patients," *NYT*, 22 December 1986, B20; James Revson, "They Mean to Live with AIDS," *Newsday*, 15 April 1987, II-4.

72. Michael Hirsch. "PWA Coalition Begins PWA/ PWARC Apartment Sharing Referrals," *Newsline*, December 1986, 5–6; Schiro, "Haven for AIDS Patients"; Bree Scott-Hartland and Larry Bee, "Debra Provenzano: Make-Up Artist/Volunteer Extraordinaire," *Newsline,* January 1990, 43–45.

73. PWA Coalition board minutes, 22 December 1986, PWAC Papers, Box 79.

74. List of support groups meeting at the Living Room, 26 April 1988, PWAC Papers, Box 22.

75. Letter from Christopher Babick to Roxanne Andrews, 22 February 1988, PWAC Papers, Box 8.

76. Michael Callen, "Survivors Column: Phil Lanzaratta," *Newsline*, June 1985, 14.

77. Max Navarre, "Survivors: A Profile of Bill Tynes," *Newsline*, February 1986, 3.

78. Michael Callen, "Remarks at the American Public Health Association Annual Meeting," *AIDS: Cultural Analysis, Cultural Activism*, ed. Douglas Crimp (Cambridge, MA: MIT Press, 1987), 161–166.

79. The Roving Reporter, "How Has Being HIV Positive Affected Your Relationships with Friends and Family Who Are HIV Negative?" *Body Positive*, May 1991, 16–17.

80. Ken Wein and Diego Lopez, *G.M.H.C. Crisis Intervention Training Handbook* (New York: Gay Men's Health Crisis, 1983), 13, author's files.

81. Gregg Bordowitz and Jean Carlomusto, "PWA Power: Life After Diagnosis," GMHC Living with AIDS Show, 1988.

82. Letter to the editor from Rodger Pettyjohn, *Newsline*, November 1990, 6.

83. Navarre, "What to Do."

84. Meredith B. McGuire, *Ritual Healing in Suburban America* (New Brunswick, NJ: Rutgers University Press, 1988).

85. Michael Ellner interview, 15 February 2001.

86. Fred E. Cantaloupe, "While We Wait," *Native*, 24 October 24–6 November 1983, 25.

87. "AIDS 'Cure' Quackery Worries Officials," *San Diego Union-Tribune*, 6 September 1987, A40.

88. D. M. Eisenberg et al. "Unconventional Medicine in the United States: Prevalence, Costs, and Patterns of Use," *New England Journal of Medicine*, no. 328 (1993): 246–252; K. M. Fairfield et al., "Patterns of Use, Expenditures, and Perceived Efficacy of Complementary and Alternative Therapies in HIV-Infected Patients," *Archives of Internal Medicine*, no. 159 (1999): 1143–1144.

89. Barry Adkins, "AIDS Organization Announces Programs for PWAs," *Native*, 25 November–1 December 1985, 15; "New York AIDS Action," *Newsline*, July 1985, 13; Alan Burns, "Reiki for AIDS," *Newsline*, March 1986, 17.

90. Max Navarre, "Get Different," *Newsline*, February 1986, 19.

91. Callen, "People with AIDS."

92. Michael Callen and Dan Turner, "A History of the PWA Self-Empowerment Movement," in *Surviving and Thriving: Collected*, 290.

Chapter 3: The Invention of Safe Sex

1. Richard Berkowitz, *Stayin' Alive: The Invention of Safe Sex—A Personal History* (Boulder, CO: Westview Press, 2003), 177; Tim Sweeney interview, 1 April 1997.

2. Lawrence Mass, "Cancer in the Gay Community," *Native*, 27 July–9 August 1981, 1, 22.

3. Gerald M. Oppenheimer, "In the Eye of the Storm: The Epidemiological Construction of AIDS." in *AIDS: The Burdens of History*, ed. Elizabeth Fee and Daniel Fox (Berkeley and Los Angeles: University of California Press, 1988), 267–300.

4. David Nimmons, *Soul Beneath the Skin: The Unseen Hearts and Habits of Gay Men* (New York: St. Martin's, 2002), 68.

5. Indyk and Rier, "Grassroots."

6. Keewhan Choi, "Assembling the AIDS Puzzle," in *AIDS: Facts and Issues*, ed. Victor Gong and Norman Rudnick (New Brunswick, NJ: Rutgers University Press, 1986), 17; D. Peter Drotman and James W. Curran, "AIDS: An Epidemiological Overview," in *AIDS*, ed. Friedman-Kien and Laubenstein, 279–286.

7. The study also found that many of the cases were heterosexuals with histories of intravenous drug use. See Mass, "The Epidemic," ch. 5.

8. Michael Marmor, "Epidemic Kaposi's Sarcoma and Sexual Practices among Male Homosexuals," in Friedman-Kien and Laubenstein, ed., *AIDS*, 291–296.

9. Drotman and Curran, "AIDS"; "A Cluster of Kaposi's Sarcoma and Pneumocystis carinii Pneumonia among Homosexual Male Residents of Los Angeles and Orange Counties, California." *MMWR* 31 (1982): 305.

10. Daniel C. William, "The Changing Life-styles of Homosexual Men in the Last Fifteen Years," in Friedman-Kien and Laubenstein, ed., *AIDS*, 261.

11. Daniel Fox, "AIDS and the American Health Polity," in Fee and Fox, *AIDS*, 318.

12. "Opportunistic Diseases: A Puzzling New Syndrome Afflicts Homosexual Men," *Time*, 21 December 1981, 68.

13. Bopper Deyton and Walter Lear, "A Brief History of the Gay/Lesbian Health Movement in the U.S.A.," in *The Sourcebook on Lesbian/Gay Health Care*, ed. Michael

Shernoff and William A. Scott (Washington, DC: National Lesbian/Gay Health Foundation, 1988), 15–19; Altman, *AIDS*, 46.

14. Larry Kramer, GMHC oral history interview, 25 July 1990.

15. Marty Levine, "Fearing Fear Itself," *GMHC Newsletter*, no. 1, July 1982, 15.

16. Reprinted in Larry Kramer, *Reports from the Holocaust: The Making of an AIDS Activist* (New York: St. Martin's Press, 1989), 14.

17. Ibid., 33–51.

18. Richard Goldstein, "Kramer's Complaint," *Village Voice*, 2 July 1985, 20.

19. Shilts, *Band*, 26–27.

20. Kramer interview, 25 July 1990.

21. Enno Porsch, GMHC oral history interview.

22. Quadland interview.

23. Shilts, *Band*, 179; "Report on the AIDS Forum in Dallas," *Native*, 13–26 September 1982, 22.

24. "Opportunistic Diseases."

25. Michael Callen and Richard Berkowitz, with Richard Dworkin, "We Know Who We Are: Two Gay Men Declare War on Promiscuity," *Native*, 8–21 November 1982, 23, 25, 27.

26. Ibid.; Peter Seitzman, "Good Luck, Bad Luck: The Role of Chance in Contracting AIDS," *Native*, 8–21 November 1982, 22.

27. Peter Seitzman, "Guilt and AIDS," *Native*, 3–16 January 1983, 23.

28. Dan William, "If AID Is an Infectious Disease . . . a Sexual Syllogism," *Native*, 16–29 August 1982, 33.

29. Ibid. 33.

30. Levine, "Fearing Fear Itself."

31. Lawrence Mass, "Basic Questions and Answers about AIDS," *GMHC Newsletter*, no. 2, January 1983, 18.

32. "Prevention of Acquired Immune Deficiency Syndrome (AIDS): Report of Interagency Recommendations," *MMWR* (4 March 1983): 102.

33. "A Letter from Your Gay Men's Health Crisis," *Native*, 25 October–7 November 1982, 20.

34. Dennis Altman, "Legitimation through Disaster: AIDS and the Gay Movement," Fee and Fox, *AIDS*, 301–315.

35. Jeffrey Levi, "Public Health and the Gay Perspective: Creating a Basis for Trust," in *AIDS: Facts and Issues*, 188.

36. Bob Bailey interview, 11 November 1993.

37. Chris Collins et al., "Who Knows What about Us?" author's files.

38. The black men who had been involved in the Tuskegee study were told that they had "bad blood," the colloquial term for syphilis.

39. Martin P. Levine, "Bad Blood: The Health Commissioner, the Tuskegee Experiment, and AIDS Policy," *Native*, 28 March–10 April 1983, 19, 21, 23.

40. Edward King, *Safety in Numbers: Safer Sex and Gay Men* (New York: Cassell, 1993), 3–4.

41. Collins, "Who."

42. Interview, 23 June1990.

43. "Majority Favor Quarantine," *NYT*.

44. Barry Adkins, "Civil Liberties Crisis Coalition Sponsors Conference," *Native*, 2–16 December 1985, 15.   .

45. Levi, "Public Health," 188.

46. Ron Vachon, "Lesbian and Gay Public Health: Old Issues, New Approaches," in *The Sourcebook on Lesbian/Gay Health Care*, ed. Michael Shernoff and William A. Scott (Washington, DC: National Lesbian/Gay Health Foundation, 1988), 20–23.

47. "New York Physicians Organize at Last," *Native*, 29 March 29–11 April 1982, 13.

48. Richard Berkowitz and Michael Callen, *"How to Have Sex in an Epidemic: One Approach* (New York: News from the Front Publications, 1983), 36.

49. Michael Shernoff interview, 5 January 1998; Altman, *AIDS*, 161; Ron Vachon, "Risks and Responsibilities of Recreational Sex: Healthful Guidelines for Gay Men," *Native*, 26 April–9 May, 1982, 11, 30; Bay Area Physicians for Human Rights, "Guidelines for AIDS Risk Reduction," author's files.

50. Berkowitz and Callen. *How*, 3, 37.

51. Shernoff interview.

52. Letter from Federico Gonzalez to Michael Callen, 29 November 1983, Callen Papers, Box 7, Folder 207; Seymour Kleinberg, "Challenges of AIDS," *Native*, 21 November–4 December 1983, 10.

53. "Reaching Out," *Native*, 12–25 March 1984, 12.

54. Davidson interview.

55. "GMHC Update," *Native*, 21 May–3 June 1984, 16, and 2–13 July 1985, 15.

56. "I Have AIDS," *Native*, 24 April–6 May 1984, 9.

57. Morgenthau et al., "Gay," 30.

58. McFarlane, GMHC oral history interview.

59. Michael Shernoff and Luis Palacios-Jimenez, "AIDS Prevention Is the Only Vaccine Available: An AIDS Prevention Educational Program," *Journal of Social Work and Human Sexuality* 6, no. 2 (1988): 141.

60. Mervyn F. Silverman, "The Public Health Response," Gong and Rudnick, *AIDS*, 159; David Harris, "Ad Hoc Group Discusses AIDS Education," *Native*, 16–29 January 1984, 8.

61. Luis Palacios-Jimenez and Michael Shernoff, *Facilitator's Guide to Eroticizing Safer Sex: A Psychoeducational Workshop Approach to Safer Sex Education* (New York: Gay Men's Health Crisis, 1986).

62. Mark Aurigemma, "AIDS Education Trail Blazers: Michael Shernoff and Dan Bloom," *Volunteer* 8 (March/April 1991), 1.

63. Shernoff interview.

64. Leonard Lambert interview, 24 February 1998.

65. David McWhorter, "Sexual Impact on Dating in the Gay Community," *AIDS and Patient Management: Legal, Ethical, and Social Issues*, Michael E. Whitt, ed. (Owings Mills, MD: National Health Publishing, 1986), 125–127; Nimmons, *Soul*, 58–59.

66. King, *Safety*, 41; Jane Gross, "Homosexuals Stepping Up AIDS Education," *NYT*, 22 September 1985, 1, 56; Daniel Weiss, "Study: Gay Men Using Precautions," *Newsday*, 22 November 1985, 11.

67. Dan William, "The Prevention of AIDS by Modifying Sexual Behavior," *Annals of the New York Academy of Sciences* 437 (1984): 283–285.

68. "Don't Risk Your Life and the Lives of Your Brothers," *Native*, 21 November–4 December, 1983, 33.

69. Gross, "Homosexuals."

70. Letter from Centers for Disease Control "to Gay Men with AIDS," 7 December 1983; letter from Frederico Gonzales, Gay Men's Health Crisis, to Michael Callen, Callen Papers, Box 7, Folder 208.

71. Safer Sex Committee of New York, letter to James Curran, 27 July 1984, author's files.

72. Nimmons interview, 31 January 2002.

73. Nimmons interview, 24 October 2002.

74. Coalition for Sexual Responsibility, "Interim Report," 14 October 1985, Nimmons Papers.

75. Michael Callen, "Some Thoughts on the Issue of Bathhouse/Backroom Closure during the AID Epidemic," 16 June 1984, Callen Papers, Box 7, Folder 207.

76. Michael Callen, "Controlling the Baths and the Backroom Bars," *Village Voice*, 12 March 1985, 36.

77. Bruce Lambert Jr., "Health Officials: AIDS Virus Infects 10 Percent of City Adults," *Newsday*, 31 October 1985, 7.

78. James Kinsella, *Covering the Plague: AIDS and the American Media* (New Brunswick, NJ: Rutgers University Press, 1989), 102.

79. Jason Andrew Kaufman, "Politics as Social Learning: Policy Experts, Political Mobilization, and AIDS Prevention Policy," *Journal of Policy History* 10 (1998): 304.

80. Bayer, *Private Acts*, 50–51.

81. Saul Friedman, "AIDS Panel: Regulate Bathhouses," *Newsday*, 10 October 1985, 19; Maurice Carroll, "State Permits Closing of Bathhouses to Cut AIDS," *NYT*, 25 October 1985, A1.

82. Scott Bronstein, "4 New York Bathhouses Still Operate under City's Program of Inspection." *NYT*, 3 May 1987, 58.

Chapter 4: Fighting AIDS is Everyone's Business

1. "For the New Year, They Resolve," *NYT*, 27 December 1992, F6.

2. GMHC, *Annual Report 1987/88*.

3. Tom Morgenthau et al., "Future Shock," *Newsweek*, 24 November 1986, 30.

4. Jennet Conant, "The Fashionable Charity," *Newsweek*, 28 December 1987, 54.

5. David Gelman with Michael Reese, "AIDS Strikes a Star," *Newsweek*, 5 August 1985, 68–69; Gerald Clarke and Denise Worrell, "The Double Life of an AIDS Victim," *Time*, 14 October 1985, 106; Paula Treichler, "AIDS, Gender, and Biomedical Discourse," Fee and Fox, *AIDS*, 205.

6. Gerald Clarke, Elaine Dutka, and Barbara Kraft, "AIDS: A Spreading Scourge," *Time,* 5 August 1985, 50.

7. New York City Department of Health, Office of AIDS Surveillance, *AIDS Surveillance Update* (New York: New York City Department of Health, January 1998). Claudia Wallis, "AIDS: A Spreading Scourge." *Time*, 5 August 1985, 50.

8. "Statement of Mr. Mel Rosen, Gay Men's Health Crisis, New York City, to the Subcommittee on Intergovernmental Relations and Human Resources on Government Operations, August 1, 1983," in Siegel, *AIDS*, 201.

9. "AIDS Resource Center—ARC," *Native*, 20 June–3 July 1983, 25.

10. Daniel Shenk interview, 22 October 1999; AIDS Resource Center tax returns, 1984 and 1985, author's files.

11. William R. Greer, "New York to Expand Subsidy for a Shelter for Victims of AIDS," *NYT*, 9 September 1985, B7; Report of the Institute of Public Service Performance Study for the AIDS Shelter Project, PWAC Papers, Box 13.

12. Barry Adkins, "City Announces AIDS Hospice," *Native*, 25 November–1 December 1985, 21.

13. Jilian Mincer, "Move of AIDS Patients Raises Fears," *NYT*, 21 July 1985, A26;

Ronald Sullivan, "Parishioners Block Archdiocese's AIDS Shelter," *NYT*, 31 August 1985, A25.

14. "Mother Theresa Opens Hospice in New York for Dying AIDS Patients," *Seattle Times*, 25 December 1985, A6.

15. Susan M. Chambré, "The Changing Nature of 'Faith' in Faith-Based Organizations: Secularization and Ecumenicism in Four AIDS Organizations in New York City," *Social Service Review* 75 (2001): 435–455.

16. Randy Frame, "The Church's Response to AIDS," *Christianity Today*, 22 November 1985, 50–51.

17. "In Service, Prayer, Religious Communities Seek Role," *AIDSline*, fall 1991, 1.

18. Robert Lindsey, "AIDS among Clergy Presents Challenges to Catholic Church," *NYT*, 2 February 1987, A15.

19. "Billy Graham Retracts Statement on AIDS as God's Judgment," United Press International, 9 October 1993, 4B; AIDS National Interfaith Network, *Annual Report 1: July 1991–1 July 1992* (Washington, DC: AIDS National Interfaith Network, 1992).

20. James E. D'Eramo, "Notables Come Out for AIDS Symposium," *Native*, 24 April–8 May 1983, 18; Steven C. Arvanette, "NYC Archbishop Condemns Homosexuality," *Native*, May 21–3 June 1984, 7.

21. Rt. Rev. Paul Moore Jr., Statement for AIDS Press Conference, 23 June 1983. Author's files.

22. "Cuomo Pledges AID for Victims of AIDS," *NYT*, 15 March 1984, B5.

23. Michael D'Antonio, "The AIDS Ministry," *Newsday*, 9 September 1986, 3.

24. Barry Adkins, "Unitarian Church Sponsors AIDS Forum: Panel Member Critical of Church Response," *Native*, 14–20 October 1985, 14.

25. "Dignity AIDS Ministry Groups" and "AIDS Prayer Group at St. Vincent's Chapel," *Newsline*, February 1986, 23; "All Are Welcome to Attend a Service of Hope at the Gay Synagogue," *Newsline*, March 1987, 9–10.

26. Toby Axelrod, "Silent Mercy: AIDS Foundation Focusing on the Orthodox Quietly Reaches Out to Patients and Their Families," *Jewish Week*, 10 May 1996, 40–41.

27. Michael Doyle, "Peter Avitabile: Man of Action," *Newsline,* September 1985, 14–15.

28. Interview, 17 May 1993.

29. Mike Salinas, "Feeding PWAs at St. Peters," *Native*, 16 March 1987, 8.

30. Doyle, "Peter Avitabile," 14–15.

31. Ed Sederbaum, "Volunteer Profile: Phyllis Haynes," *Volunteer*, July/August 1987.

32. "St. Peter's Church Expands Programs and Locations," *Newsline*, December 1988, 18.

33. See Courtney Bender, *Heaven's Kitchen: Living Religion at God's Love We Deliver* (Chicago: University of Chicago Press, 2003), 26–27.

34. Ganga Stone, "Message from Ganga: The More It Changes," *The Good News Letter*, September/October 1991, 2.

35. Ed Sederbaum, "Have It Your Way," *Volunteer*, January 1987, 5.

36. Trish Hall, "Solace and Sustenance for AIDS Patients," *NYT*, 14 October 1987, C3; GLWD Client Demographics, May 1990, March 1993, March 1995; GLWD Fact Sheet, http://www.aidsnyc.org/glwd/fact.html; author interview with Keith Berg, God's Love We Deliver, 7 September 1999.

37. Joy A. Tomchin, "Nathan Kolodner, 1951–1989" *Volunteer*, November/December 1989, 3.

38. "Nathan Kolodner, 38, Ex–AIDS Group Head," *NYT*, 30 August 1989, B5.

39. Kayal, "Volunteer," author's files; Ouelette et al., "GMHC."

40. Derreth Duncan interview, 21 January 1997.
41. Georgia Dullea, "AIDS Mothers' Undying Hope," NYT, 20 April 1994, C1.
42. Judith Stone, "AIDS Volunteers," *Glamour*, March 1987, 288–289, 332–335; Barbara Grande LeVine, "A Board Member Speaks: First-Time Volunteer," *Volunteer* 7, May/June 1990, 5.
43. Daniel Shaw, "Crossing Over," *New York Magazine*, 13 October 1986, 42–43; Nadine Brozan, "A Compassionate Force in the AIDS Battle," *NYT*, 13 April 1987, B6.
44. "Joan Tisch: Donor, Board Member, and Volunteer," GMHC, *Annual Report 1991/1992*, 24–25.
45. Joan Tisch, "A Board Member Speaks: Getting Emotionally Involved," *Volunteer*, May/June 1989, 2.
46. Georgia Dullea, "A Charity's 1,000 Parties to Benefit AIDS Victims," *NYT*, 20 December 1988, B2.
47. "Board of Directors Elects Richard Feldman Chair," *The Good News Letter*, winter 1992, 1, 4.
48. Michael Seltzer interview, 2 November 1992; GMHC, *Annual Report 1987/88*.
49. GMHC Benefactors Project fundraising letter, author's files.
50. "1987 AIDS Walk Set," *Native*, 6–20 April 1987, 11; Richard Laermer, "AIDS Walk New York Raises $1.6 Million," *Native*, 1–15 June 1987, 11.
51. "AIDS Dance-A-Thon: Reaching Out to New Audiences," *Volunteer*, March/April 1991, 9.
52. Francie Ostrower, *Why the Wealthy Give* (Princeton, NJ: Princeton University Press, 1995), 29.
53. Ganga Stone, lecture at Institute for Noetic Sciences, New York City, 20 May 1990.
54. Kim Neely, "Arista Sets AIDS Benefit," *Rolling Stone*, 29 November 1989, 22.
55. Stephen Holden, "AIDS Benefit Show at the Met Opera," *NYT*, 4 November 1985, C15.
56. Judy Kleimsrud, "Dr. Mathilde Krim: Focusing Attention on AIDS Research," *NYT*, 3 November 1984, A48.
57. Lindsay Van Gelder, "The Socialite Scientist," *Daily News Magazine*, 28 December 1985, 6–9, 20.
58. "The AIDS Medical Foundation," *Native*, 26 September–9 October 1983, 22.
59. AIDS Medical Foundation tax return, 1984 and 1985.
60. "American Foundation for AIDS Research News," 26 September 1985, author's files.
61. "A Special Campaign of the American Foundation for AIDS Research," fundraising letter, 20 May 1988, author's files.
62. Loren Renz et al., *Foundation Giving: Yearbook of Facts and Figures on Private, Corporate, and Community Foundations* (New York: Foundation Center, 1995), 58.
63. B. J. Stiles, "AIDS: How a Problem Became a Priority," *Foundation News*, March/April 1986, 49.
64. Kinsella, *Covering*.
65. Michael S. Seltzer and Katherine M. Galvin, "Organized Philanthropy's Response to AIDS," *The Nonprofit and Voluntary Sector Quarterly* 20 (1991): 249–326.
66. Michael Seltzer, *Meeting the Challenge: Foundation Responses to Acquired Immune Deficiency Syndrome* (New York: The Ford Foundation, 1987); Susan M. Chambré, "The HIV/AIDS Grants Economy in New York City, 1983–1992," *Health Affairs* 15 (1996): 250–260.
67. Seltzer, *Meeting the Challenge*.
68. Stiles, "AIDS."

69. Kathleen Teltsch, "Ford Foundation Leads Delayed Philanthropic Response to AIDS," *NYT*, 24 April 1988, A26.

70. Carol Levine, "The Citizens Commission on AIDS: A Private-Sector Response to an Epidemic," *Nonprofit and Voluntary Sector Quarterly* 20 (1991): 329–350.

Chapter 5: The Changing Face of AIDS

1. Catherine Woodard, "AIDS Fight Moves to Street Corner," *Newsday*, 4 September 1989, 8; Jonathan Mandell, "Latinos Battle AIDS Virus, Poverty," *Newsday*, 28 October 1991, 6; Edith Springer interview, 8 April 1997.

2. Elizabeth Fee and Nancy Krieger, "Understanding AIDS: Historical Interpretations and the Limits of Biomedical Individualism," *American Journal of Public Health* 83 (1993): 1477–1486.

3. Malcolm Gladwell, "Kimberly Bergalis' Ride of Rage," *Washington Post*, 26 September 1991, D1; Bruce Lambert, "One Victim's Campaign Changes Image of AIDS," *NYT*, 18 May 1989, B5.

4. Judith Randal, "City AIDS Carriers Put at 400,000," *NY Daily News*, 22 February 1985, 2.

5. Cathy Cohen, *The Boundaries of Blackness* (Chicago: University of Chicago Press, 1999); Ernest Quimby and Samuel R. Friedman, "Dynamics of Black Mobilization against AIDS in New York City," *Social Problems* 36 (1989): 403–415; Merrill Singer et al., "Owning AIDS: Latino Organizations and the AIDS Epidemic," *Hispanic Journal of Behavioral Sciences* 12 (May 1990): 196–211.

6. Susan M. Chambré, "Civil Society, Differential Resources, and Organizational Development: HIV/AIDS Organizations in New York City, 1982–1992," *Nonprofit and Voluntary Sector Quarterly* 26 (1997): 466–488.

7. Henry Masur et al., "An Outbreak of Community-Acquired Pneumocystis Carinii Pneumonia," *New England Journal of Medicine* 305 (1981): 1431–1438; Jerry E. Bishop, "New, Often-Fatal Illness in Homosexuals Turns Up in Women, Heterosexual Males," *Wall Street Journal*, 25 February 1982, 8.

8. David Sencer, "Tracking a Local Outbreak," in *The AIDS Epidemic*, ed. Kevin Cahill (New York: St. Martin's, 1983), 20–23.

9. Roger Bakeman et al., "The Incidence of AIDS among Blacks and Hispanics," *Journal of the National Medical Association* 79 (1987): 923.

10. "AIDS Cases by Borough of Residence, December 1983, *Native*, 30 January–12 February 1984, 19.

11. Ernest Drucker, "Communities at Risk: The Social Epidemiology of AIDS in New York City," in *AIDS and the Social Services: Common Threads*, ed. Richard Ulack and William F. Skinner (Lexington: University of Kentucky Press, 1991), 51–52.

12. *AIDS in New York State through 1989* (Albany: New York State Department of Health, n.d.), 24.

13. Don C. Des Jarlais et al., "AIDS among IV Drug Users: Epidemiology, Natural History, and Therapeutic Community Experiences," *AIDS and IV Drug Abusers: Current Perspectives*, ed. Robert P. Galea et al., (Owings Mills, MD: National Health Publishing, 1988), 53.

14. Rand L. Stoneburner et al., "A Larger Spectrum of Severe HIV-1-Related Disease in Intravenous Drug Users in New York City," *Science* (11 November 1988): 916–919.

15. Sencer, "Tracking," 22.

16. New York City Department of Health AIDS Surveillance, "The AIDS Epidemic in New York City, 1981–1984," *American Journal of Epidemiology* 123 no. 6: 1016.

17. Tom Morgenthau et al., "The New Panic in Needle Park: AIDS," *Newsweek*, 13 April 1987, 63; Charles R. Schuster, "Intravenous Drug Use and AIDS Prevention," *Public Health Reports* 103 (May/June 1988): 261–266.

18. Mary E. Guinan and Ann Hardy, "Epidemiology of AIDS in Women in the United States: 1981 through 1986," *JAMA* 257 (1987): 2039–2042.

19. Ellie E. Schoenbaum and Mayris P. Webber, "The Underrecognition of HIV Infection in Women in an Inner-City Emergency Room," *American Journal of Public Health* 83 (1993): 363–368.

20. Ibid.

21. "The AIDS Epidemic," 1016.

22. Miryea Navarro, "Diversity but Conflict under Wider AIDS Umbrella," *NYT*, 2 May 1993, B1.

23. Susan M. Chambré, "Being Needful: Family, Love, and Prayer among AIDS Volunteers," in *Research in the Sociology of Health Care*, ed. Jennie Jacobs Kronfeld, (Westport, CT: JAI Press, 1995), 113–139.

24. Dowd, "For Victims," B1; David Birth and David W. Dunlap, "Help for AIDS Patients Goes beyond Group's Name," *NYT*, 28 July 1986, B2; Davidson interview.

25. Letter from Marilyn Auerbach and Joanne E. Mantell, "Women's AIDS Project," GMHC, 22 April 1987; GMHC, "Women and AIDS: Safer Sex Guidelines for Women," 5 April 1987, author's files; Sara Rimer, "Volunteers Comfort Lonely AIDS Children," *NYT*, 27 February 1986, B1; statement of Mark S. Senak in *AIDS Issues, Part 2, Hearings before the Subcommittee on Health and the Environment of the Committee on Energy and Commerce, House of Representatives* (Washington, DC: U.S. Government Printing Office, 1988), 650–653.

26. Colin Robinson, "53 Percent Is No Minority," *Volunteer* 3, 7 (1986), 1, 16–17; David W. Dunlap, "Three Black Members Quit AIDS Organization Board," *NYT*, 11 January 1996, B2; Masha Gessen, "New York Lesbians Demand AIDS Care from GMHC," *Advocate*, 9 April 1991, 55; Ronald Johnson interview, 22 September 2003.

27. Michael Callen, "The PWA Coalition and People of Color—An Update," *Newsline*, April 1987, 1–2; National AIDS Network, *AIDS Education and Support Services to Minorities: A Survey of Community-Based AIDS Service Providers* (Washington, DC: National AIDS Network, 1987), A7.

28. *Momentum News*, 9 September 1998, 1; "St. Peter's Church Expands Programs and Locations," *Newsline*, December, 1988, 18.

29. Ganga Stone, "Who We Are," *The Good News Letter*, September, 1988, 1.

30. The Momentum Project, Inc., "Site Rules," author's files.

31. John F. Kennedy School of Government, Harvard University, "Bailey House," 1989, 2.

32. "Bailey House," 13–15.

33. Memo from Bill Brevoort to PWA Coalition board, 23 August 1991, PWA Coalition Papers, Box 82.

34. Miryea Navarro, "Diversity but Conflict under Wider AIDS Umbrella," *NYT*, 28 May 1993, B1.

35. "New York State AIDS Bill," in Siegel and Siegel, *AIDS*, 175–177.

36. Memo from Mel Rosen to local community AIDS Institute Task Force members, 4 October 1983; request for proposals, Community Services Programs, New York State Department of Health AIDS Institute, 1 December 1983, Lawrence Papers.

37. Robert Moroney, "(800)-462–1844: State AIDS Hotline," *Native*, 9–22 April 1984, 12; New York State Department of Health, *AIDS: New York's Response—A 5-Year Interagency Plan* (Albany, NY: New York State Department of Health, 1989), 98.

38. New York State Assembly, Task Force on Women's Issues, *Report of the Public Hearing on AIDS, Its Impact on Women, Children, and Families: Summary of Testimony* (Albany, NY: New York State Division for Women, 1988), 9.
39. "Haitians Removed from AIDS Risk List," Associated Press, 10 April 1985, Lexis/Nexis.
40. Ditte Nexo, "Black Gay Forum Offers AIDS Help," *Native*, 27 February–11 March 1984, 8–9.
41. Cohen, *Boundaries of Blackness*, ch. 9.
42. Mireya Navarro, "In Hispanic Community, Many Ignore AIDS," *NYT*, 29 December 1989, B4.
43. Minutes, Hispanic AIDS Forum, 23 September, 21 October, and 6 December 1985, author's files.
44. Letter from the Council of Churches of the City of New York, 12 November 1985, author's files.
45. Philip M. Boffey, "Blacks Alerted on Risks of AIDS," *NYT*, 23 November 1985, B4.
46. Author interview, 2 June 1993.
47. Author interview, 3 January 1995.
48. Author interview, 2 June 1993.
49. Michael E. Howard, "A Tiger in the House: Gay Black Men Take on AIDS," *Village Voice*, 27 December 1988, 15.
50. William Hawkeswood, *One of the Children: Gay Black Men in Harlem*, Alex W. Costly, ed. (Berkeley and Los Angeles: University of California Press, 1996), 169.
51. Mindy Thompson Fullilove and Robert E. Fullilove III, "Stigma as an Obstacle to AIDS Action: The Case of the African American Community," *American Behavioral Scientist* 42 (1999): 1118.
52. Erik Eckholm, "Poll Finds Many AIDS Fears That the Experts Say Are Groundless," *NYT*, 12 September 1985, B11.
53. James H. Jones, *Bad Blood: The Tuskegee Syphilis Experiment* (New York: Free Press, 1993).
54. Jones, *Bad*, 228–231.
55. Stephen B. Thomas and Sandra Crouse Quinn, "The Tuskegee Syphilis Study, 1932–1972: Implications for HIV Education and AIDS Risk Education Programs in the Black Community," *American Journal of Public Health* 81 (1991): 1498–1505.
56. Jason DeParle, "Talk of Government Being Out to Get Blacks Falls on More Attentive Ears," *NYT*, 29 October 1990, B7.
57. Gregory M. Herek and John P. Capitanio, "Conspiracies, Contagion, and Compassion: Trust and Public Reactions to AIDS," *AIDS Education and Prevention* 6, 4 (1994): 365–375.
58. Edna Negron, "Focus on AIDS: Targeting the Hispanic Community," *Newsday*, 23 February 1988, 11.
59. Presentation by Ruth Rodriguez, *Women in Crisis Presents Minority Women and AIDS: Conference Proceedings* (New York: Women in Crisis, 1990), 7.
60. Rafael M. Díaz, *Latino Gay Men and HIV: Culture, Sexuality, and Risk Behavior* (New York: Routledge, 1998), 7.
61. Guillermo Vasquez, "The Impact of the Epidemic on the Hispanic Community," presentation to the National Academy of Sciences Panel on the Social Impact of the AIDS Epidemic, 2 April 1990, New York, NY.
62. Interview, 4 January 2000.
63. Gerardo Marin, "AIDS Prevention among Hispanics: Needs, Risk Behaviors, and Cultural Values," *Public Health Reports* 104 (September–October, 1989): 411–415.

64. Carmen Medina, "Latino Culture and Sex Education," SIECUS Report 15, January–February 1987: 60.

65. George DeStefano, "Are Gay Men Having Safer Sex?" *Outweek*, 18 February 1990, 42.

66. "In a Gay Haven, a Sense of Community Builds," *NYT*, 4 December 1994, 13–9; *Fighting Back: Puerto Ricans Respond to the AIDS Epidemic* (Washington, DC: Puerto Rican Coalition, 1992), 15.

67. Ari L. Goldman, "AIDS Patients in Dire Need Finding Solace," *NYT*, 12 December 1987, 33

68. Minority Task Force on AIDS tax returns, author's files.

69. "Commission on AIDS," *Amsterdam News*, 1 October 1988, 11; presentation by Deborah Fraser-Howze, United Hospital Fund Conference, 4 November 1990.

70. E. R. Shipp and Miryea Navarro, "Reluctantly, Black Churches Confront AIDS," *NYT*, 18 November 1991, A1.

71. Bill Bahlman, "NAACP Conference Addresses AIDS Epidemic," *Native*, 3–17 August 1987, 10; "Sullivan Warns AIDS Plague Will Ravage Black America," *Jet*, 5 August 1991, 4; Cohen, *Boundaries*, ch. 8.

72. Cohen, *Boundaries*, p.149.

73. Natalie Hopkinson, "Black Caucus Calls for AIDS Emergency," *Pittsburgh Post-Gazette*, 12 May 1998, A3.

74. 2 June 1993 interview.

75. Marin, "AIDS," 414.

76. Michael Howard, "Have the Black and Latino Media Dropped the Ball on Covering AIDS?" *AIDS Patient Care* 5 (April 1991): 54–55.

77. Fullilove and Fullilove, "Stigma," 1118.

78. Elaine B. Sharp, *The Dilemma of Drug Policy in the United States* (New York: HarperCollins, 1994), 15.

79. Richard Goldstein, "AIDS and Race," *The Village Voice*, 10 March 1987, 23.

80. Harlon Dalton, "AIDS in Blackface," *Daedalus* 118, summer 1989, 217.

81. Interview, 6 December 1999.

82. Crystal Nix, "More and More AIDS Cases Found among Drug Abusers," *NYT*, 20 October 1985, A51; Lawrence K. Altman, "Drug Abusers Try to Cut AIDS Risk," NYT, 18 April 1985, B11.

83. Don C. Des Jarlais, "Stages in the Response of the Drug Abuse Treatment System to the AIDS Epidemic in New York City," *Journal of Drug Issues* 20 (1990): 335–347.

84. Anthony Scro interview, 13 May 1997.

85. d'Adesky, "Minority."

86. "ADAPT Update," memo from Anthony Scro to Charles LaPorte, Scro Files.

87. "Minutes—AIDS meeting, 11/27/85," author's files.

88. "Dear Program Administrator, Staff, and Clients," April 1986, author's files.

89. "Heroin Addicts in Jail: New York Tries Methadone Treatment Program," *Corrections Today*, August 1989, 24, 130–131.

90. Letter from David Patterson to Roger Paris, 20 March 1986, author's files.

91. Joseph interview.

92. Marianne Arneberg, "AIDS Inmates Protest Treatment," *Newsday*, 3 June 1986, 21; Edith Springer interview; Joseph interview.

93. Richard H. Needle et al., "HIV Prevention with Drug-Using Populations—Current Status and Future Prospects: Introduction and Overview," *Public Health Reports* (June 1998): 2.

94. Frank Tardalo interview, 13 May 1997.

95. Springer interview.

96. Mike McAlary, "Group Warns Addicts: 'Don't Share the Spike,'" *New York Newsday*, 14 April 1986, 2.

97. Springer interview.

98. Peter Schmeisser, "Zeroing In on AIDS with Street Smarts," *National Journal*, 5 March 1988, 615.

99. McAlary, "Group."

100. Lee Smith, "Throwing Money at AIDS," *Fortune*, 13 August 1987, 67.

101. Kathy Dobie, "Yolanda Serrano," *Ms.*, January/February 1989, 79–83; Heidi Evans, "Spread Word—Not Disease: Fighting AIDS in the Street," *NY Daily News*, 4 October 1987, 29.

102. Sandra Bodovitz, "Reaching the Hard-to-Reach: Aid for Addicts," *NYT*, 12 July 1987, A20

103. "Request to the New York Foundation for a Start-Up, General-Support Grant for ADAPT, the Association for Drug Abuse Prevention and Treatment," n.d., author's files.

104. ADAPT, minutes, 1 May 1986; ADAPT, 1986 tax return; letter from Madeline Lee to Yolanda Serrano, 20 October 1986; letter from Yolanda Serrano to Community Service Society, 1 July 1986. Author's files.

105. Memo from Richard Marx to Charles La Porte, 27 December 1985, Scro Files; letter from Elaine Ehrlich to Yolanda Serrano, 26 August 1986, author's files; New York City Department of Health, "Request for Proposals for AIDS Educational Services," 12 May 1986, author's files.

106. Letter from Ravinia Hayes-Crozier, 13 August 1986; letter from Zuhirah Sabreen Shabazz to Yolanda Serrano, 26 March 1987; letter from George W. Clifford to Yolanda Serrano, 15 June 1987; Springer interview. Author's files.

107. Nicholas Freudenberg and Urayoana Trinidad, "The Role of Community Organizations in AIDS Prevention in Two Latino Communities in New York City," *Health Education Quarterly* 19 (1992): 219–232; Nicholas Freudenberg et al., "How Black and Latino Community Organizations Respond to the AIDS Epidemic: A Case Study in One New York City Neighborhood," *AIDS Education and Prevention* 1 (1989): 12–21.

108. George W. Clifford, AIDS in New York City: 1981–1990 (unpublished Ph.D. dissertation, SUNY at Albany, 1992), 419.

109. New York City Office of Management and Budget, *Actual and Projected Appropriations for AIDS in New York City* (New York: New York City Office of Management and Budget, 1990).

110. Elaine J. Ehrlich and Paul A. Moore, "Delivery of AIDS Services: The New York State Response," *Social Work* 35 (March 1990): 175.

111. Barbara Goldsmith, "Women on the Edge," *New Yorker*, 26 April 1993, 64–81.

112. Dooley Worth, "Sexual Decision-Making and AIDS: Why Condom Promotion among Vulnerable Women Is Likely to Fail," *Studies in Family Planning* 20 (November/December 1989): 306.

113. "The Woman and AIDS Project," *Focus on AIDS in New York State* (October 1990): 9.

114. Author's database on foundation funding, obtained from the Foundation Center records; WARN tax return for 1989, author's files.

115. "Women and AIDS Resource Network," *Newsline*, June 1989, 15–16.

116. "Woman and AIDS Project," 8

117. Barbara Draimin et al., "AIDS and Its Traumatic Effects on Families," in *International Handbook of Multigenerational Legacies of Trauma,* Yael Danieli, ed. (New York: Plenum, 1998), 587–601.

118. Mary Talbot, "The AIDS Mother's Dilemma," *NY Daily News,* 27 February 1994.

119. Mary Jane Rotheram-Borus et al., "The Impact of Illness Disclosure and Custody Plans on Adolescents Whose Parents Live with AIDS," *AIDS* 11 (1997): 1159–1164.

120. "Health Force: Women and Men against AIDS" and "Life Force: A History of the Organization, Area, and Population Served," author's files.

121. "Manhattan 'Women Living with AIDS Day,'" *Newsline,* January/February 1991, 11.

122. Mary Reinholz, "Sisters in Arms," *NY Daily News,* 16 October 1989, 1, 34.

123. Locke McKelvey, presentation at the United Jewish Appeal (UJA) Federation Conference on AIDS Services, 25 March 1993.

124. Nicholas Freudenberg et al., "Reaching Low-Income Women at Risk of AIDS: A Case History of a Drop-in Center for Women in the South Bronx, New York City," *Health Education Research* 9 (1994): 119–132.

125. "Family-Centered HIV Services," Visiting Nurse Service of New York, brochure, author's files; Angela Gonzales, "Self-Help Community Services," presentation at the UJA Federation Conference on AIDS Services, 25 March 1993.

126. Halina Maslanka et al., "An Evaluation of Community-Based HIV Services for Women in New York State," *Journal of the American Women's Medical Association* 50 (May/August 1995): 123.

Chapter 6: The "New Calcutta"

1. Art Levine et al., "The Uneven Odds," *U.S. News and World Report,* 13 October 1986, 31–32.

2. The local groups included the Interagency Task Force on AIDS, the New York City AIDS Task Force, the Citizen's Commission on AIDS, the New York City AIDS Fund, the Mayor's AIDS Task Force, and the New York State AIDS Task Force. See Citizen's Commission on AIDS for New York and Northern New Jersey, "A Guide to the Plans," March 1989, author's files.

3. "Head of AIDS Commission Pledges Quick Reorganization of Panel," *NYT,* 11 October 1987, A45; David Whitman, "How Reagan Judges Dismantled AIDS Agenda," *Wall Street Journal,* 11 August 1988, accessed from Factiva; Sandra G. Boodman, "Chairman Steering AIDS Panel Away from Rancor," *Washington Post,* 28 March 1988, A13; "PBS' Portrayal of an Epidemic," *Boston Globe,* 8 March 1989, 18; Bernard E. Trainor, "James David Watkins: A Compassionate Pragmatist," *NYT,* 4 June 1988, A7.

4. Susan Jenks, "Commission to Goad Government," *Medical World News,* 28 August 1989, 57; "U. of Michigan Dean Chosen to Head U.S. Panel on AIDS," *NYT,* 5 August 1989, A8.

5. "Americans Consider AIDS Nation's Worst Problem," *Wall Street Journal,* 23 August 1988.

6. *Report of the Presidential Commission on the Human Immunodeficiency Virus Epidemic* (Washington, DC: U. S. Government Printing Office, 1988), 93. A search of major newspapers in the United States in the Lexis/Nexis database indicated that not one major newspaper article published between 1984 and 1986 contained both the words "AIDS" and "underclass" anywhere in the text. In contrast, this combination was found in forty-four articles published between 1988 and 1990.

7. Chambré, "Civil."

8. Daniel M. Fox and Emily H. Thomas, "AIDS Cost Analysis and Social Policy," *Law, Medicine, and Health Care* 15 (1987): 186–211.

9. New York State Department of Health, *AIDS: New York's Response: A 5-Year Inter-agency Plan* (Albany, NY: New York State Department of Health, 1989), v.

10. Hilary MacKenzie, "200,000 in U.S. Exposed to AIDS, Disease Study Says," *The Globe and Mail*, 20 July 1984, M6; Donald Ian Macdonald, "Coolfont Report: A PHS Plan for Prevention and Control of AIDS and the AIDS Virus," *Public Health Reports* 101 (July/August 1986): 341–348.

11. Peter S. Arno et al., "Economic and Policy Implications of Early Intervention in HIV Disease," *JAMA* 262 (1989): 1493–1498.

12. Anthony Giddens, *The Third Way: The Renewal of Social Democracy* (Cambridge, UK: Polity Press, 1998).

13. Bruce Lambert, "Task Force Increases Projections of Care Needed by AIDS Patients," *NYT*, 23 February 1989, B5.

14. New York City AIDS Fund, *AIDS: Community Needs and Private Funding: A Needs Assessment for New York City* (New York: New York Community Trust, 1988), 17.

15. *AIDS: New York's Response.*

16. Interagency Task Force on AIDS, "New York City: Strategic Plan for AIDS" (New York: Interagency Task Force on AIDS, 1988).

17. The Citizens' Commission on AIDS, press release, 6 March 1989, author's files.

18. Bruce Lambert, "AIDS Drives Jobs Away, Report Says," *NYT*, 7 March 1989, B1

19. Clarence Stone, *Regime Politics: Governing Atlanta, 1946–1988* (Lawrence: University Press of Kansas, 1989), 1.

20. Bruce Lambert, "Business Leaders Agree to Seek Money for AIDS," *NYT*, 6 April 1989, 3; Bruce Lambert, "AIDS in a Deficit Year: More Plans Than Money," *NYT*, 23 April 1989, E24.

21. John H. Ellis, *Yellow Fever and Public Health in the New South* (Lexington: University Press of Kentucky, 1992).

22. Howard Kurtz, "Koch's Rivals Say Big Apple Is Rotting: Mayor Calls New York Envy of the World," *Washington Post*, 11 August 1989, A3.

23. Colin McCord and Harold Freeman, "Excess Mortality in Harlem," *New England Journal of Medicine* 322 (1990): 173; Stephen W. Nicholas and Elaine J. Abrams, "Boarder Babies with AIDS in Harlem: Lessons in Applied Public Health," *American Journal of Public Health* 92 (February 2002): 163–165.

24. Michel Marriot, "Needs Strain Social Services and Budgets," *NYT*, 14 September 1988, B1.

25. Jane Gross, "First Look at Homeless: A Raw Sight for Tourists," *NYT*, 9 November 1987, B1.

26. Elaine Sharp, *The Dilemma of Drug Policy in the United States* (New York: Harper-Collins, 1994), 15.

27. Gillian Walker, "Supportive Counseling for HIV-Infected Drug-Using Women," *Focus* 10 (September 1995): 1–4.

28. Peter Kerr, "Babies of Crack Users Fill Hospital Nurseries," *NYT*, 25 August 1986, B1.

29. U.S. General Accounting Office, *Foster Care: Parental Drug Abuse Has Alarming Impact on Young Children* (Washington, DC: U.S. General Accounting Office, 1994), 2.

30. Craig Wolff, "Youths Rape and Beat Central Park Jogger," *NYT*, 21 April 1989, B1.

31. Paul Boyer, *Urban Masses and Moral Order in America: 1820–1920* (Cambridge, MA: Harvard University Press, 1978).

32. Kenneth Lipper, "What Needs to Be Done?" *NYT*, 31 December 1989, F28; John Leo, "The Heartbreak That Is New York," *U.S. News and World Report*, 24 September 1990, 37; Malcolm Gladwell, *The Tipping Point: How Little Things Can Make a Big Difference* (Boston: Little, Brown, 2000), 132–137.

33. Deborah A. Stone, "Causal Stories and the Formation of Policy Agendas," *Political Science Quarterly* 104 (1989): 281–300.

34. Stephen S. Caizza, "Will New York Become Plague City?" *Native*, 11–24 February 1985, 17.

35. Randy Shilts, "AIDS Overwhelms N.Y. Health System," *San Francisco Chronicle*, 14 February 1985, 1.

36. Kristin Loomis, "AIDS: Numbers Game," *New York*, 6 March 1989, 48.

37. Thomas Killip, "Hospitals in New York City: A System under Stress," in *Public and Professional Attitudes toward AIDS Patients*, ed. David E. Rogers and Eli Ginzburg (Boulder, CO: Westview, 1989), 76.

38. "Hospitals Fear Burden of Unpaid AIDS Bills," *NYT*, 3 November 3, 1985, A1.

39. Ann H. Hardy et al., "The Economic Impact of the First 10,000 Cases of Acquired Immunodeficiency Syndrome in the United States," *JAMA* 255 (1986): 209–211.

40. Statement by Jo Ivey Boufford, M.D., acting president, New York City Health and Hospitals Corporation before the Subcommittee on Health and the Environment, Committee on Energy and Commerce, United States House of Representatives, 8 November 1985, 3, author's files.

41. Jesse Green et al., "The $147,000 Misunderstanding: Repercussions of Overestimating the Cost of AIDS," *Journal of Health Politics, Policy, and Law* 19 (1994): 69–90; Joseph A. Cimino, "Integrated Services for AIDS Patients: Comments and Cautions," in John Griggs, ed., *AIDS: Public Policy Dimensions. New York: United Hospital Fund*, 1987, 194.

42. Peter S. Arno, "The Nonprofit Sector's Response to the AIDS Epidemic: Community-Based Services in San Francisco," *American Journal of Public Health* 76 (1986): 1325–1330.

43. New York State Senate Majority Task Force on AIDS, *The AIDS Crisis in New York: A Legislative Perspective and Agenda for Study* (Albany, NY: Senate Majority Task Force, 1987), 116.

44. New York State AIDS Advisory Council minutes, 19 May 1988, Callen Collection, Box 2, Folder 56.

45. Ruby P. Hearn, "Overview of AIDS Programs Receiving Support from the Robert Wood Johnson Foundation," in *Proceedings: AIDS Prevention and Services Workshop*, ed. Vivian E. Fransen (Princeton, NJ: Robert Wood Johnson Foundation, 1990), 10.

46. *AIDS Service Demonstration Programs: Three-Year Report, 1987–1989* (Washington: U.S. Department of Health and Human Services, 1990), 7.

47. Systemetrics McGraw-Hill, Inc., *Evaluation of AIDS Service Demonstration Projects: Executive Summary, Part 1*, 10 October 1989, 5.

48. Interagency Task Force on AIDS, The City of New York, *Report to the Mayor*, April 1987, 50.

49. AIDS Service Delivery Consortium, "Annual Progress Report, Year One," PWA Coalition Papers, Box 1.

50. David J. Sencer and Victor E. Botnick, *Report to the Mayor: New York City's Response to the AIDS Crisis*, December 1985, 53.

51. Peter S. Arno and Robert G. Hughes, "Local Policy Responses to the AIDS Epidemic: New York and San Francisco," *New York State Journal of Medicine* 87 (May 1987): 267.

52. Jo Ivey Boufford, "AIDS in New York City: Program and Costs," *AIDS: Public Policy Dimensions*, ed. John Griggs (New York: United Hospital Fund, 1987), 224.

53. Kenneth Raske, "The Impact of AIDS on New York's Not-For-Profit Hospitals," in Imperato, *Acquired Immunodeficiency Syndrome*, 82–84.

54. Loomis, "AIDS," 44–49.

55. Bruce C. Vladeck, "Worst-Case Scenarios," president's letter, United Hospital Fund, February 1990, 2.

56. "AIDS Crisis in New York," 119.

57. Loïc J. D. Wacquant, "The New Urban Color Line: The State and Fate of the Ghetto in PostFordist America," in *Social Theory and the Politics of Identity*, ed. Craig Calhoun (Cambridge, MA: Blackwell, 1994), 231–276.

58. Ronald Mincey and Erol Ricketts, "Growth of the Underclass: 1970–1970," *Journal of Human Resources* 25 (1990): 137–147.

59. William Julius Wilson, *The Truly Disadvantaged: The Inner City, the Underclass, and Public Policy* (Chicago: University of Chicago Press, 1987); Jonathan Crane, "The Epidemic Theory of Ghettoes and Neighborhood Effects on Dropping Out and Teenage Childbearing," *American Journal of Sociology* 96 (1991): 1226–1259.

60. Christopher Jencks, *The Homeless* (Cambridge, MA: Harvard University Press, 1994); Herman Joseph, "Substance Abuse and Homelessness within the Inner Cities," in *Substance Abuse: A Comprehensive Textbook*, ed. Joyce Lowinson et al. (New York: Williams and Wilkins, 1992), 875–889.

61. Risa Denenberg, "Childhood Sexual Abuse as an HIV Risk Factor in Women," *Treatment Issues* (July/August 1997): 5.

62. Richard Berkowitz, "Newsline Interviews Joyce Wallace, M.D.," *Newsline*, December 1992, 25.

63. Anitra Pivnick, "Loss and Regeneration: Influences on the Reproductive Decisions of HIV-Positive, Drug-Using Women," *Medical Anthropology* 16 (1994): 51.

64. Sherry Deren et. al., "Behavior-Change Strategies for Women at High Risk for HIV," *Drugs and Society* 7, no. 3–4 (1994): 123.

65. Lawrence M. Mead, "The Rise of Paternalism," in *The New Paternalism: Supervisory Approaches to Poverty*, ed. Lawrence M. Mead (Washington, DC: Brookings Institution Press, 1997), 2.

66. United States Senate, *The American Health Care Crisis: A View from Four Communities. Hearings of the Committee on Labor and Human Resources, December 11, 12, 13 and 14, 1989* (Washington: U.S. Government Printing Office, 1990), 2.

67. U.S. Congress, Committee on the Budget, *Hospitals in Crisis* (Washington: U.S. Government Printing Office, 1990), 4.

68. Mayor Edward I. Koch, "Why We Need More Federal AIDS Funding," *Native*, 27 October–9 November 1986, 16.

69. Juan Williams, "Hard Times, Harder Hearts," *Washington Post*, 2 October 1988, C1; Mead, *New Paternalism*, 16.

70. Sarah Schulman, "Thousands May Die in the Streets," *The Nation*, 10 April 1989, 480.

71. Scott Harris, "Society Pays for AIDS: The Cost of Compassion is Soaring," *Los Angeles Times*, 8 December 1986, 1–1; Shawn Hubler and Victor F. Zonana, "An Escalation of Need—Epidemics of AIDS, Homelessness Are Converging," *Los Angeles*

Times, 29 April 1990, A3; Philip Seib, "Health Care Is a Problem for Homeless," *Dallas Morning News*, 9 August 1989, 15A.

72. Steven K. Paulson, "Public Hospital Administrators Say Hospital Care Deteriorating," Associated Press, 10 March 1989, Lexis/Nexis.

73. "Urban Health Status Deteriorating," *PR Newswire*, 12 June 1990, Factiva.

74. Gwen Ifill, "Sympathy Wanes for Homeless," *Washington Post*, 21 May 1990, A1; Linda Greenhouse, "Ban Is Left Intact on Subway Begging," *NYT*, 27 November 1990, A1.

75. United States Conference of Mayors, "The Impact of AIDS upon America's Cities," *AIDS Information Exchange*, April 1990, 1, 3.

76. Presentation by Rhoda White, Bronx AIDS Services, Mayor's Voluntary Action Center AIDS Taskforce, 17 March 1993; Chambré, "Civil."

77. *Report of the Presidential Commission*, 17.

78. Bruce Lambert, "AIDS Services: A Disjointed Network," *NYT*, 5 May 1989, B1.

79. "Swamped by Surge in AIDS: GMHC Forced to Curtail Caseload," *Outweek*, 17 October 1990, 16; Bruce Lambert, "AIDS Groups Feel the Fiscal Crisis," *NYT*, 6 May 1990, A38.

80. Bruce Lambert, "AIDS Program Fails Many, Patients Say," *NYT*, 21 October 1989, A27.

81. U.S. House of Representatives, "Statement of Pat Christen, Acting Executive Director, San Francisco AIDS Foundation," *Treatment and Care for Persons with HIV Infection and AIDS* (Washington: U.S. Government Printing Office, 1990), 170; Marilyn Chase, "Noble Experiment: Volunteers' Distress Cripples Huge Effort to Provide AIDS Care," *Wall Street Journal*, 12 March 1990, A1; Helen Schietinger, "Coordinated Community-Based AIDS Treatment," in *What to Do about AIDS*, ed. L. McKusick (Berkeley and Los Angeles: University of California Press, 1986), 18.

82. Hubler and Zonana, "An Escalation."

83. Cities where more than .0025 percent of the population had been diagnosed with AIDS could also qualify (Patricia D. Siplon, *AIDS and the Policy Struggle in the United States* [Washington, DC: Georgetown University Press, 2002], 96–97).

84. "Bush Reluctantly Signs AIDS Measure," *1990 CQ Almanac*, 583.

85. Letter from Ted Weiss, 15 March 1985, Lawrence Papers.

86. Cynthia Cannon Poindexter, "Promises in the Plague: Passage of the Ryan White Comprehensive AIDS Resources Emergency Act as a Case Study for Legislative Action," *Health and Social Work* 24 (1999): 35–42.

87. "U.S. Housing Programs Overhauled," *1990 CQ Almanac*, 640.

88. Poindexter, "Promises."

89. "Ryan White Comprehensive AIDS Emergency Act—Conference Report" (Senate, 4 August 1990), www.thomas.gov, accessed 19 June 2003.

90. Mark C. Donovan, *Taking Aim: Target Populations and the Wars on AIDS and Drugs* (Washington, DC: Georgetown University Press, 2001), 62–63.

91. This was documented in 1987 Gallup polls and a 1991 Roper poll, Lexis/Nexis.

92. Committee on the Ryan White CARE Act, *Measuring What Matters: Allocation, Planning, and Quality Assessment for the Ryan White CARE Act* (Washington, DC: National Academies Press, 2004), 2; Robert Pear, "Congress Authorizes $875 Million to Fight AIDS in Hard-Hit Areas," *NYT*, 4 August 1990, A1; Catherine Woodard, "$16 M to Fight AIDS in 20 Neighborhoods," *Newsday*, 12 February 1991, 8.

93. Richard A. Rettig, "The Policy Debate on Patient Care Financing for Victims of End-Stage Renal Disease," *Law and Contemporary Problems* 40 (1976): 196–230.

94. "Bush Reluctantly," 582.

95. Michael Lipsky and Steven Rathgeb Smith, "When Social Problems Are Treated as Emergencies," *Social Service Review* (March 1989): 6.

96. GAO, *Ryan White Care Act: Access to Services by Minorities, Women, and Substance Abusers* (Washington, DC: GAO, 1995); GAO, *HIV/AIDS: Use of Ryan White CARE Act and Other Assistance Grant Funds* (Washington, DC: GAO, 2000); "Decreasing Hospital Use for HIV," National Center for Health Statistics, www.cdc.gov/nchs/products/pubs/pubd/hestats/hosphiv.htm, accessed 21 July 2005.

97. Craig Horowitz, "A South Bronx Renaissance," *New York*, 21 November 1994, 54–59; Tamar Jacoby and Fred Siegel, "Growing the Inner City?" *New Republic*, 23 August 1999.

98. "Teenage Birthrate Falls to Lowest Point in 60 Years," *Washington Post*, 9 August 2000, A5; Alfred Blumstein and Joel Wallman, *The Crime Drop in America* (New York: Cambridge University Press, 2000); Fox Butterfield, "Number of People in State Prisons Declines Slightly," *NYT*, 13 August 2001, A1; "The Innovation Issue: New Initiatives in New York Child Welfare," *Child Welfare Watch* (summer 2005): 1.

99. G. Thomas Kingsley and Kathryn L. S. Pettit, "Concentrated Poverty: A Change in Course," *Neighborhood Change in Urban America* 2 (May 2003), 1, www.urban.org/uploadedPDF/310790_NCUA2.PDF, accessed on 3 December 2005.

100. R. Andrew Parker, "A Stealth Urban Policy in the U.S.? Federal Spending in Five Large Metropolitan Regions, 1984–93," *Urban Studies* 34 (1997): 1831–1850.

Chapter 7: Our Place at the Table

1. Sweeney interview; Peter Blauner, "Trying to Live with the AIDS Plague," *New York Magazine*, 17 June 1985, 51.

2. Dick Thompson, "The AIDS Political Machine," *Time*, 22 January 1990, 24–26.

3. Paul Burstein and April Linton, "The Impact of Political Parties, Interest Groups, and Social Movement Organizations on Public Policy: Some Recent Evidence and Theoretical Concerns," *Social Forces* 81 (2002): 381–408.

4. William A. Maloney, Grant Jordan, and Andrew W. McLaughlin, "Interest Groups and Public Policy: The Insider/Outsider Model Revisited," *Journal of Public Policy* 14 (1994): 17–38; Wayne A. Santoro and Gail M. McGuire, "Social Movement Insiders: The Impact of Institutional Activists on Affirmative Action and Comparable Worth Policies," *Social Problems* 44 (1997): 503–529.

5. "ACT UP Marks Tenth Anniversary Founding at Center," *Center Voice*, April/May 1997, 4.

6. John Moore, presentation at "Whatever Happened to AIDS?" Baruch College, New York, NY, 17 March 1994; speech by Nilsa Gutierrez, New York State AIDS Institute Conference, Albany, NY, 13 November 1993.

7. Altman, *AIDS*, 86.

8. Fundraising letter, National Gay Task Force, author's files; Virginia Apuzzo, presentation at "Two Activists, Two Decades," Lesbian and Gay Community Services Center, New York, NY, 10 February 1999.

9. Sweeney interview; Joyce Wadler, "Lobbyist Finds Gay Rights an Uncomfortable Issue on Hill," *Washington Post*, 29 August 1980, A17; "Task Force History," www.thetaskforce.org/aboutus/history.cfm, accessed on 26 July 2005; Neil Miller, *In Search of Gay America* (New York: Atlantic Monthly Press, 1989), 266.

10. Cindy Patton, *Sex and Germs: The Politics of AIDS* (Boston: South End Press, 1985), 147.

11. Lawrence Mass, "Time for Prevention: Devising Ways of Evading AID," *Native*, 16–20 August 1982, 31–32.

12. "Where Are We Now?" reprinted in Kramer, *Reports*, 27.

13. Martin Levine interview, June 1990; Martin Levine, "The Life and Death of Gay Clones," in *Gay Culture in America: Essays from the Field*, ed. Gilbert Herdt (Boston: Beacon Press, 1991), 68–86.

14. Richard De Thuin, "CS People: Mel Rosen," *Christopher Street.* 23 February 1983, 12.

15. Michael Spector, "Gay Groups Mobilize against AIDS," *Washington Post*, 2 August 1985, A1.

16. Morgan, "Amid AIDS," *NYT*; "Words from Leonard Bloom," *Volunteer*, July/August 1990, 10.

17. Lisa Levitt Ryckman, "Gay Community Mobilizes to Battle AIDS," *Associated Press*, 13 September 1985, accessed from Factiva.

18. Morgan, "Amid AIDS"; Lisa Leff, "Gay Cause Is Gaining Attention," *Washington Post*, 26 August 1986, A4.

19. Anne-Christine d'Adesky, "Mass Turnout for Gay Rights," *Native*, 26 October 1987, 6.

20. Leff, "Gay Cause."

21. "Fear of AIDS Has Red Cross Discouraging Certain Donors," *NYT*, 7 March 1983, B7; Lawrence Mass, "Blood and Politics: An AIDS Notebook," *Native*, 14–27 February 1983, 23.

22. Callen, "A History."

23. Letter from Keith Lawrence to Dr. David Sencer, author's files.

24. Sweeney interview.

25. Kinsella, *Covering*, 69.

26. "The AIDS Network Letter to Mayor Koch," repr. in Kramer, *Reports*, 52–57.

27. Lawrence Mass, "City Opens Gay Health Office," *Native*, 28 March–10 April 1983, 15.

28. Richard Kaye, "Koch Meets with AIDS Network," *Native*, 9–22 May 1983, 7.

29. Leonard R. Brown, "AIDS Network Update," *Native*, 20 June–3 July 1983, 25; "Report on Visit," 2.

30. Andrew L. Yarrow, "'Day without Art' to Mourn Losses from AIDS," *NYT*, 29 November 1989, C15; Eleanor Blau, "With Art and Without, a Day for Calling Attention to the AIDS Crisis," *NYT*, 29 November 1990, B4.

31. Anne-Christine d'Adesky and Phil Zwickler, "The Names Project: The Quilt That Woke Up America," *Native*, 26 October 1987, 6.

32. Cleve Jones and Jeff Dawson, *Stitching a Revolution: The Making of an AIDS Activist* (San Francisco: Harper, 2000).

33. Yarrow, "'Day Without Art'" *NYT*; Blau, "With Art and Without."

34. "NGTF Urges People with AIDS to Apply for Social Security Benefits," *Native*, 29 August–11 September 1988, 71.

35. Rodger McFarlane, "Where Have All the Activists Gone?" *Journal of the International Association of Physicians in AIDS Care* 1 (1995): 10–13.

36. Larry Bush, "Reagan Response Blasted in AIDS Hearings," *Native*, 15–28 August 1983, 14–15; Jeff Levi and Judy Burns, "NGTF Meets with Dr. Brandt; Heckler Announces $22.2 Million Increase in AIDS Funding Requests," *Task Force Report*, September/October 1983, 1.

37. "Federation of AIDS-Related Organizations (FARO)," *Native*, 29 August–11 September 1983, 71; Altman, *AIDS*, 105.
38. David Shribman, "Seeking Research Funds for AIDS," *NYT*, 27 December 1983, B6.
39. John Wallace, "Lobbying Intensifies for AIDS Research Funding," *Native*, 6–19 December 1982, 9; "GMHC Update," *Native*, 4–17 June 1984, 18.
40. Jeffrey M. Berry, "Citizen Groups and the Changing Nature of Interest Group Politics in America," *Annals of the American Academy of Political and Social Science* 528 (July 1993): 30–41; David S. Meyer and Douglas R. Imig, "Political Opportunity and the Rise and Decline of Interest Group Sectors," *Social Science Journal* 30, 3 (1993): 253–270.
41. Dave Taylor, "$300,000 AIDS Education Media Campaign," *Newsline*, November 1986, 1–2.
42. "GMHC News," *Native*, 4–17 June 1984, 18.
43. "Malkin and Ross: GMHC Advocates in Albany," *Volunteer*, May/June 1990, 7; Larry Caputo, "A Meeting with the Governor," *Newsline*, January 1986, 1–2.
44. "GMHC Action Update" and "Policy," *Volunteer*, September/October 1989, 9, 11.
45. GMHC, *Annual Report, 1987/1988*.
46. "Coop Board Sued," Peter Lewis Allen, *The Wages of Sin: Sex and Disease, Past and Present* (Chicago: University of Chicago Press, 2000), 138.
47. Peter Freiberg et al., "Thousands March Nationwide to Demand Federal Action on AIDS," *Advocate*, 9 June 1983, 8–9; Steven C. Arvanette, "Thousands in Vigil Demand Millions for AIDS," *Native*, 23 May–5 June 1983, 9–10.
48. Kramer, *Reports*, 58.
49. Lindsey Gruson, "1,500 Attend Central Park Memorial Service for AIDS Victim," *NYT*, 14 June 1983; Edward D. Sargent, "1,500 March to Hill Seeking Funds to Fight AIDS," *Washington Post*, 9 October 1983, B1; "Demonstration Called for June 27," *Newsline*, May 1985, 1.
50. David E. Brown, "Striking Back," *Native*, 2 December 1985, 23.
51. Clendinen and Nagourney, *Out*, 524–525.
52. Joyce Purnick, "A Protest Erupts outside Hearing on an AIDS Bill," *NYT*, 16 November 1985, A31; David Summers, "How I Went to Testify before the New York City Council and Ended Up Getting Arrested," *Newsline*, January 1986, 9; Jane Rosett, "The Buddy Line," *Poz*, March 1997, 40.
53. Cleniden and Nagourney, *Out*, 525.
54. Maxine Wolfe, "The AIDS Coalition to Unleash Power : A Direct Model of Community Research for AIDS Prevention," in *AIDS Prevention and Services: Community-Based Research*, ed. Johannes P. Van Vugt (Westport, CT: Bergun and Garvey, 1994), 219; Alan Finder, "Police Halt Rights Marchers at Wall St.," *NYT*, 5 July 1986, A32.
55. Wolfe, "AIDS Coalition," 219.
56. "GLAAD Meets with *New York Times*," *Native*, 16 March 1987, 9, 41; "Buckley Retracts 'AIDS Tattoo' Proposal," *Native*, 8 December 1986, 6.
57. Chuck Steward, *Gay and Lesbian Issues: A Reference Handbook* (Santa Barbara, CA: Clio, 2003), 14.
58. Bob Lederer, "Lavender Hill Protests CDC, 'Timid' Gay Groups," *Gay Community News*, 22–28 March 1987, 3.
59. Lederer, "Lavender Hill."
60. Kramer, *Reports*, 128, 135–136.
61. Sweeney interview.
62. Mike Salinas, "Kramer, Mob, Others Call for Traffic Blockade," *Native*, 30 March 1987, 6.

63. Peter S. Arno and Douglas Shenson, "From AIDS to HIV Disease: Transformation of an Epidemic," in *Community-Based Care of Persons with AIDS: Developing a Research Agenda* (Rockville, MD: National Center for Health Services Research and Health Care Technology Assessment, 1989), 97–104.

64. "A Failure Led to Drug against AIDS," *NYT*, 28 September 1986, 38.

65. Salinas, "Kramer, Mob, Others," 6.

66. Interview, 1 April 1997.

67. Joyce Rothschild-Whitt, "The Collectivist Organization: An Alternative to Rational Bureaucratic Models," *American Sociological Review* 44 (1979): 509–527.

68. Gilbert Elbaz, "Beyond Anger: The Activist Construction of the AIDS Crisis," *Social Justice* 22, 4 (1995): 47.

69. Mike Salinas, "Wall Street Closed for 15 Minutes by Angry Gays," *Native*, 16 April 1987, 9; Clifford, *AIDS Epidemic*, 223; Larry Kramer, "The FDA's Callous Response to AIDS," repr. in Kramer, *Reports*, 40.

70. Flyer of the First Action, 24 March 1987, Wall Street, New York City. http://www.actupny.org\1stFlyer.htm, accessed on 15 September 2000.

71. Salinas, "Kramer, Mob, Others,"; Michael Specter, "Public Nuisance," *New Yorker*, 13 May 2001, 56–65.

72. Salinas, "Wall Street Closed"; Clifford, *AIDS Epidemic*, 223.

73. Donna Minkowitz, "ACT UP at a Crossroads," *The Village Voice*, 5 June 1990, 1.

74. Josh Gamson, "Silence, Death, and the Invisible Enemy: AIDS Activism and Social Movement 'Newness,'" *Social Problems* 36 (1989): 351–367.

75. Phil Zwickler, "AIDS Activists Convene," *Native*, 25 October 1987, 11; Phil Zwickler, "ACT NOW Plans Spring Actions," *Native*, 4 April 1988, 11.

76. Paula Span, "Getting Militant about AIDS," *Washington Post*, 28 March 1989, D1; Victor F. Zonana, "New Fronts in the AIDS War," *Los Angeles Times*, 4 April 1,1989, 5–1.

77. Kenneth Hausman, "'AIDS Panic' Brings Lonely Life to Patients, Gays," *Psychiatric News* (19 August 1983): 25.

78. B. D. Colen, "AIDS Suicides Drop," *Newsday*, 21 October 2002, 30.

79. "Thinking about Death," GMHC Video.

80. J. G. Rabkin, R. Remien, et al., "Suicidality in AIDS Long-Term Survivors: What Is the Evidence?" *AIDS Care* 5, no. 4 (1993): 409.

81. Eric Steward and Rona S. Weinstein, "Volunteer Participation in Context: Motivations and Political Efficacy within Three AIDS Organizations," *American Journal of Community Psychology* 25, no. 6 (1997): 821.

82. Robert Remien, presentation at Mental Health Issues and the HIV Epidemic conference, New York Academy of Medicine, 6 April 1994.

83. Lon G. Nungasser, *Epidemic of Courage: Facing AIDS in America* (New York: St. Martin's, 1986), 29.

84. David Handelman, "ACT UP in Anger," *Rolling Stone*, 8 March 1990, 82.

85. Cynthia Crossen, "Shock Troops: AIDS Activist Group Harasses and Provokes to Make Its Point," *Wall Street Journal*, 7 December 1989, A9; Robert Ariss, "Performing Anger: Emotion in Strategic Response to AIDS," *Australian Journal of Anthropology* 4, no. 1 (1993): 18–30; Deborah Gould, "Life during Wartime."

86. Vito Russo, "A Test of Who We Are as a People, " in *Surviving and Thriving: Collected*, 280–282.

87. Wolfe, "AIDS Coalition," 222.

88. Sal Licata, "Taking It to the Streets: Fighting for Treatments," *Newsline*, May 1987, 1–3.

89. Michael Callen,"Getting Arrested," *Newsline*, July/August 1987, 40–41.; Sal Licata, "Protesting at the International AIDS Conference," *Newsline*, July/August 1987, 2–3.

90. Philip J. Hilts, "82 Held in Protest on Pace of AIDS Research," *NYT*, 22 May 1990, C2.

91. Bruce Lambert, "3,000 Assailing Policy on AIDS Ring City Hall," *NYT*, 29 March 1989, B3.

92. Abigail Hacli, "The AIDS Activist Movement," *Sociology Review* 10 (2001): 28–32.

93. Phil Zwickler, "Send in the Clowns: Group Zaps D'Amato, Civil Rights Commission," *Native*, 6 June 1988, 6.

94. Thomas Morgan, "Mainstream Strategy for AIDS Group," *NYT*, 22 July 1988, B1.

95. Handelman, "ACT UP," 82.

96. Phil Zwickler, "Community Activists Meet with Members of AIDS Commission," *Native*, 31 August 1987, 8; Phil Zwickler, "AIDS Commission Meets in Washington," *Native*, 21 September 1987, 8.

97. N. Offen et al., "From Adversary to Target Market: The ACT-UP Boycott of Philip Morris," *Tobacco Control* 12 (June 2003): 203–208.

98. Chris Nealon, "Day of Inspiration," *Gay Community News*, 28 January–3 February 1991, 1, 7,

99. Paul Taylor, "AIDS Guerillas," *New York*, 12 November 1990, 65.

100. Dinitia Smith, "Guggenheim to Show Video Series on Early Days of AIDS," *NYT*, 29 November 2000, A1; Jean Carlomusto, "Focusing on Women: Video as Activism," in *Women, AIDS, and Activism*, ed. Women's Handbook Group (Boston, MA: South End Press, 1990), 215–218.

101. Handelman, "ACT UP," 82.

102. Ibid., 85; merchandise catalogue, author's files.

103. "Ashes of AIDS Casualties Tossed over White House Fence," *NYT*, 14 October 1996, A11

104. Irene Elizabeth Stroud, "Faith and Life (and Death) in ACT UP," *Christianity and Crisis*, 4 January 1993, 52, 420–22.

105. Kevin Michael DeLuca, "Unruly Arguments: The Body Rhetoric of ACT UP, Earth First! and Queer Nation," *Argumentation and Advocacy* 36 (1999): 9–21.

106. Thomas Morgan, "Mainstream Strategy for AIDS Group," *NYT*, 22 July 1988, B1; Crossen, "Shock Troops."

107. Stephen C. Joseph, *Dragon within the Gates: The Once and Future AIDS Epidemic* (New York: Carroll and Graf, 1992); Bruce Lambert, "Health Chief and AIDS: A Chant of Critics amid Praise," *NYT*, 30 August 1988, B1.

108. Handelman, "ACT UP," 90; "Angry AIDS Activists Rally near Convention," *Christian Science Monitor*, 16 July 1992, 7; author's fieldnotes.

109. Jane Gross, "11 Are Arrested in Gay Protest at St. Patrick's," *NYT*, 7 December 1987, B1.

110. Ed Magnuson, "In a Rage over AIDS," *Time*, 25 December 1989, 33; Manuel Perez-Rivas and Ji-Yeon Yu, "Protest Siege at St. Pat's," *Newsday*, 11 December 1989, 3; "Anti-Catholics," *Economist*, 16 December 1989, 23.

111. Larry Gutenberg, "A New Decade, A New Dilemma," *Newsline*, 52, February 1990, 26–27. The author has changed the order of these thoughts.

112. Jason DeParle, "Rude, Rash, Effective, Act-UP Shifts AIDS Policy," *NYT*, 3 January 1990, B1.

113. David Handelman, "ACT UP," 116.

114. Minkowitz, "ACT UP."

115. Stephen C. Joseph, *Dragon Within the Gates*, 169.

116. Shilts, "Politics Confused," A4.

117. Martin Kasindorf and Catherine Woodard, "AIDS Activists to Protest INS Rule," *Newsday*, 19 June 1990, 15; Marilyn Chase, "Big AIDS Conference Will Be Show-case for Activists' Discontent with U.S. Policy," *Wall Street Journal*, 18 June 1990, A12; Gina Kolata, "Advocates' Tactics on AIDS Issues Provoking Warnings of a Backlash," *NYT*, 11 March 1990, 4–5.

118. Victor F. Zonana, "Did AIDS Protest Go Too Far?" *Los Angeles Times*, 2 July 1990, A3.

119. Jesse Heiwa Loving, "ACTing UP All Over," *POZ*, March 1997, 47; "Activist Groups and PWA Coalitions, U.S. and Canada," January 1997, http://www.thebody.com/atn/263.html, accessed on 21 April 1999.

120. Minkowitz, "ACT UP"; John Gallagher, "When the Spotlight Dims," *The Advocate*, 12 January 1993, 57; James S. Rosen, "Whatever Happened to ACT UP?" *Westsider*, 22 June 1995, S6; Frank Bruni, "ACT UP Doesn't Much Anymore," *NYT*, 21 March 1997, B1.

121. John Weir, "Rage, Rage," *New Republic*, 13 February 1995, 11.

122. Frederick M. Biddle, "ACT UP's Last Act?" *Boston Globe Magazine*, 5 September 1993, 13.

123. Michael Specter, "Public Nuisance," *New Yorker*, 13 May 2001, 65.

124. Minkowitz, "ACT UP," 1; DeParle, "Rude, Rash, Effective"; contact sheet for 6 March 1995, author's files.

125. Mark Golden, "ACT UP REDUX," *QW*, 11 October 1992, 23.

126. Larry Gutenburg, "Letter to the Editor," *Newsline*, January/February 1991, 9.

127. "Voices from the Front," 1992 video produced by Testing the Limits.

128. Gilbert Elbaz, "Measuring AIDS Activism," *Humanity and Society* 20, 3 (1996): 50.

129. Catherine Woodard, "The Struggles Go On for AIDS Activists," *Newsday*, 18 June 1990,

130. Jeffrey Goodell, "The AIDS Civil War," *7 Days*, 14 February 1990, 11, 13–15.

131. Form letter to Miguelina Maldonado, 28 January 1991; dollar bill and poster in the author's files.

132. Letter from Pablo Ruiz-Salamon to the members of the Latino/Latina Caucus of ACT UP, 31 January 1991, author's files.

133. Janis Astor del Valle, "Latino AIDS Group Comes under Angry ACT UP Fire," *Outweek*, 13 March 1991, 12–13, 64.

134. Letter from Amy Herman, Ron Johnson, and Tim Sweeney to other AIDS organizations, PWA Coalition Papers, Box 28a; letter from Rod Sorge to Yolanda Serrano, 26 February 1991, author's files.

135. Chris Norwood, "New York Forum about Health," *Newsday*, 7 March 1990, 54.

136. David Handelman, "ACT UP in Anger," *Rolling Stone, 8* March 1990, 116.

137. Catherine Woodard, "AIDS in 1989," *Newsday*, 24 June 1989, 1.

138. "The Albany AIDS March Organizers," obtained by the author at the New York State AIDS Institute Conference, 15 November 1993; W. Henry Lambright and Mark J. O'Gorman, "New York State's Response to AIDS: Evolution of an Advocacy Agency," *Journal of Public Administration Research and Theory* 2 (1992): 174–198.

139. Author interview, 11 November 1999.

140. Rachel Pepper, "Schism Slices ACT UP in Two: San Francisco Chapter Splits in Debate Over Focus," *Outweek*, 10 October 1990, 12.

141. Minkowitz, "ACT UP."

142. Jeffrey Edwards, "AIDS, Race, and the Rise and Decline of a Militant Oppositional Lesbian and Gay Politics in the U.S.," *New Political Science* 22 (2000): 485–505; Michael Cunningham, "If you're queer and you're not angry in 1992, you're not paying attention," *Mother Jones*, May/June 1992, 60–68.

143. "Out and About," *Economist* 320, 27 July 1991, A21; Larry Black, "A Gay Backlash: Queer Nation Is Waging War on Homophobia," *Maclean's* 103, 10 September 1990, 48.

144. Sally Chew, "ACT UP Zaps Cosmo," *Native*, 1 February 1988, 4; Women's Handbook Group, *Women, AIDS, and Activism*.

145. "Terry McGovern–Bio," author's files; Chris Nealon, "Actions Focus on Women with AIDS/HIV," *Gay Community News*, 7–13 October 1990, 1, 7.

146. "Rally for Homeless AIDS Patients," *NYT*, 26 November 1988, 27.

147. Sheila McKenna, "Manhattan Profile: Charles King," *Newsday*, 25 September 1992, 28.

148. Ginger Thompson, "Turning Up the Volume on AIDS," *NYT*, 1 November 1999, B5.

149. Nichole E. M. Christian, "Court Tells City to Improve Services for AIDS Victims," *NYT*, 19 December 2001, D2.

150. Gabriel Rotello, "Cityscape: How City Hall Saved Money, and Lives," *Newsday*, 12 May 1994, A42.

151. Gilbert Elbaz, "Measuring AIDS Activism," 54.

Chapter 8: Finding a Cure

1. Peg Byron, "Self-Help Research AIDS Group Sets Example for Other Diseases," *UPI*, 21 December 1988; Philip M. Boffey, "New Initiative to Speed AIDS Drugs Is Assailed," *NYT*, 5 July 1988, C1.

2. Michael Specter, "Pressure from AIDS Activists Has Transformed Drug Testing," *Washington Post*, 2 July 1989, A1.

3. Robert M. Wachter, "AIDS, Activism, and the Politics of Health," *New England Journal of Medicine* 326 (1992): 128.

4. Bert Hansen, "America's First Medical Breakthrough: How Popular Excitement about a French Rabies Cure in 1885 Raised New Expectations for Medical Progress," *American Historical Review* 103 (1998): 373–419.

5. Edwin N. Brandt Jr., "The Concentric Effects of the Acquired Immune Deficiency Syndrome," *Public Health Reports* 99 (1984): 1–2.

6. Siegal and Siegal, *AIDS*, 165.

7. Nathan Fain, "Is Our Lifestyle Hazardous to Our Health?" Mass Papers, Box 1.

8. Joseph A. Sonnabend, "Treating the Epidemic: Comments on Interferon and Plasmapheresis," *Native*, 20 December 1982–2 January 1983, 21–23.

9. James E. D'Eramo, "Incipient AIDS May Be Reversible: Encouraging New Study from St. Luke's–Roosevelt," *Native*, 24 September–9 October 1983, 24–28, 30.

10. Wallis, "AIDS," 50.

11. Jane S. Smith, *Patenting the Sun* (New York: Morrow, 1990).

12. David Dickson, *The New Politics of Science* (New York: Pantheon Books, 1984), 4.

13. Gina Kolata, "Congress, NIH Open Coffers for AIDS," *Science* (29 July 1983): 436.

14. David Perlman, "Expert Tells Why AIDS Research Is a Tough Job," *San Francisco Chronicle*, 6 February 1985, 5; Lawrence K. Altman, "The Doctor's World: AIDS Data Pour In, As Studies Proliferate," *NYT*, 23 April 1985, C3.

15. Frank J. Prial, "AIDS Program in Paris Gives Hope to Americans," *NYT*, 31 July 1985, A10.

16. Walter Sullivan, "New Drug Appears to Curb AIDS Virus," *NYT*, 9 February 1985, A6.

17. Peter S. Arno and Karyn L. Feiden, *Against All Odds: The Story of AIDS Drug Development, Politics, and Profits* (New York: Harper Collins, 1992), ch. 6 and 7; Jack Sirica, "Drugs for AIDS Funneled from Mexico to City," *Newsday*, 15 October 1985, 5.

18. Howard Wolinsky, "Underground AIDS 'Clinics' Springing Up," *Chicago Sun-Times*, 29 March 1987, 1.

19. Philip M. Boffey, "FDA. Will Allow AIDS Patients to Import Unapproved Medicines," *NYT*, 24 July 1988, A1.

20. "Underground AIDS Clinics Give Experimental Drugs," *Associated Press*, 29 March 1987.

21. "AL721: Experimental AIDS Treatment," *AIDS Treatment News* (11 April 1986): 1–4.

22. M. L., "My Illness," *Newsline*, December 1986, 22.

23. Thomas Hannan, "Egg Lecithin to Be Offered by the PWA Health Group," *Newsline*, April 1987, 19; Mike Salinas, "PWA Health Group Takes Charge: AL 721 to Be Distributed by Private Collective," *Native*, 4 May 1987, 5.

24. Paula Span, "Pharmacy for the Desperate," *Washington Post*, 8 April 1992, D1.

25. Derek Hodel, "Notes from the Underground," *Newsline*, October 1989, 49–51; Gina Kolata, "AIDS Patients and Their Above-Ground Underground," *NYT*, 10 July 1988, D32.

26. "PWA Health Group Price List Effective September 1993," author's files.

27. Michael Ravitch, "Herbal Rinse," *Notes from the Underground*, September/October 1992, 1; minutes, PWA Health Group, 27 June 1988, Callen Papers, Box 6.

28. PWA Health Group, "Welcome to the PWA Health Group," http://www.aidsinfonyc.org/pwahg/welcome.html, 12 February 1998.

29. PWA Health Group brochure, 1993, author's files.

30. Katherine Bishop, "Authorities Act against AIDS 'Cures,'" *NYT*, 30 August 1987, A1.

31. "Focus on AIDS Drugs from 'Guerilla Clinics,'" *Newsday*, 24 November 1987, 15.

32. Jean Latz Griffin, "The Fight against AIDS," *Seattle Times*, 13 December 1991, A3.

33. Warren J. Blumenfeld, "FDA, Buyers' Clubs Negotiate New Relationship," *Advocate*, 19 November, 1991, 62.

34. Sabin Russell, "FDA Hoping to Halt Profiteering on AIDS Drug," *San Francisco Chronicle*, 5 September 1991, A15.

35. "FDA Urges Buyers Clubs to End Sales of Underground DDC," http://www.fda.gov/bbs/topics/answers/ans00377.html, accessed on 25 August 2005.

36. John S. James, "ddC: Buyers' Clubs Discontinue Sales after Potency Variations Found," *AIDS Treatment News* (21 February 1992), http://www.aids.org/atn/a-145–01.html, accessed on 25 August 2005.

37. Jean Latz Griffin, "Thousands to Get AIDS Drug Free from Hoffman LaRoche," *Journal of Commerce*, 5 March 1992: 7A.

38. John Schwartz, "FDA Issues Warning about AIDS Drugs from 'Buyers' Clubs,'" *Washington Post*, 26 May 1993, A3.

39. "Thalidomide Clinical Trials in HIV Patients," *Antiviral Agents Bulletin* (1 March 1997): Factiva; "Cryptosporidiosis: NTZ Available at Buyers' Club," *AIDS Treatment News* (5 July 1996), http://www.aids.org/atn/a-250–01.html.

40. Arno and Feiden, *Against All Odds*, 40.

41. Marilyn Chase, "Dedicated Soldier: In War against AIDS, Samuel Broder Serves as General and Private," *Wall Street Journal*, 17 October 1986, Factiva.

42. Brian O'Reilly, "The Inside Story of the AIDS Drug," *Fortune*, 5 November 1990, 112–119.

43. Denise Grady, "'Look Doctor, I'm Dying. Give Me the Drug," *Discover*, August 1986, 79–80; Nussbaum, *Good Intentions*, ch. 7.

44. Margaret A. Fischl et al., "The Efficacy of Azidothymidine (AZT) in the Treatment of Patients with AIDS and AIDS-Related Complex: A Double-Blind, Placebo Controlled Trial," *New England Journal of Medicine* 317 (23 July 1987): 185–191.

45. Larry Thompson, "Progress against AIDS: Work Proceeds amid Guarded Optimism," *Washington Post*, 30 December 1986, Z6.

46. Erik Eckholm, "AIDS Drug Is Raising a Host of Thorny Issues," *NYT*, 28 September 1986, A38.

47. Erik Eckholm, "Panel Backs Licensing of AIDS Drug," *NYT*, 17 January 1987, A32.

48. Marlene Cimons, "AIDS Funds: Tardy but Catching Up," *Los Angeles Times*, 26 November 1985, 1.

49. Bob Wyrick, "Major Test of 6 AIDS Drugs Near," *Newsday*, 21 July 1986, 7.

50. Erik Eckholm, "$100 Million for AIDS Drug Testing," *NYT*, 1 July 1986, C1.

51. George J. Annas, "The Changing Landscape of Human Experimentation: Nurenberg, Helsinki, and Beyond," *Health Matrix* 2 (1992): 119.

52. Erik Eckholm, "Should the Rules Be Bent in an Epidemic?" *NYT*, 13 July 1986, D30.

53. Mathilde Krim, "Let AIDS Patients Use Experimental Drugs," *Newsday*, 11 June 1986, 77.

54. Bill Ervolino, "Club Medicine: Underground Pharmacies Dispensing Experimental Drugs to Patients Who Cannot Wait," *Bergen Record*, 11 January 1993, D1.

55. James F. Braun et al., "A Guide to Underground AIDS Therapies," *Patient Care* (15 August 1993): 53–64.

56. Larry Kramer, "Read This and Live," *The Village Voice*, 27 June 27, 1989, 24.

57. "A Failure Led to Drug against AIDS," *NYT*, 28 September 1986, 38.

58. Bruce Nussbaum, *Good Intentions: How Big Business and the Medical Establishment Are Corrupting the Fight against AIDS* (New York: Atlantic Monthly Press, 1990), 222.

59. Joseph Sonnabend et al., "Community Treatment Initiative: A Proposal for the Prevention of AIDS," *Newsline*, December 1986, 2–3.

60. Colin B. Begg et al., "Participation of Community Hospitals in Clinical Trials," *New England Journal of Medicine* 306 (6 May 1982): 1076–1080; Sharon Begley et al., "Desperation Drugs," *Newsweek*, 7 August 1989, 48.

61. Steven Epstein, *Impure Science: AIDS, Activism, and the Politics of Knowledge* (Berkeley and Los Angeles: University of California Press, 1996), 216–217.

62. Thomas Hannan, "Community Research Initiative Established," *Newsline*, April 1987, 2.

63. Sonnabend et al., "Community Treatment Initiative,"

64. "Statement of Thomas Hannan," Committee on Government Operations, *Therapeutic Drugs for AIDS: Development, Testing, and Availability* (Washington, DC: U.S. Government Printing Office, 1988), 183.

65. Phil Zwickler, "CRI Announces AIDS Drug Trials," *Native*, 4 January 1988, 10.

66. Gena Kolata, "Doctors and Patients Take AIDS Drug into Their Own Hands," *NYT*, 15 March 1988, C3.

67. *Report of the Presidential Commission*, 56.

68. Nussbaum, *Good Intentions*, ch. 13.; Catherine Woodard, "AIDS Community-Based Trials," *Newsday*, 23 May 1989, 5; Barbara Whitaker, "Feds Snub NY Group on AIDS Funding," *Newsday*, 4 October 1989, 19.

69. Memo from Mike Callen to CRI Board, 2 September 1989, Callen Papers, Box 4.

70. "Community Research Initiative, Estimated 1990 Income and Expenses," Callen Papers, Box 4.

71. Mark Harrington, "The Community Research Initiative (CRI) of New York: Clinical Research and Prevention Treatments," in *AIDS Prevention and Services: Community-Based Research*, ed. Johannes P. Van Vugt (Westport, CT: Bergin and Garvey, 1994), 173.

72. AIDS Community Research Initiative of America, 2003 Annual Report, http://www.acria.org/about/annual_reports/acria_annua103.pdf.

73. Tamar Jacoby with Tim Padgett, "Desperation Drugs," *Newsweek*, 7 August 1989.

74. Jean L. Marx, "The Trials of Conducting AIDS Trials," *Science* (26 May 1989): 916.

75. Philip M. Boffey, "Trial of AIDS Drug in U.S. Lags as Too Few Participants Enroll," *NYT*, 28 December 1987, A1.

76. John D. Arras, "Noncompliance in AIDS Research," *Hastings Center Report* 20, September–October 1990: 24–33.

77. Elliot Marshall, "Quick Release of AIDS Drugs," *Science* (28 July 1989): 345.

78. Dale E. Brashers et al., "Collective AIDS Activism and Individuals' Perceived Self-Advocacy in Physician-Patient Communication," *Human Communication Research* 26, no. 3 (July 2000): 372–402.

79. Arras, "Noncompliance"; Rachel Nowak, "AIDS Researchers, Activists Fight Crisis in Clinical Trials," *Science* (22 September 1995): 1666.

80. 'Wayne,' "Lying and Cheating to Get in a Protocol," *Newsline*, June 1989, 37–38.

81. Gina Kolata, "A Critique of Pure Reason, A Passion to Survive," *NYT*, 21 October 1990, D4.

82. See Epstein, *Impure Science*, 440.

83. Dennis Wyss, "The Underground Test of Compound Q," *Time* 134, 9 October 1989, 18–20; "Compound Q's First Tests Encouraging," *San Francisco Chronicle*, 25 September 1991, A15.

84. David J. Rothman and Harold Edgar, "AIDS, Activism, and Ethics," in *AIDS: Problems and Prospects*, ed. Lawrence Corey (New York: Norton, 1993), 145–155.

85. David Vogel, "When Consumers Oppose Consumer Protection: The Politics of Regulatory Backlash," *Journal of Public Policy* 10 (October–December 1990): 458.

86. William M. Wardell et al., "The Rate of Development of New Drugs in the United States, 1963 through 1975," in *The Food and Drug Administration's Process for Approving New Drugs: Hearings before the Subcommittee on Science, Research, and Technology of the Committee on Science and Technology, U.S. House of Representatives* (Washington, DC: U.S. Government Printing Office, 1979), 543–563.

87. Comptroller General of the United States, *FDA Approval: A Lengthy Process That Delays the Availability of Important New Drugs* (Washington, DC: U.S. Government Accounting Office, 1980).

88. Thomas C. Hayes, "The Drug Business Sees a Golden Era Ahead," *NYT*, 17 May 1981, C1.

89. Comptroller General, *FDA Approval*, 7.

90. Dale Gieringer, "The Safety and Efficacy of New Drug Approval," *Cato Journal* 5, spring/summer 1985, 178, 188.

91. Morton Mintz, "HEW Panel Urges Changes in Federal Regulation of Drugs," *Washington Post*, 31 May 1977, A2.

92. Cynthia Gornely, "Large-Scale Update in FDA Regulations Urged by Califano," *Washington Post*, 6 October 1977, A14.

93. Robert Reinhold, "Senate Panel Assails 'Red Tape' in Approvals of Prescription Drugs, *NYT*, 30 April 1982, A12; "FDA Chief Seeks to Speed Up Drug Approval Process," *Wall Street Journal*, 12 August 1981, Factiva; "Aid Urged for Drug Industry," *NYT*, 5 September 1983, A31; "New Drug Approval Record Set in 1985 by FDA: Bowen," *Public Health Reports* (March/April 1986): 223–224.

94. Michael deCourcy Hinds, "Speeding FDA. Drug Review," *NYT*, 22 September 1982, C1; "FDA Easing Clearance of New Drugs," *Globe and Mail*, 10 February 1983, B9; "U.S. to Speed Up Licensing of Drugs," *Wall Street Journal*, 26 July 1985, Factiva.

95. Peter S. Arno et al., "Rare Diseases, Drug Development, and AIDS: The Impact of the Orphan Drug Act," *Milbank Quarterly* 73 (summer 1995): 231.

96. Marion J. Finkel, "The Orphan Drug Act and the Federal Government's Orphan Products Development Program," *Public Health Reports* 99 (May/June 1984): 313–316.

97. Arno et al., "Rare Diseases."

98. "Red Tape for the Dying: The Food and Drug Administration and AIDS," cited in "FDA Reform: Major New Position Paper," *AIDS Treatment News* (3 June 1988).

99. Gregg Bordowitz and Jean Carlomusto, "Seize Control of the FDA" (video).

100. Rothman and Edgar, "AIDS, Activism," 148–149.

101. "New FDA Rules for Fostering Medicine and AIDS Research," *San Francisco Chronicle*, 26 July 1985, 30.

102. Marilyn Chase, "Faster Action: FDA Rule Changes May Rush New Drugs to Very Sick Patients," *Wall Street Journal*, 5 October 1987, Factiva.

103. Frank E. Young, "The Role of the FDA in the Effort against AIDS," *Public Health Reports* 103 (May/June 1988): 242–245.

104. Boffey, "New Initiative."

105. Jim Eigo et al., "FDA Action Handbook," 12 September 1988, http://www.actupny.org/documents/FDAhandbook1.html, accessed on 4 December 2005.

106. Mike Salinas, "Sloan-Kettering Allegedly Threatens ACT UP," *Native*, 20 July 1987, 9.

107. Eigo et al., "FDA Action."

108. Coimbra M. Sirica, "176 Arrested in AIDS Drug Protest at FDA," *San Francisco Chronicle*, 12 October 1988, A1.

109. Warren E. Leary, "FDA Announces Changes to Speed Testing of Drugs," *NYT*, 20 October 1988, A1.

110. Gina Kolata, "FDA Gives Quick Approval to Two Drugs to Treat AIDS," *NYT*, 27 June 1989, A1.

111. Ron Goldberg, "Conference Call: When PWAs First Sat at the High Table," http://www.actupny.org/documents/montreal.html, accessed on 4 December 2005.

112. Fran Pollner, "Protest at NIH Dramatizes Anger over Narrow Research," *Medical World News*, 25 June 1990, 16.

113. Gina Kolata, "AIDS Researcher Seeks Wide Access to Drugs in Tests," *NYT*, 26 June 1989, A1.

114. Paul Cotton, "FDA 'Pushing Envelope' on AIDS Drug," *JAMA* 266 (14 August 1991): 757.

115. Epstein, *Impure Science*, 278–279.

116. Handelman, "ACT UP," 86.

117. Nussbaum, *Good Intentions*, 194–195.

118. Mark Harrington, "Some Transitions in the History of AIDS Treatment Activism: From Therapeutic Utopianism to Pragmatic Praxis," in *Acting on AIDS: Sex, Drugs,*

and Politics, ed. Helena Reckitt and Joshua Oppenheimer (New York: Serpent's Tail, 1997), 283.

119. Steven Epstein, "The Construction of Lay Expertise: AIDS Activism and the Forging of Credibility in the Reform of Clinical Trials," *Science, Technology, and Human Values* 20 (1995), Academic Search Premier.

120. Epstein, *Impure Science*, 232.

121. "This Side of Despair: Theo Smart Challenges the Doomsayers of Treatment Activism to Take Heart," *QW*, 13 September 1992, 43.

122. Nussbaum, *Good Intentions*, 292; Michael Shnayerson, "Kramer vs. Kramer," *Vanity Fair*, October 1992, 294.

123. Arno and Feiden, *Against the Odds*, 225.

124. "FDA Reform: Major New Position Paper," *AIDS Treatment News* (20 May 1988): 319.

125. Jim Eigo, Mark Harrington et al., "FDA Action."

126. Letter from Richard Dunne to Arnie Kantrowitz and Lawrence Mass, 17 February 1987, Mass Papers, Box 7; Epstein, *Impure Science*, 218.

127. *AIDS Issues, Part 2*, 5–26.

128. Arno and Feiden, *Against the Odds*, 173–174.

129. Michael Spector, "Pressure from AIDS Activists Has Transformed Drug Testing," *Washington Post*, 2 July 1989, A1; Paul Cotton, "Scientifically Astute Activists Seek Common Ground with Clinicians on Testing New Drugs," *JAMA* 264 (8 August 1990): 666.

130. Victor F. Zonana, "Community Research Seeks to Speed Work on AIDS Treatments," *Los Angeles Times*, 9 July 1989, 3.

131. Victor F. Zonana, "AZT Maker Gives $1 Million to Research," *Los Angeles Times*, 1 July 1992, A20.

132. David Barr, "Action on AIDS: Shaping the Federal AIDS Research Agenda," *Volunteer*, November/December 1990, 7.

133. Mark Harrington, "Homing in on Basic Research," *TAGline*, January/February 2002, http://www.aidsinfonyc.org/tag/taglines/0202.html, accessed on 9 September 2005.

134. The Renegade Caucus, "Kick the Shit Out of the System!" *Newsline*, January/February 1991, 24.

135. Harrington, "Some Transitions.," 280–281.

136. Peter Staley, "The Responsibilities of Empowerment," keynote address at Until There is a Cure 6 conference, Palmetto, Florida, 2 December 1994, author's files.

137. Bob Blanchard, "A Genius for Activism," *Progressive*, 12 December 1997, 30–31.

138. Epstein, *Impure Science*, 292.

139. "Clinton Names AIDS Panel to Speed Drug Search," *NYT*, 7 February 1994, A7; Bruce Agnew, "NIH Invites Activists into the Inner Sanctum," *Science* (26 March 1999): 1999.

140. Kiki Mason, "Manifesto Destiny," *POZ*, June–July 1996, 66.

141. "Fairness Fund Establishes AIDS Action Hotline," *Native*, 3 August 1987, 9.

142. William Booth, "AIDS Policy in the Making," *Science* (4 March 1988): 1087.

143. Robert Bazell, "Medicine Show," *New Republic*, 22 January 1990, 16.

144. Larry Kramer, "All-Out Federal Effort Needed to Defeat AIDS," *St. Petersburg Times*, 17 July 1990, A15.

145. Jon Cohen, "A 'Manhattan Project' for AIDS," *Science* (9 February 1993): 1112–1114.

146. The Barbara McClintock Project to Cure AIDS, ACT UP/New York, n.d., author's files.

147. Cohen, "Manhattan Project," 1114.

148. Gina Kolata, "Federal Study Questions Ability of AZT to Delay AIDS Symptoms," *NYT*, 15 February 1991; Phyllida Brown, "AZT and AIDS: The Doubts Persist," *New Scientist*, 26 October 1991, 20–22.

149. Tom Phillips, "Michael Callen Retires from AIDS Activism," *We the People*, June 1991, 10.

150. Mark Harrington, "Ten Texts on Saquinavir: Its Rapid Rise and Fall," 16 June 2001, http://www.aidsinfonyc.org/tag/tx/saquinavirten.html, accessed on 8 September 2005.

151. Susan Katz Miller, "AIDS Activists Change Tack on Drugs," *New Scientist*, 2 October 1993:, 4; Christine Gorman, "Let's Not Be Too Hasty: Activists Who Once Clamored for Speedier Approval of AIDS Drugs Now Favor a More Deliberate Approach," *Time*, 19 September 1994, 7.

152. Paul Cotton, "AIDS Research Coordination Abetted," *JAMA 271, no. 14* (13 April 1994): 1061.

153. William E. Paul, "Reexamining AIDS Research Priorities," *Science* 267, no. 5198 (3 February 1995): 633.

154. Harrington, "Ten Texts"; "The Other Drug War," *New Republic*, 17 October 1994, 9.

155. Harrington, *Ten Texts*.

156. David Brown, "Speedy Release of AIDS Drugs Challenged on Lack of Follow-Through," *Washington Post*, 11 September 1994, A3.

157. Lawrence Goodman, "The Problem with Protease," *POZ*, September 2002, 34.

158. Laurie Garrett, "New AIDS Arsenal Comes with a Massive Dose of Uncertainty," *Newsday*, 17 December 1996, B19; Michael Waldholz, "Trial Medicines Foil Resistance of HIV Strains," *Wall Street Journal*, 5 February 2001, B1.

159. Tom Abate, "FDA Panel Rejects HIV Drug," *San Francisco Chronicle*, 2 November 1999, C1.

160. Alan F. Holmer, "Progress against AIDS Promises to Continue with 102 New Medicines in Development," *New Medicines in Development for AIDS: 1999 Survey*; author's files; "Researchers Are Testing 79 Medicines and Vaccines for HIV and Opportunistic Infections," 30 November 2005, www.phrma.org/mediaroom/press/releases/30.11.2004.1101.cfm, accessed on 1 December 2005; David Brown, "Batch of New HIV Drugs Looks Promising," *Washington Post*, 15 February 2004, A14.

161. Richard A. Merrill, "Modernizing the FDA: An Incremental Revolution," *Health Affairs* 18, no. 2 (1999): 96–111; "FDA Sets Record in Medication Approval Times," *AORN Journal* 67 (1998): 874.

162. "Drug Safety," *CQ Researcher* (11 March 2005): 221–244; Jennifer Corbett Dooren, "Drug Makers Seen as Slow to Finish Postmarket Studies," *Wall Street Journal*, 1 June 2005, D4.

163. Gardiner Harris, "FDA. Responds to Criticism with New Caution," *NYT*, 6 August 2005, A1.

164. Gardiner Harris, "Drug Safety System Is Broken, A Top FDA Official Says," *NYT*, 9 June 2005, A4; Gardiner Harris, "FDA to Create Advisory Panel to Warn Patients about Drugs," *NYT*, 16 February 2005, A1.

165. Kurt Eichenwald and Gina Kolata, "Drug Trials Hide Conflicts for Doctors," *NYT*, 16 May, 1999, A1.

166. Jeffrey M. Pettercorn et al., "Comparison of Outcomes in Cancer Patients Treated Within and Outside Clinical Trials: Conceptual Framework and Structured Review," *Lancet* 363 (24 January 2004): 263–270.

167. Gregg Gonsalves, "Perestroika: Rebuilding Our Nation's AIDS Research Program," *The Update* (National Minority AIDS Council), January/February 1994, 7.

Chapter 9: Clean Needles Save Lives

1. Peter Schmeisser, "Zeroing in on AIDS with Street Smarts," *National Journal*, 5 March 1988, 615; interview conducted by Dana Ain Davis, September 1997.
2. The terms "needle," "syringe," and "injection equipment" were all used in discussions of increasing access to sterile equipment for injecting drugs. This discussion uses all three terms. As a rule, I use the word used by individuals and/or groups. As a rule, "needle" was used earlier and has been replaced by "syringe."
3. Warwick Anderson, "The New York Needle Trial: The Politics of Public Health in the Age of AIDS," *American Journal of Public Health* 81 (1991): 1506–1517.
4. Suzanne Golubski and Alex Michelini, "Make it Easier for Addicts to Get Needles: An AIDS Plan," *New York Daily News*, 4 September 1985, 3.
5. David Bird, "Little Success in Curbing Spread of AIDS by Addicts Is Seen," *NYT*, 1 December 1985, A1.
6. "Choosing between Two Killers," *New York Times*, 15 September 1985, D20.
7. Extensive searches of LexisNexis and Factiva yielded only one article when the legislation was passed, along with three subsequent articles about its implementation. Kenneth Lovett, "Pols: Needle Law is RX for AIDS," *New York Post*, 6 May 2000, 12.
8. Jon S. Vernick et al., "Public Opinion about Syringe Exchange Programmes in the U.S.A.: An Analysis of National Surveys," *International Journal of Drug Policy* 14 (2003): 431–435.
9. James Inciardi, "Federal Efforts to Control the Spread of HIV and AIDS among IV Drug Users," *American Behavioral Scientist* 33 (March/April 1990): 408–418.
10. Robert J. Blendon and John T. Young, "The Public and the War on Illicit Drugs," *JAMA* 279 (1998): 827–833.
11. Stanley R. Yancovitz et al., "A Randomized Trial of an Interim Methadone Maintenance Clinic," *American Journal of Public Health* 81 (1991): 1185–1191.
12. Sandra G. Boodman and Michael Isikoff, "Eased Methadone Rules Urged in AIDS Fight," *Washington Post*, 3 March 1989, A3.
13. Thomas J. Maier, "The Business of Addiction," *Newsday*, 12 June 1989, 3.
14. "AIDS Benefit in Methadone Use Is Questioned," *NYT*, 3 August 1989, B6.
15. U.S. General Accounting Office, *Methadone Maintenance: Some Treatment Programs Are Not Effective* (Washington, DC: GAO, 1990), 5, 13.
16. Charles R. Schuster, "Intravenous Drug Use and AIDS Prevention," *Public Health Reports* 103 (May/June 19880): 261–266.
17. Joseph, *Dragon* , 191.
18. The Committee on Medicine and Law, "Legalization of Nonprescription Sale of Hypodermic Needles: A Response to the AIDS Crisis," *The Record of the Association of the Bar of the City of New York*, 1986, 809; ADAPT, "Position Paper: Distribution of Hypodermic Needles and Syringes to Intravenous Substance Users," November 1986, author's files.
19. Ronald Sullivan, "Official Favors a Test Program to Curb AIDS," *NYT*, 30 May 1986, B3; Anderson, "New York Needle," 1508.
20. Institute of Medicine, *Confronting AIDS: Directions for Public Health, Health Care, and Research* (Washington, DC: National Academy of Sciences, 1986), 110.
21. John Cardinal O'Connor and Mayor Edward Koch, *His Eminence and Hizzoner: A Candid Exchange* (New York: William Morrow, 1989), 229; Ronald Sullivan,

"Health Commissioner Considers Distribution of Needles to Addicts," *NYT*, 8 November 1986, B1.

22. Ronald Sullivan, "New York State Rejects Plan to Give Drug Users Needles," *NYT*, 17 May 1987, A1.

23. Catherine O'Neill interview, 12 May 1998.

24. Bruce Lambert, "Drug Group to Offer Free Needles to Combat AIDS in New York City," *NYT*, 8 January 1988, A1.

25. Bruce Lambert, "Reaction to Needles-for-Addicts Plan," *NYT*, 9 January 1988, A7; telegram from ADAPT to Julio Martinez, New York State Division of Substance Abuse Services, 8 January 1988, author's files.

26. Lambert, "Drug Group"; Lambert, "Reaction,"

27. Peter Kerr, "Weighing of Two Perils Led to Needles-for-Addicts Plan," *NYT*, 1 February 1988, B1.

28. David Holmberg, "IV Needle Exchange Program Endorsed," *Newsday*, 6 June 1988, 9.

29. Michel Marriot, "Needle Plan Fails to Attract Drug Addicts, So It's Revised," *NYT*, 30 January 1989, A1.

30. General Accounting Office, *Needle Exchange Programs: Research Suggests Promise as an AIDS Prevention Strategy*, GAO/HRD-93–60 (March 1993): 25.

31. Michael Marriot, "Drug Needle Exchange Is Gaining but Still under Fire," *NYT*, 7 June 1989, B1; Lawrence K. Altman, "Needle Program Is a Small One to Test Concept," *NYT*, 8 November 1988, B5.

32. Suzanne Daley, "Two Addicts Seek Needles on First Day," *NYT*, 8 November 1988, B1; Marriot, "Drug Needle,"

33. Peter Kerr, "Experts Find Fault in New AIDS plan," *NYT*, 7 February 1988, E7.

34. Heidi Evans and Mike Santagelo, "O'C Blasts Addict Plan," *New York Daily News*, 1 February 1988, 5.

35. "Council Calls for End to Free-Needles Plan," *NYT*, 7 December 1988, B10.

36. "Needle Exchange Experimental Program: Why It Mustn't Be Tried," *Amsterdam News*, 15 October 1988, 15.

37. David L. Kirp and Ronald Bayer, "Needles and Race," *Atlantic*, July 1993, 1, 38–41.

38. Charles Rangel, "Needle Exchanges Hurt the Fight against Drugs," *USA Today*, 28 April 1989, 10A; Spencer Rich, "Aiding Needle Exchange Is Illegal, Rangel Says," *Washington Post*, 10 March 1989, A3.

39. Sandra G. Boodman, "N.Y. 'Needle Exchange': Curbing AIDS or Condoning Drug Use," *Washington Post*, 6 March 1989, A1; "Commission Opposes Free Needle Give-away," *Amsterdam News*, 15 October 1988, 6.

40. Bruce Lambert, "Pro and Con: Free Needles for Addicts to Help Curb AIDS?" *NYT*, 20 December 1987, D20.

41. "Statement of Roy Innes," in *AIDS Issues, Part 1, Hearings before the Subcommittee on Health and the Environment of the Committee on Energy and Commerce, House of Representatives* (Washington, DC: U.S. Government Printing Office, 1989), 534.

42. New York City Department of Health, *The Pilot Needle Exchange Study in New York City: A Bridge to Treatment* (New York: Author, 1988), 6, 10–11, 16.

43. Todd S. Purdum, "Dinkins to End Needle Plan for Drug Abusers," *NYT*, 14 February 1990, B1.

44. Bruce Lambert, "Myers Opposes Needle Projects to Curb AIDS," *NYT*, 10 April 1990, B4.

45. Letter from Elizabeth Holtzman to Dr. Woodrow Myers, 14 May 1990; letter from Andrew Stein to Dr. Woodrow Myers, 10 May 1990; ADAPT board minutes, 3 May 1990, author's files.
46. Letter from Dr. Woodrow Myers to Frank Tardalo, 3 May 1990.
47. "Press Briefing," 10 May 1990, author's files.
48. Johnson interview; Gina Kolata, "Black Group Assails Giving Bleach to Addicts," *NYT*, 17 June 1990, A1.
49. Minority Task Force on AIDS, "Press Briefing Statement," author's files.
50. Bruce Lambert, "Dinkins Reexamines AIDS Pact," *NYT*, 11 May 1990, B2.
51. Bruce Lambert, "AIDS Battler Gives Needles Illicitly to Addicts," *NYT*, 20 November 1989, A1.
52. Mike Spiegel, "Preparing and Conducting a 'Necessity' Defense," In *ACLU Briefing Book*, ed. Ruth Harlow and Rod Sorge (New York: ACLU, 1994), 542–549.
53. Catherine Woodard, "Needle Giveaway to Invite Arrest," *Newsday*, 2 March 1990, 3, 27; Bruce Lambert, "10 Seized in Demonstration as They Offer New Needles," NYT, 7 March 1990, B3.
54. Peg Byron, "AIDS Activists Go on Trial for Handing Out Hypodermics," United Press International, 8 April 1991.
55. "Dead Addicts Don't Recover," *Newsline*, April 1991, 18.
56. Catherine Woodard, "Needle Providers Wrestle Law, Demand," *Newsday*, 9 October 1990, 25.
57. Maia Szalavitz, "Stick Shift," *The Village Voice*, 20 November 1990, 16; New York State Department of Health, AIDS Institute, *Annual Report of the New York State–Authorized Needle Exchange Programs*, August 1992 through September 1993, 10.
58. Richard Elovich and Rod Sorge, "Toward a Community-Based Needle Exchange for New York City," *AIDS and Public Policy* 6 (1991): 168.
59. "Notes and Comment," *New Yorker*, 16 September 1991, 23; Elovich and Sorge, 169.
60. Letter from Loren Siegel and William Rubenstein, American Civil Liberties Union, to presiding judge, Manhattan Criminal Court, 7 June 1990, *ACLU Briefing Book*, 499.
61. Spergel, 546–548; Emily Sachar, "Activists Helped, Court Told," *Newsday*, 10 April 1991, 36.
62. "Decision and Order: The People of the State of New York against Gregg Bordowitz et al.," 8, author's files.
63. Ronald Sullivan, "Needle-Exchangers Had Right to Break Law, Judge Rules," *NYT*, 26 June 1991, B1.
64. Dana Ain Davis interview with Rod Sorge, September 1997.
65. "Decision and Order," 28.
66. Memo from ACT UP/NY Needle Exchange to New York City Department of Health; ADAPT press release, 19 August 1991, author's files; "MTFA Policy Statement on Needle Exchange as a Way to Prevent the Spread of HIV/AIDS" (approved December 1991), PWA Coalition Papers, Container 16.
67. Miryea Navarro, "Needle Swap Programs Gain Wider Acceptance," *NYT*, 30 October 1991, B1.
68. "Remarks by Mayor Dinkins at Press Conference to Announce the Findings of the Needle Exchange Working Group," 7 November 1991, author's files.
69. Memo from Margaret A. Hamburg to Hon. David N. Dinkins "re: Needle Exchange," 1 November 1991; Elaine O'Keefe et al., "City of New Haven Needle Exchange Program: Preliminary Report," 31 July 1991, author's files.

70. Miryea Navarro, "Dinkins Panel Is Moving to Revive Needle Exchange to Combat AIDS," *NYT*, 29 October 1991, A1; "Policy Statement on Drugs, HIV/AIDS, and Needle Exchange," press release from Manhattan Borough president Ruth Messinger, 28 October 1991, author's files.

71. Letter from Velmanette Montgomery to Hon. Dale Volker, 27 June 1991, author's files.

72. Letter from John C. Daniels to Rod Sorge, 21 August 1990, author's files.

73. Miryea Navarro, "Needle Swaps to Be Revived to Curb AIDS," *NYT*, 14 May 1992, A1.

74. Norman Bauman, "In a State of Denial," *New Scientist*, 7 October 1995, 12.

75. Lee M. Kochems et al., "The Transition from Underground to Legal Syringe Exchange: The New York City Experience," *AIDS Education and Prevention* 8, no. 6 (1996): 478.

76. Navarro, "Needle Swaps."

77. "Chart of U.S. Needle Exchange Arrests and Their Disposition," *ACLU Briefing Book*, 747–748; Donna Leusner, "Stuck with the Consequences: AIDS Crusader Paying the Price," *Newark Star Ledger*, 26 October 1998, 13; Wendy Ruderman, "AIDS Activist Who Broke the Law Says the State Broke Her Spirit," Associated Press, 18 December 1998.

78. "Syringe Exchange in the United States: 1995 Update," HIV Capsule Report, February 1996; "Update: Syringe Exchange Programs—United States, 2002," *MMWR* (15 July 2005): 673–676.

79. For an overview, see Edith Springer, "Effective AIDS Prevention with Active Drug Users: The Harm Reduction Model," in *Counseling Chemically Dependent People with HIV Illness*, ed. Michael Shernoff (New York: Harrington Park Press, 1991), 141–157; See "Principles of HIV Prevention in Drug-Using Populations: A Research-Based Guide," National Institute on Drug Abuse, March 2002, www.Nida.nih.gov/pdf/pohp.pdf, accessed on 1 September 2005.

80. Richard Elovich and Michael Cowing, "Recovery Readiness: Strategies that Bring Treatment to Addicts Where They Are," in *Harm Reduction and Steps toward Change* (New York: Gay Men's Health Crisis, n.d.),1.

81. Lewis Yablonsky, *Synanon: The Tunnel Back* (Baltimore, MD: Penguin, 1965).

82. Yankovitz et al., "Randomized Trial," 1187.

83. Ernst C. Buning et al., "Amsterdam's Drug Policy and Its Implications for Controlling Needle Sharing," in *Needle Sharing among Intravenous Drug Abusers: National and International Perspectives*, ed. Robert J. Battjes and Roy W. Pickens (Rockville, MD: National Institute on Drug Abuse, 1988), 61.

84. John Strang, "Harm Reduction for Drug Users: Exploring the Dimensions of Harm, Their Measurement, and Strategies for Reductions," *AIDS and Public Policy Journal* 7, no. 3 (fall 1992): 145–152; James O. Prochaska et al., "In Search of How People Change: Applications to Addictive Behaviors," *American Psychologist* 47 (1992): 1102–1114.

85. Joanna Herrod et al., "Cleaning Injection Equipment: A Message Gone Wrong?" *British Medical Journal* 299 (2 September 1989): 601; Joanna E. Siegel et al., "Bleach Programs for Preventing AIDS among IV Drug Users: Modeling the Impact of HIV Prevalence," *American Journal of Public Health* 81 (1991): 1273–1279.

86. U.S. Department of Health and Human Services, *HIV/AIDS Prevention Bulletin*, 19 April 1993; C. B. McCoy et al., "Compliance to Bleach Disinfection Protocols among Injecting Drug Users in Miami," *Journal of Acquired Immune Deficiency Syndromes* 7, no. 7 (1994): 773–776.

87. Stephen Titus et al., "Bleach Use and HIV Seroconversion among New York City Injection Drug Users," *Journal of Acquired Immune Deficiency Syndromes* 7: 700–704.

88. Jacques Normand et al., eds., *Preventing HIV Transmission: The Role of Sterile Needles and Bleach* (Washington, DC: National Academy Press, 1995), 5.

89. David R. Gibson et al., "Effectiveness of Syringe Exchange Programs in Reducing HIV Risk Behavior and HIV Seroconversion among Injecting Drug Users," *AIDS* 15 (2001): 1329–1341.

90. Sandro Galea et al., "Needle Exchange Programs and Experience of Violence in an Inner-City Neighborhood," *Journal of Acquired Immune Deficiency Syndromes* 28, no. 3 (2001): 282–288.

91. For a list of endorsements, see http://www.dogwoodcenter.org/science/20science. html, accessed on 8 August 2005.

92. Peter Lurie et al., *The Public Health Impact of Needle Exchange Programs in the United States and Abroad: Summary, Conclusions, and Recommendations* (Berkeley, CA: University of California, School of Public Health, 1993); Philip Coffin, "Syringe Availability as HIV Prevention: A Review of Modalities," *Journal of Urban Health* 77 (2000): 306–330.

93. "Contrasting AIDS Views," *USA Today*, 30 July 1992, 3A, Factiva.

94. Laurie Garrett, "Needle Exchange Debate: Shalala Releases an Inconclusive Report," *Newsday*, 19 February 1997, A19.

95. John W. Fountain, "Protest at Agency Targets Rule on Needle Exchange," *Washington Post*, 18 September 1997, A17.

96. Rick Weiss, "President's AIDS 'Strategy' Offers Call to Arms, Few New Weapons," *Washington Post*, 17 December 1996, A4.

97. Gibson, "Effectiveness," 1338.

98. John F. Harris and Amy Goldstein, "Puncturing an AIDS Initiative: At Last Minute, White House Political Fears Killed Needle Funding," *Washington Post*, 23 April 1998, A1; Amy Goldstein, "Clinton Supports Needle Exchanges but not Funding," *Washington Post*, 21 April 1998, A1.

99. Kathy Kiely, "AIDS Activists Storm Office," *N.Y. Daily News*, 21 July 1998, 16.

100. Kevin Krajick, Damage Control: Needle Exchange Programs Make Sense and Save Lives (Ford Foundation, summer 2002), http://www.fordfound.org/publications/ ff_report/view_ff_report_detail.cfm?report_index=350, accessed on August 20, 2002.

101. Hopkinson, "Black Caucus."

102. Christopher Wren, "One Million Pledged for Needle Exchanges," *NYT*, 24 April 1998, A14; "Update: Syringe Exchange Programs," 675.

103. Robert Heimer, "Syringe Exchange Programs: Lowering the Transmission of Syringe-Borne Diseases and Beyond," *Public Health Reports* 113 (1998): 67–74.

104. John Tierney, "The Big City: The Needle Trade," *NYT*, 5 October 1997, 6–46.

105. John E. Anderson et al., "Needle Hygiene and Sources of Needles for Injection Drug Users: Data from a National Survey," *Journal of Acquired Immune Deficiency Syndromes and Human Retrovirology* 18 (July 1998): S147.

106. Ruth Finkelstein and Amanda Vogel, *Towards a Comprehensive Plan for Syringe Exchange in New York City* (New York: New York Academy of Medicine, 2000), 36.

107. Anderson et al., "Needle Hygiene," S148; Carl A. Latkin and Valerie L. Forman, "Patterns of Needle Acquisition and Sociobehavioral Correlates of Needle Exchange Program Attendance in Baltimore, Maryland, U.S.A," *Journal of Acquired Immune Deficiency Syndromes* 27 (2001): 398–404.

108. Michael Cooper, "So How Bad Is Albany? Well, Notorious," *NYT*, 22 July 2004, B1.

109. For estimates of the number of infections associated with a lack of SEPs in the United States, and of the impact of ESAP on health costs, see Peter Lurie and Ernest Drucker, "An Opportunity Lost: HIV Infections Associated with Lack of National Needle-Exchange Programme in the U.S.A.," *Lancet* 349 (1997): 604–608; Franklin N. Laufer, "Cost Effectiveness of Syringe Exchange as an HIV Prevention Strategy," *Journal of Acquired Immune Deficiency Syndromes* 28, no. 3 (2001): 273–278; Samuel R. Friedman, Theresa Perlis, and Don C. Des Jarlais, "Laws Prohibiting Over-the-Counter Syringe Sales to Injection Drug Users: Relations to Population Density, HIV Prevalence, and HIV Incidence," *American Journal of Public Health* 91 (2001): 791–793.

110. Scott Burris et al., "The Legality of Selling or Giving Syringes to Injection Drug Users," *Journal of the American Pharmaceutical Association* 42 (2002): S13–S18.

111. Princeton Survey Research Associates poll, August–October 2000, LexisNexis.

112. Phillip O. Coffin et al., "New York City Pharmacists' Attitudes toward Sale of Needles/Syringes to Injection Drug Users before Implementation of Law Expanding Syringe Access," *Journal of Urban Health* 77 (2000): 781–793.

113. Susan J. Klein et al., "Mobilizing Public and Private Partners to Support New York's Expanded Syringe Access Demonstration Program," *Journal of the American Pharmaceutical Association* 42, no. 6, supp. 2 (2002): S28–29; Phillip O. Coffin et al., "More Pharmacists in High-Risk Neighborhoods of New York City Support Selling Syringes to Injection Drug Users," *Journal of the American Pharmaceutical Association* 42, no. 6, supp. 2: S62–67; Celeste Katz, "Needle Access Difficult in Rx: Most Drugstores Shun Program," *N.Y. Daily News*, 20 June 2002, 3; New York Academy of Medicine, *New York State Expanded Syringe Access Demonstration Program Evaluation* (New York: New York Academy of Medicine, 2003), 15–16.

114. Sherry Deren et al., "Impact of Expanding Syringe Access in New York on Sources of Syringes for Injection Drug Users in Harlem and the Bronx, N.Y.C., U.S.A.," *International Journal of Drug Policy* 14 (December 2003): 373–379.

115. R. Rockwell and D[on] C. Des Jarlais, "Geographic Proximity, Policy, and Utilization of Syringe Exchange Programmes," *AIDS Care* 11 (1999): 437–442.

Chapter 10: HIV Stops with Me

1. Stephen Joseph, "Breaking the AIDS Connection: New York City's Approach," *AIDS Patient Care* 1 (December 1987): 7; Jennifer Lin, "Jackson Urges Wider HIV Testing," *Philadelphia Inquirer*, 1 March 2005, B4.

2. "HIV and AIDS—United States, 1981–2000," *MMWR* (1 June 2001): 430–440.

3. "Access to Care for HIV Patients—Robert S. Janssen, M.D.," Congressional Testimony by Federal Document Clearinghouse, 23 June 2005, Factiva; *HIV Strategic Plan through 2005* (Atlanta: Centers for Disease Control and Prevention, 2001), 2.

4. "The Twentieth Year of AIDS: A Time to Reenergize Prevention," *MMWR* (1 June 2001): 444–445.

5. Marshall H. Becker and Jill G. Joseph, "AIDS and Behavioral Change to Reduce Risk: A Review," *American Journal of Public Health* 78 (1988): 394–410; John M. Karon et al., "HIV in the United States at the Turn of the Century: An Epidemic in Transition," *American Journal of Public Health* 91 (2001): 1060–1069.

6. Mollyann Brodie et al., "AIDS at 21: Media Coverage of the HIV Epidemic, 1981–2002," http://www.kff.org/kaiserpolls/7023.cfm, accessed on 8 September 2005.

7. Jeffrey Schmaltz, "Whatever Happened to AIDS?" *NYT*, 28 November 1993, 6–58.

8. Andrew Sullivan, "When Plagues End: Notes on the Twilight of an Epidemic," *NYT*, 10 November 1996, 6–52.

9. David Sanford, "Back to a Future," *Wall Street Journal*, 8 November 1996, A1.

10. "AIDS Update," *CQ Researcher* (4 December 1998).

11. John Gallagher, "The New Crisis Facing AIDS Organizations: Adapt or Die," *Advocate*, 27 May 1997, 35–42; Gay Men's Health Crisis, Form 990, accessed from www.guidestar.org, 3 January 2004.

12. Ana Oliviera interview, 14 November 2003.

13. Michael Warner, "Unsafe: Why Gay Men Are Having Unsafe Sex Again," *The Village Voice*, 31 January 1995, 32; Sarah Miles, "And the Bathhouse Plays On," *Out*, July/August 1995, 87–90, 128–134; "CDC Stats Show Unsafe Sex Practices Are Increasing," *AIDS Alert* (1 April 1999): 43.

14. Samantha Marshall, "HIV's New York Comeback," *Crain's New York Business*, 11 March 2002, 1.

15. Harvey Fierstein, "The Culture of Disease," *NYT*, 31 July 2003, A25.

16. Ronald O. Valdisserri, "Mapping the Roots of HIV/AIDS Complacency: Implications for Program and Policy Development," *AIDS Education and Prevention* 16 (2004): 426–439.

17. Craig Demmer, "Impact of Improved Treatments on Perceptions about HIV and Safer Sex among Inner-City HIV-Infected Men and Women," *Journal of Community Health* 27 (February 2002): 63–74; Waimar Tun et al., "Attitudes toward HIV Treatments Influence Unsafe Sexual and Injection Practices among Injecting Drug Users," *AIDS* 17 (2003): 1953–1962.

18. "Curbing the Increase in Rates of STDs," *AIDS Weekly* (9 December 1991): 9–11.

19. David Kirby, 'risky business," *Advocate*, 13 April 1999, 40.

20. New York Academy of Medicine, *New York State Expanded*, 11.

21. Erika Check et al., "AIDS at 20," *Newsweek*, 11 June 2001, 35–37; David Brown, "U.S. Survey Indicates Blacks Hardest Hit by HIV Infection," *Washington Post*, 26 February 2005, A3.

22. CDC: National Center for HIV, STD, and TB Prevention, "HIV/AIDS among U.S. Women: Minority and Young Women at Continuing Risk," www.cdc.gov/hiv/pubs/facts/women.htm, accessed on 8 January 2004.

23. Bob Herbert, "Young, Poor, Positive," *NYT*, 7 December 1997, 4–17.

24. Thomas A. Birkland, *After Disaster: Agenda Setting, Public Policy, and Focusing Events* (Washington, DC: Georgetown University Press, 1997).

25. Thomas Shevory, *Notorious HIV* (Minneapolis, MN: University of Minnesota Press, 2004).

26. Justin Bergman, "Pataki Signs HIV Partner Notification Bill into Law," Associated Press Newswires, 10 July 1998, Factiva.

27. Lynda Richardson, "Wave of Laws Aimed at People with HIV," *NYT*, 25 September 1998, B2.

28. "GMHC Statement on HIV Surveillance," *www*.gmhc.org/aidslib/monitor.html, accessed on 12 February 1998; Jim Yardley, "Counselors Battle Spread of Infection—and Despair," *NYT*, 25 January 1998, 27.

29. "GMHC Blunder Pushes HIV Name Reporting Forward," *New York AIDS Issues Update*, 16 January 1998, 1.

30. "'Refuse and Resist': What the HIV/AIDS Community Can Do to Mitigate the Negative Impact of the Mayersohn Legislation," *New York AIDS Issues Update*, 10 July 1998, 1.

31. "New Surveillance Law Takes Effect," *Body Positive*, July 2000, www.thebody.com/ bp.ju100/nystate.html, accessed on 1 September 2005.

32. Lynda Richardson, "AIDS Groups Stunned by Vote for Partner Notification," *NYT*, 20 June 1998, B2.

33. Lawrence O. Gostin and James G. Hodge Jr., "The 'Names Debate': The Case for National HIV Reporting in the United States," *Albany Law Review* 61 (spring 1998): 679–743.

34. Marlene Cimons and Harry Nelson, "Bush Is Booed as He Defends AIDS Proposals," *Los Angeles Times*, 2 June 1987, 1–1.

35. Barry Adkins, "CDC AIDS Program Head Visits GMHC," *Native*, 20–26 January 1986, 12.

36. Erik Eckholm, "Screening of Blood for AIDS Raises Civil Liberties Issues," *NYT*, 30 September 1985, A1.

37. Ronald Bayer, "Clinical Progress and the Future of HIV Exceptionalism," *Archives of Internal Medicine* 159 (1999): 1042; Gostin and Hodge, "'Names Debate.'"

38. Lawrence O. Gostin, "Public Health Strategies for Confronting AIDS," *JAMA* 261 (1989): 1621–1630.

39. William E. Dannemeyer and Michael G. Franc, "The Failure of AIDS-Prevention Education," *Public Interest* 96 (summer 1989): 47–60.

40. Robin Goldstein, "Once Soloist on AIDS, Dannemeyer Now Joined by Conservative Chorus," *Orange County Register*, 18 April 1987, A1; Jeff Weir, "Rep. Dannemeyer Calls for Expulsion of Frank, Lukens from the House," *Orange County Register*, 4 November 1989, A1; Robin Goldstein, "Dannemeyer Dissents, Deep Kissing Might Transmit AIDS," *Orange County Register*, 5 May 1988, A1.

41. Ronald Bayer and Kathleen E. Toomey, "HIV Prevention and the Two Faces of Partner Notification," *American Journal of Public Health* 82 (1992): 1158–1164.

42. Bruce Lambert, "New York City Will Test for AIDS in Autopsies to Trace Its Spread," *NYT*, 15 December 1989, A1.

43. Joseph, *Dragon*, 89.

44. Bruce Lambert, "Health Board Backs Move to Trace AIDS," *NYT*, 15 November 1989, B1.

45. Ronald Bayer, "Public Health Policy and the AIDS Epidemic: An End to HIV Exceptionalism?" *New England Journal of Medicine* 324 (1991): 1500–1504.

46. Karon et al., "HIV in the United States,"

47. Richardson, "Wave of Laws."

48. Michael A. Stoto, Donna A. Almario, and Marie C. McCormick, eds., *Reducing the Odds: Preventing Perinatal Transmission of HIV in the United States* (Washington, DC: National Academies Press, 1999).

49. Samuel Maull, "HIV Law Project Asks Court to Require Baby AIDS Test Results in 72 Hours," Associated Press Newswires, 14 May 1998, Factiva.

50. Tracey E Wilson and Howard Minkoff, "Mandatory HIV Testing of Infants and Rates of Follow-up Care," *American Journal of Public Health* 89 (1999): 1583.

51. Ravinia Hayes-Cozier, "HIV Legislation is a Bad 'Quick-Fix,'" *Amsterdam News*, 25 June 1998, 12.

52. For an empirical study, see Karen H. Rothenberg and Stephen J. Paskey, "The Risk of Domestic Violence and Women with HIV Infection: Implications for Partner Notification, Public Policy, and the Law," *American Journal of Public Health* 85 (1995): 1569, Proquest.

53. Chris Norwood, "Mandated Life versus Mandatory Death: New York's Disgraceful

Partner Notification Record," *Journal of Community Health* 20 (April 1995): 161–170.

54. Chris Norwood, "Testing, Testing," *Newsday*, 23 June 1989, 83; Norwood, "Mandated Life."

55. Dannemeyer and Franc, "Failure."

56. S. J. Rogers et al., "Partner Notification with HIV-Infected Drug Users: Results of Formative Research," *AIDS Care* 10 (August 1998): 415–430.

57. "Interventions to Prevent HIV Risk Behaviors," National Institutes of Health Consensus Development Conference Statement, 11–13 February 1997, www.consensus.nih.gov/cons/104/104_Intro.htm, accessed on 28 August 2005.

58. Institute of Medicine, *No Time to Lose: Getting More from HIV Prevention* (Washington, DC: National Academy Press, 2001), 4, 6, 26, 54, 163.

59. *HIV Strategic Plan.*

60. Richard J. Wolitski et al., "Are We Headed for a Resurgence of the HIV Epidemic among Men Who Have Sex with Men?" *American Journal of Public Health* 91 (June 2001): 883–888.

61. "HIV Incidence among Young Men Who Have Sex with Men—Seven U.S. Cities, 1994–2000," *MMWR* (1 June 2001): 440–444.

62. Robert S. Janssen et al., "The Serostatus Approach to Fighting the HIV Epidemic: Prevention Strategies for Infected Individuals," *American Journal of Public Health* 91 (2001): 1019–1024.

63. "SAFE, A Serostatus Approach to Fighting the HIV/AIDS Epidemic," NCHSTP Program Briefing 2001, www.cdc.gov/nchstp/od/program_brief_2001/AIDS%20Epidemic.htm, accessed on 5 January 2004.

64. Jansen et al., "Serostatus Approach," 1023.

65. "HIV Stops with Me," *Being Alive*, May 2000, www.aegis.org/pubs/bala/2000/BA00501.html, accessed on 18 August 2003.

66. "HIV Stops with Me! Positive Prevention in Los Angeles County: Your Energy and Ideas Are Needed!" *Being Alive*, October 2000, www.aegis.org/pubs/bala/2000/BA0011002.html, accessed on 18 August 2003.

67. Chris Collis et al., "Designing Primary Prevention for People Living with HIV," www.ari.ucsf.edu/primaryprevention.pdf, accessed on 10 March 2004.

68. David Tuller, "New Tactics to Prevent AIDS Spread," *NYT*, 13 August 2002, F5.

69. "Julie Gerberding's Remarks at the National Press Club Conference—The State of the CDC: Fiscal Year 2004, Protecting Health for Life," 22 February 2005, Centers for Disease Control Documents, Factiva.

70. Christopher Heredia, "AIDS Cases Increase Slightly in U.S," *San Francisco Chronicle*, 29 July 2003, A2.

71. "HIV Diagnoses among Injection-Drug Users in States with HIV Surveillance: 25 States, 1994—2000," *MMWR* (11 July 2003): 634–636; Nicholas M. Christian, "Syphilis Cases in the City Rise by 55 Percent, Health Officials Say," *NYT*, 10 January 2003, B3.

72. "CDC Deputy Chief Says Trend 'Very Worrisome': U.S. Far From Goal to Cut New Infections by Half," *AIDS Alert* (June 2003): 75–78.

73. "Advancing HIV Prevention: New Strategies for a Changing Epidemic—United States, 2003," *MMWR* (18 April 2003): 329–332.

74. "CDC Deputy Chief."

75. "Advancing HIV Prevention."

76. Yee, "AIDS Activists."

77. Esther Kaplan, "Political Science," *POZ* (January 2004), www.poz.com/articles/151_178.shtml, accessed on 18 August 2005.

78. "Reports from the 2003 National CDC Prevention Conference," *News From Albany*, www.nyaidscoalition.org/cgi-bin/iowa/nyac/news/albany/425.html, accessed on 14 August 2003.

79. Letter from Terje Anderson to Julie Gerberding, n.d., www.papwa.org/pdf/030418.pdf, accessed on 8 January 2004.

80. Daniel Yee, "AIDS Activists Jeer Senior Bush Health Official," Associated Press, 29 July 2003, Factiva.

81. Mary Lynn Hemphill, "The CDC's 2003 National HIV Prevention Conference," *Survival News*, www.thebody.com/asp/septoct03/cdc_prev_conf.html, accessed on 10 March 2004.

82. "Thousands Protest Abstinence-Only HHS Official Sent to Speak at National HIV Prevention Conference," www.aidschicago.org/about_afc/07_31_2003.php, accessed on 24 August 2005.

83. "HIV/AIDS Prevention Today," www.cdcnpin.org/scripts/hiv/prevent.asp, accessed on 10 March 2004.

84. "The Track Record on the Bush Administration on HIV/AIDS," www.actupny.org/reports/bush_reportcard.pdf, accessed on 24 August 2005.

85. "Thousands Protest."

86. "Here is How Obscenity Issue Was Raised," *AIDS Alert* (March 2002): 36–38; Ceci Connolly, "U.S. Warns AIDS Group on Funding," *Washington Post*, 14 June 2003, A14.

87. Robert Stacy McCain, "Stricter Rules for AIDS Funds Written," *Washington Times*, 18 June 2004, A4.

88. Thomas Frieden, "HIV/AIDS in New York City: Collaborative Capacity Building Is the Key to Success," presentation at New York AIDS Coalition Conference on Collaborative Capacity Building, New York City, 29 April 2004.

89. Letter from NORA to Dr. Robert Janssen, 31 July 2003, www.Aidsaction.org/legislation/nora/nora_cdc_initiative.response.pdf, accessed on 10 March 2004.

90. Joseph P. McGowan et al., "Risk Behavior for Transmission of Human Immunodeficiency Virus (HIV) among HIV-Seropositive Individuals in an Urban Setting," *Clinical Infectious Diseases* 38 (2004): 122–127; Seth C. Kalichman et al., "Effectiveness of an Intervention to Reduce HIV Transmission Risks in HIV-Positive People," *American Journal of Preventive Medicine* 21, no. 2: 84–92.

91. Robert Klitzman and Ronald Bayer, *Mortal Secrets: Truth and Lies in the Age of AIDS* (Baltimore, MD: Johns Hopkins University Press, 2003).

92. "How to Have Sex," 214.

93. Gina Kolata, "Targeting Urged in Attack on AIDS," *NYT*, 7 March 1993, A1.

94. Todd Simmons, "Farewell Gingrich . . . Signorile?" *Advocate*, 16 September 1997, 43–45.

95. "House Approves More AIDS Funds."

96. National Research Council Panel on Monitoring the Social Impact of the AIDS Epidemic, *The Social Impact of AIDS in the United States* (Washington, DC: National Academy of Sciences, 1993), 6–7.

97. David E. Rogers and June E. Osborn, "AIDS Policy: Two Divisive Issues," *JAMA* 270 (28 July 1993): 494–495.

98. Richard Goldstein, "AIDS and Race: The Hidden Epidemic," *The Village Voice*, 10 March 1987.

99. Charles R. Caulfield, "Zip Code Genocide," *San Francisco Sentinel*, 11 March 1993, www.aegis.com/pubs/bala/1993/ba930421.html, accessed on 21 December 1999.

100. "Gay and Black Leaders Demand AIDS Funding," *Native*, 16–30 December 1985, 17.

101. Enoch Williams, "The Changing Face of AIDS," *Amsterdam News*, 16 May 1992, 21.

102. Richard Peréz-Peña, "State Overlooks Minority-Run AIDS Groups, a Report Finds," *NYT*, 23 January 2001, B1.

103. Robert Ratish, "Boros Need AIDS Funds—Coalition," *NY Daily News*, 7 October 1996, Suburban-1.

104. Stephanie A. Robert, "Socioeconomic Position and Health: The Independent Contribution of Community Socioeconomic Context," *Annual Review of Sociology* 25 (1999): 489–516.

105. Balm in Gilead, "Our Church Lights the Way," www.balmingilead.org/programs/tested, accessed on 24 August 2005.

106. "Harlem Center Focuses on Prevention for Positives," *AIDS Alert* (February 2005): 20–21.

107. Lin, "Jackson Urges"; Linda Tarrant-Reid, "A Leader in the War on AIDS," *NY Daily News*, 21 February 2005, *nydailynews.com*, accessed on 28 February 2005.

108. Letter from Robert S. Janssen to Jessica Tytel, 23 October 2003, author's files.

109. David Wahlberg, "U.S. Shifts Strategy to Curb HIV's Spread," *Atlanta Journal-Constitution*, 22 May 2004, A5.

110. A. Carballo-Dieguez et al., "Intention to Notify Sexual Partners about Potential HIV Exposure among New York City STD Clinics' Clients," *Sexually Transmitted Diseases* 29 (2002): 465–471.

111. Susan J. Klein et al., "A Public Health Approach to 'Prevention with Positives': The New York State HIV/AIDS Service Delivery System," *Journal of Public Health Management and Practice* 11 (2005): 7–18.

112. *Report of the New York City Commission on HIV/AIDS*, 31 October 2005, 1–2, www.nyc.gov/html/doh/downloads/pdf/ah/ah-nychivreport.pdf, accessed on 1 December 2005.

113. Presentation by Thomas Frieden, Conference on Collaborative Capacity Building, New York AIDS Coalition, 29 April 2004, New York City; presentation by Scott Kellerman, 8 June 2005, FITA Conference, New York City.

114. Paul von Zielbauer, "Rapid-Result HIV Testing Will Be Offered in City Jails," *NYT*, 12 December 2003, B6; D. Bell, "Testing, Testing," *City Limits*, 2 May 2005, www.citylimits.org/content/articles/weeklyView.cfm?articlenumber=1716, accessed on 2 May 2005; James Withers, "It's Raining Condoms," *NY Blade Online*, www.nyblade.com/2005/5–27/news/localnews/condoms.cfm, accessed on 4 December 2005.

115. Lynette Clemetson, "First the Free Test, Then the Free Tunes," *NYT*, 14 March 2004, A28.

116. Daniel Yee, "Study: Doctors Not Doing Enough HIV Counseling in Some Cities," Associated Press, 27 July 2004, Factiva.

Chapter 11: The Politics of Disease

1. Jeff Getty's statement "We changed the course of the disease," in Margie Mason, "Activist AIDS Group ACT UP Comes to a Crossroads after Early Successes," Associated Press, accessed from LexisNexis.

2. Richard Zeckhauser, "Procedures for Valuing Lives," *Public Policy* 23 (1975): 419–464.

3. Robert Putnam, *Making Democracy Work: Civic Tradition in Modern Italy* (Princeton, NJ: Princeton University Press, 1993).

4. Jeffrey Berry with David Arons, *A Voice for Nonprofits* (Washington, DC: Brookings Institution Press, 2003).

5. Theda Skocpol, "Advocates without Members: The Recent Transformation of American Civic Life," in *Civic Engagement in American Democracy*, ed. Theda Skocpol and Morris Fiorina (Washington, DC: Brookings Institution Press, 1999), 461–509.

6. J. Craig Jenkins, "Nonprofit Organizations and Policy Advocacy," in *The Nonprofit Sector: A Research Handbook*, ed. Walter W. Powell (New Haven, CT: Yale University Press, 1987), 296–318.

7. Peter Katel, "Lobbying Boom," *CQ Researcher* (22 July 2005); Kay Lehman Schlozman, "What Accent the Heavenly Chorus? Political Equality and the American Pressure System," *Journal of Politics* 46 (1984): 1006–1032.

8. E. E. Schattschneider, *The Semisovereign People: A Realist's View of Democracy in America* (Hinsdale, IL: Dryden Press, 1975), 35.

9. Jane Gross, "Turning Disease into Political Cause: First AIDS, and Now Breast Cancer," *NYT*, 7 January 1991, A12; Malcolm Gladwell, "Beyond HIV: The Legacies of Health Activism, " *Washington Post*, 15 October 1992, A29; Arno and Feiden, *Against the Odds*, 243.

10. Abigail Riggs Spangler, "Health-Related Social Movement in the United States: Motivations for Mobilization," *Research in Social Policy* 4 (Greenwich, CT.: JAI Press, 1996), 55–95.

11. Rettig, "The Policy Debate," 220.

12. Carolyn H. Asbury, *Orphan Drugs: Medical versus Market Value* (Lexington, MA: Lexington Books, 1985), 164–165.

13. Patrick Fox, "From Senility to Alzheimer's Disease: The Rise of the Alzheimer's," *Milbank Quarterly* 67: 59, 91.

14. Ken Kollman, *Outside Lobbying: Public Opinion and Interest Group Strategies* (Princeton, NJ: Princeton University Press, 1998), 18; Michael Lipsky, "Protest as a Political Resource," *American Political Science Review* 62 (1968): 1144–1158.

15. Robert J. Ross, "Generational Change and Primary Groups in a Social Movement," in *Social Movements of the Sixties and Seventies*, ed. Jo Freeman (New York: Longmans, 1983), 177–189.

16. Gregg Gonsalves, "You Can't Always Get What You Want (And Sometimes You Can't Even Get What You Need)," *Treatment Issues*, January/February 2003, 16.

17. Curtis L. Taylor, "Mayor: City Will Retool Its AIDS Policy, Services," *Newsday*, 14 March, 2003, A16.

18. Bob Roehr, "AIDS Watch in DC," *Windy City Times*, 11 May 2005, www.windycitymediagroup.com, accessed on 12 May 2005.

19. Author interview, 6 November 2003.

20. U.S. Department of Health and Human Services, Office of Inspector General, *Audit of Outreach and Risk Reduction Programs Funded by the New York Eligible Metropolitan Area under Title I of the Ryan White Comprehensive AIDS Resources Emergency Act of 1990*, February 1997, 1, http://www.oig.hhs.gov/oas/reports/region2/29602502.pdf, accessed on 4 December 2005.

21. Terje Anderson, "Aspects of Bush Proposal for Ryan White CARE Act Threaten Hard-Won Gains and Future Progress in HIV/AIDS Care and Treatment," 1 August 2005, www.napwa.org/pdf/analysis.pdf, accessed on 6 September 2005; letter from Joe Pressley, 15 August 2005; www.nyaidscoalition.org/binary-data, accessed on 6 September 2005.

22. Malcolm Gladwell, "Pediatric AIDS Studies at Adults' Exprense: Congress Focuses

40 Percent of NIH Drug-Testing Budget on 2 Percent of Cases," *Washington Post*, 5 October 1992, A1.

23. Cary P. Gross et al., "The Relation between Funding by the National Institutes of Health and the Burden of Disease," *New England Journal of Medicine* 340 (17 June 1999): 1882–1887.

24. Beatrix Hoffman, "Health Care Reform and Social Movements in the United States," *American Journal of Public Health* 93 (2003): 75–85.

25. Cynthia French et al., "State Implementation of the Breast and Cervical Cancer Prevention and Treatment Act of 2000: A Collaborative Effort among Government Agencies," *Public Health Reports* 119 (May–June 2004): 279–286.

26. Robert Guy Matthews, "Recovery Bypasses Many Americans," *Wall Street Journal*, 31 August 2005, A2.

27. Kevin Cullen, "An Act of Empowerment," *Boston Globe*, 1 July 1990, 1.

28. Advertisement in *NYT*, 12 February 2003, A33.

29. "Coalition for Health Funding," http://www.aamc.org/advocacy/healthfunding/start.htm, accessed on 5 September 2005.

30. Lawrence K. Altman, "More Living with HIV but Concerns Remain," *NYT*, 14 June 2005, F7.

31. Richard Pérez-PeÀa, "New Drug Promises Shift in Treatment for Heroin Addicts," *NYT*, 11 August 2003, A1; "Bupe Gets a Boost," *Housing Works AIDS Issues Update*, 9 August 2005, www.hwadovacy.com/update/archieves/2005/08/bupe_gets_boo.html, accessed on 8 August 2005; "Growing Number of Drug Resistant Strains Dominates at Retroviruses Conference," *AIDS Alert* (1 May 2005), accessed from Health Reference Center–Academic; Betsey McKay, "U.S. Backs Limited Use of Emergency HIV Regimen," *Wall Street Journal*, 21 January 2005, B2.

32. Jeff Graham, "The Campaign to End AIDS Has Begun," *AIDS Survival Project*, July/August 2005, www.thebody.com/asp/julaug05/campaign.html?m107h, accessed on 25 July 2005.

Index

ACT NOW, 123

ACT UP (AIDS Coalition to Unleash Power), 5, 6; on Bush Sr. administration and AIDS, 188; decline of, 129–133; demonstrations by, 125–129; divergence between TAG and, 155–156; drug access/treatment and, 153–154; on drug companies/FDA, 150; founding of, 122; growth of, 123–124; needle exchange and, 167–168, 173–174; relationship with minorities, 131–132

ACT UP-New York, 125–126, 129, 133, 152, 156–157

ACT UP-San Francisco, 133

ADAP (AIDS Drug Assistance Program), 146–147

ADAPT (Association for Drug Abuse Prevention and Treatment), 84, 85–88, 90, 163, 164, 167, 169

Ad Hoc Committee of Black Gay Activists, 79

Advancing HIV Prevention (AHP), 186–187, 189, 190–194

advocacy, AIDS, 6; collaboration among health advocacy organizations, 200–201; disease-related advocacy, 200; increasing national, 117; march/demonstration, 118–120, 122–128; organization for (see *individual organization*); predecessors of, 197. *See also* treatment advocacy, AIDS

Advocate, the, 113

Aerosol Pentamidine, 144

African American community: AIDS activism in, 79; AIDS in, 74, 75, 76; disproportionate number of AIDS cases in, 80; drug use/AIDS in, 84; HIV prevalence in, 179–180; HIV testing and, 192–193; opposition to needle exchange by, 165–166; response to AIDS epidemic, 80–82, 83–84; stigma of homosexuality in, 80, 84; support of needle exchange program by, 166, 170

AIDS Action, 41

AIDS Action Baltimore, 158

AIDS Action Council, 117

AIDS Action Pledge, 123

AIDS/AIDS-Related Complex case rate: growth in, 14, 28, 29; in New York City, 4

AIDS Clinical Trial group, 156–157

AIDS community, overview of: disease-related advocacy, 200; diversity of, 57–58, 73–78; funding and, 198–199; growing influence of, 111; influence on advocacy groups, 196–197; members of, 2, 6–7; move from social movement to interest group, 197–200; summary of impact on AIDS policy, 195

AIDS Community Research Initiative of America, 144

AIDS Drug Assistance Programs, 146

AIDS exceptionalism, 183

AIDS Health Services Program, 69–70, 98

AIDS hotline, 30

AIDS Institute (AI; New York State), 5, 78, 98, 116, 133, 171

AIDS Mastery workshop, 41

AIDS Medical Foundation (AMF), 66–67, 143

AIDS movement, 6

AIDS National Interfaith Network, 60

AIDS Network, 34, 114–115

AIDS organizations, 5; fragmentation/redundancy among, 200; promotion of citizen advocacy/awareness, 116. See also *individual organization*

AIDS quilt, 116

AIDS-related organizations: growth in, 88–89. See also *individual organization*

AIDS Resource Center (ARC), 58–60, 62

AIDS Service Demonstration Project, 98

AIDS stigma, 7, 24, 29, 31, 33

AIDS Task Force, New York City, 94

AIDS Task Force, of Unitarian Church of All Souls, 61

About the Author

Susan M. Chambré is a professor of sociology at Baruch College, City University of New York. She is the author of *Good Deeds in Old Age* and numerous articles on the nonprofit sector's response to the HIV epidemic.